D1563657

FAMILY ASSESSMENT: A GUIDE TO METHODS AND MEASURES

Harold D. Grotevant
Division of Child Development and Family Relationships
University of Texas at Austin

Cindy I. Carlson
Department of Educational Psychology
University of Texas at Austin

The Guilford Press
New York   London

*Dedicated to the families
from whom we have learned—
both our own and those
with whom we have worked
in research and therapy*

© 1989 The Guilford Press
A Division of Guilford Publications, Inc.
72 Spring Street, New York, N.Y. 10012

Printed in the United States of America

Last digit is print number: 9 8 7 6 5 4 3 2 1

Library of Congress Cataloging in Publication Data

Grotevant, Harold D.
    Family assessment: A guide to methods and measures / Harold D. Grotevant, Cindy
    I. Carlson.
       p. cm.
    Bibliography: p.
    Includes indexes.
    ISBN 0-89862-733-8
    1. Family. 2. Psychometrics. 3. Behavioral assessment.
    I. Carlson, Cindy I., 1949– . II. Title.
    HQ518.G75 1989
    306.8′5—dc19   88–12041
                                                            CIP

PREFACE

In the past decade, the study of the family has become a truly interdisciplinary enterprise. Initially within the purview of sociology and anthropology, family scholars now span the fields of psychology, psychiatry, linguistics, communications, home economics, nursing, and social work.

Although there is widespread acknowledgment that it is important to understand the role of the family in the development of individuals, consensus about the most productive approaches to take is only slowly beginning to emerge. Theoretical perspectives on the family are diverse. Major traditions that contribute to family theory include family sociology, family therapy (i.e., systems and communication theory), developmental psychology, and social learning theory (Gottman, 1979; Jacob, 1987). When the theoretical views are so varied, it should not be surprising that issues of family measurement are similarly divergent.

Several attempts have been made to bring together information about family measurement in a systematic way. Most notable is *Family Measurement Techniques: Abstracts of Published Instruments, 1935–1974* (Strauss & Brown, 1978), which includes brief descriptive abstracts of more than 800 measures. *Tests and Measurements in Child Development* (O. G. Johnson, 1976), though focusing primarily on intrapersonal psychological measures (e.g., personality, cognitive abilities, self-concept), also contains abstracts of some measures of parental attitudes toward children and social interaction of parents and children. Although these resources are valuable, they are both dated, and they contain only sketchy information on a wide variety of measures.

The impetus for writing this book grew out of our own need for a more comprehensive resource to use in our family research, our teaching about family interaction and assessment, and our clinical work with families. Thus, our purpose in writing this book is to provide an up-to-date reference manual for family clinicians and researchers who are either users or consumers of measures that involve the coding of family interaction, the global rating of family processes, or self-reports of perceptions of family functioning.

In writing the book, we had several goals in mind. First, we wanted it to be reasonably comprehensive in its inclusion of the best current measures in the broad field of family studies. Second, we wanted it to include both detailed descriptions and critiques of the measures. Finally, we wanted the book to put

the theoretical and measurement issues in the field into perspective for its au-
dience of clinicians, researchers, students, and other family scholars. We hope
that this resource will assist in the selection of appropriate measures for research questions or for clinical screening, diagnosis, and treatment evaluation
and will facilitate integration of research findings across studies and communication among clinicians.

Family Assessment focuses primarily on instruments that concern whole-family functioning or the functioning of multiple family relationships. Because of
the availability of other resources (e.g., Filsinger, 1983a, 1983b; Filsinger &
Lewis, 1981), measures that focus solely on marital interaction and functioning
are not reviewed in this book.

PROCEDURES USED IN PREPARING THIS BOOK

A search of the literature was accomplished through the automated data bases
of Psychological Abstracts and the National Council on Family Relations. In
addition, other review articles that included measures of family functioning
were examined. Selected family and child development journals were searched.
Finally, colleagues of the authors were asked to nominate measures for inclusion. Measures developed for dissertations or theses were not included unless
they subsequently resulted in published work.

Authors of the measures were contacted and asked to provide the most current information available for their measures. When authors did not respond to
inquiries, evaluation was based on the publications that were available. Measures were omitted from the review if the authors so requested. (This happened
in only a very few instances, usually with measures that were outdated or
undergoing major revision.)

Measures were evaluated using a standard outline that facilitated comparisons of theoretical perspectives, physical properties, administrative procedures,
evidence for reliability and validity, and discussion of clinical and research
utility. Once the review was completed on each measure, it was sent to the
author for comments and corrections. In many cases, this round of communication elicited new information or articles, which were then incorporated into a
revised outline. Authors were also invited to contribute 150-word comments
concerning the current states of their measures and plans for their futures. The
final outlines and authors' comments are included in Part Two of *Family Assessment*. In addition to the abstracts, other features of this book that enhance
its usefulness include an index of variables and constructs by measure, an index
of authors by measure, and an index of titles of measures.

EVALUATION CRITERIA

Although several different types of measures were included in this book, they
were all reviewed in terms of common criteria. Remarks on each of these criteria are included in the abstracts of the instruments.

General descriptive information includes the author of the measure, its date of publication, its availability, and a brief description of the measure and its theoretical base.

The physical description of the measure was tailored to the type of measure. For obsrvational coding schemes and rating scales, information was included concerning the task and setting used to elicit behavior, the unit of study, the unit of coding and analysis, the organization of the code, the manual, and standardization and norms. For self-report measures, information concerning the physical features of the measure and the identity of the respondent was also included.

Administrative procedures of each measure were also examined. For observational measures, information concerning the equipment needed for the observation, training of data collectors and coders, data transcription and reduction, and scoring procedures was included. For self-report measures, information on test directions, ease of use, and training of administrators and scorers was also included.

Reliability of the measures was considered in light of the types of reliability most appropriate to each type of measure. *Validity* evidence was sought concerning content validity, criterion-related validity, and construct validity, whenever available. Each measure was also evaluated in terms of its usefulness and appropriateness for both clinicians and researchers.

ORGANIZATION OF THE BOOK

Family Assessment is divided into two major parts: Part One contains three sections: an overall introduction (Section I), discussions of observational measures (Section II), and discussions of self-report measures (Section III). Part Two contains abstracts of the measures (Sections IV–VIII) and indexes of the abstracts (Section IX).

In Part One, the chapters in Section II concern observational measures—those that involve assessment of the family by outsiders. Following an introduction (Chapter 2) to issues in observational methodology, Chapter 3 presents a comparative discussion of 13 family interaction coding schemes, and Chapter 4 presents a discussion of 8 global rating scales of family functioning. The chapters in Section III concern self-report measures—those that assess the self-perceptions of family members. Chapter 5 introduces the section; Chapter 6 includes a review of 17 measures of whole-family functioning; Chapter 7 reviews 9 measures of family stress and coping; and Chapter 8 presents discussions of 19 self-report measures of parent–child relationships.

The organization of the book mirrors an important distinction that has been made in the family assessment literature between "insider" and "outsider" perspectives. Olson (1977) noted that different theoretical traditions tended to rely more strongly on one strategy than another. For example, family sociology relied more heavily on "insiders'" (usually wives') reports concerning their family, whereas social psychology relied more heavily on observational techniques. Currently, it is fair to say that most family scholars recognize that both self-report and observational techniques have their strengths and limitations, and many investigators now incorporate both strategies into their research designs. Advocates of observational methods point out that family members are often inaccurate informants about their own behavior and that they also have difficulty describing family behavior at the process level (Markman & Notarius, 1987). On the other hand, advocates of self-report methods note that the "inside" individual's perception of the family is at least as important as what an outsider would observe. In addition, observers' inferences about family functioning may be inaccurate because of the idiosyncratic shared meanings that families sometimes develop (Larzelere & Klein, 1986).

ACKNOWLEDGMENTS

The initial review of measures included in this book was supported in part by a research grant from the University Research Institute of the University of Texas at Austin. We are indebted to a number of our colleagues at the University of Texas at Austin (Mark Bickhard, Catherine Cooper, Ted Huston, Paul Kelley, and Beeman Phillips), who graciously reviewed parts of the manuscript, as well as to several anonymous reviewers and our colleagues within the field who have been supportive of our venture. We are especially indebted to the authors of the measures included in the book, who took time to respond to requests for materials and to review our abstracts of their measures for accuracy. We have been assisted in this project by many students in our family assessment, family psychology, and family intervention courses, including our research assistant, JoAnn Seymour; by our chapter co-authors, Margaret Koranek, Paul Miller, and Rhonda Hauser; and by our secretaries, Sarah Kear and Debbie Finn. We are grateful to *Family Process* and to the *Journal of Family Psychology* (Sage Publications) for their permission to include revisions of our published works in this book. Finally, we acknowledge the support of our editor at Guilford Press, Sharon Panulla.

We began this project with the goals of gaining mastery of the family assessment field and sharing that mastery with others. At its onset, neither the complexity nor the duration of this project was evident to us. Given the rapid and continuous change in the field of family research and assessment, and the conceptual and methodological diversity of the field, mastery proved to be an illusive goal. However, we have delighted in becoming more informed scientists and consumers, challenged to find solutions to methodological problems and to contribute to the advancement of family theory. It is our hope that this book will inform and challenge others.

Harold D. Grotevant
Cindy I. Carlson

CONTRIBUTORS

Cindy I. Carlson, PhD, Department of Educational Psychology, University of Texas at Austin, Austin, Texas

Harold D. Grotevant, PhD, Division of Child Development and Family Relationships, University of Texas at Austin, Austin, Texas

Rhonda K. Hauser, MA, Division of Child Development and Family Relationships, University of Texas at Austin, Austin, Texas

Margaret Koranek, Department of Educational Psychology, University of Texas at Austin, Austin, Texas

Paul Miller, PhD, Department of Psychology, Arizona State University–West Campus, Phoenix, Arizona

CONTENTS

PART ONE

REVIEW AND DISCUSSION OF FAMILY ASSESSMENT MEASURES

Section I
Introduction

1

FAMILY ASSESSMENT: PAST, PRESENT, AND FUTURE

Attempting to review the domain of family assessment brings to mind the metaphor of the hydra from Greek mythology. The hydra was a nine-headed monster that Hercules was challenged to slay. But whenever anyone managed to cut off one of the hydra's heads, two new heads grew in its place. The state of affairs in the family assessment field evokes this metaphor because, like the hydra's heads, measures and specialized theories in family studies have proliferated rapidly and in an uncoordinated fashion. New coding schemes and measures surface frequently, often without sufficient regard for theoretical underpinnings, psychometric quality, or careful development of linkages between theory and assessment. Like good dragon-slayers, we have attempted to impose some order on this unruly field, but our ability to do so has been limited by the nature of the field itself.

Family assessment has developed in a laissez-faire manner: measures spring up and are tested, and the fittest survive. This slow, inefficient process, however, contributes to a great deal of disorder in the field. The time now seems right for some reflective consolidation in both the family theory and assessment domains.

THEORY AND METHOD

Three issues concerning theory and method deserve the best attention professionals in the field can provide. One issue is the lack of theoretical consensus in the field (Cowan, 1987). Of course, it is naive to expect that any one theory will ever be comprehensive enough to order fully our understanding of the complex systems we call families. At a minimum, such a theory would have to integrate the perspectives of anthropology, sociology, psychology, and biology.

An examination of the shifts in major theoretical perspectives over the past 30 years reflects the need for multiple lenses to understand family functioning (Broderick, 1971; Burr, Hill, Nye, & Reiss, 1979; Hill & Hansen, 1960; Holman & Burr, 1980). Although some family scholars and clinicians mourn the lack of a general family theory, others acknowledge that some theories are better suited than others to explicating certain aspects of family functioning (Holman & Burr, 1980). Regardless of one's preferences, it is clear that the emergence of an all-encompassing, unified family theory is nowhere in sight. In the meantime, we must do the best we can with our "theories of the middle range" (Merton, 1945).

What does this state of affairs mean for family assessment? Given the plurality of family theories, it should not be surprising that family assessment devices have proliferated as well. Although the development of some measures has been theory-driven and the development of others intervention-driven, still others have grown up outside a clear theoretical context. As Cowan (1987) has suggested, we may be putting the cart before the horse if we develop reliable measures before facilitating their emergence out of theory. Thus, one key issue for family researchers to address is the development and validation of theories of family process.

A second important issue concerns the linkages between family theory and measurement. An obvious but often overlooked criterion is that measures should correspond to the theoretical constructs for which they were developed (Schumm, 1982). Later in this book, a number of instances are cited in which scales that have the same title have dramatically different item content or observed behavior. As Larzelere and Klein (1986, p. 125) have observed: *"What* we know about families is largely determined by *how* we know what we know." Clearly defined theoretical constructs will enhance both "how" and "what" we know about families.

Third, as Schumm (1982) has noted, attention must be paid to the links between measurement and data analysis. Computer programs are just as willing to analyze data from poorly constructed measures as from good ones. If the measure is invalid, however, the analyses are not meaningful. The following statistical issues merit consideration in constructing, selecting, and using family assessment measures (Schumm, 1982). Statistical problems such as lack of variance, skewness, kurtosis, and low reliability can undermine the usefulness of measures. The level of measurement (e.g., nominal, ordinal, interval) at which data are collected is directly related to the types of statistics that may be used. Unequal intervals between item response choices can produce analytic problems. In addition, traditional statistical assumptions about linearity may not pick up curvilinear effects in data. Finally, theoretical perspectives on the family will influence analytic decisions about examining family structures or sequential patterning of interaction (Steinglass, 1987).

Given these problems, researchers and clinicians who are interested in family measurement are faced with the challenge of adapting to life with the hydra. Because of the complexity of these theoretical and methodological issues, they cannot work in a vacuum and must participate together in the construction of links among theory, assessment, and intervention. Advances on all three fronts will occur more rapidly when practitioners and researchers work together to understand the interrelatedness of their efforts. Despite the need to work together, however, distinctive issues also emerge for clinicians and researchers. It is to these issues that we now turn.

IMPLICATIONS FOR CLINICIANS

An important recent development in the clinical field is that practitioners are more frequently being called on to evaluate family functioning in addition to individual functioning. Traditionally, the clinical psychologist's role was to assess an individual's functioning and to develop a treatment approach for improving that functioning. As behaviorism gained acceptance, psychologists were admonished to assess the context of individual functioning and to consider variations in functioning across settings as well. Attention to context in mental health has been extended further by the adoption of a systems perspective, which has had profound implications for the ways in which psychologists view and intervene in individual psychopathology. Problems no longer reside only within the individual; they may be symptoms of other problems in the family or the broader environment. Furthermore, systems theory emphasizes that the source of functional or dysfunctional behavior lies in the relational patterns within and across systems. Failure to evaluate the role of family relationships not only may limit the effectiveness of interventions (Patterson & Fleischman, 1979), but may also ensure the continuation of the problem (C. I. Carlson, 1987). Adoption of the systems perspective means that practitioners who formerly specialized in individual assessment and intervention must now understand both individual and family assessment.

Clinical and research assessment differ in an important way. In a typical research project, the investigator has one or more questions in mind at the beginning of the study and collects data from families to answer those questions or test related hypotheses. The researcher should also have access to the necessary instruments, equipment, and space to use appropriate measures with participants. In the clinical setting, the therapist must be a detective, first, to identify the central issues or questions, as the "presenting" problem may not be the "real" problem. A key goal of the clinician, then, is to use assessment techniques to identify the client's issues, formulate a treatment plan, and evaluate progress. Unlike researchers who are collecting observational data, clinicians may be limited in their access to expensive equipment and may lack the necessary training, staff, time, and computer facilities to analyze the results of observational data. Because of these inherent differences between the research and clinical settings, the practice of assessment in these two settings has often looked very different. We argue, however, along with Cromwell, Olson, and Fournier (1976), that the same criteria apply to effective assessment in any setting.

Family assessment measures used in the clinical setting to make consequential decisions about families and children should meet more rigorous psychometric standards than are typically required with research instruments. Clinical uses of measurement include screening, diagnosis, and treatment evaluation. High reliability is necessary, of course, when decisions regarding people are based on measurement outcomes. Family measures designed for clinical use are also limited by the lack of validity studies. In many studies, validity is ascertained by discrimination between a clinical and a nonclinical group. Although such a design may be adequate for screening instruments, it provides no information that is useful in the essential process of differential diagnosis. Thus, a particularly pressing need regarding the clinical use of family assessment measures is the establishment of differential predictive validity—that is, which measures and which dimensions within measures reliably predict and discriminate among types of dysfunctions. Our review of the family assessment field indicates that although measurement development is promising, most measures are not yet adequately refined for clinical decision making.

A second clear limitation of the current status of the family assessment field is the lack of test development for clinical use with children. In this volume, only one nonprojective measure of family functioning (the Children's Version of the Family Environment Scale) was identified for elementary school–age children. The cognitive ability of young children to understand the qualities of the family in an interpretable and meaningful way is as yet unknown. However, this is a critical question given the mental health needs of children, the crucial role of family process in child problems, and the frequent access to family dysfunction through identification of child behavior and learning problems in settings beyond the family. In addition to the development of family assessment measures for children, evaluation of the criterion-related validity of existing measures for childhood problems is important.

Concern about systems functioning also has direct implications for assessment. Systems-oriented clinicians are likely to want to know whether their interventions have affected the client, his or her dyadic relationships, and the functioning of the family as a whole (Gurman & Kniskern, 1981a); however, assessment at every level may be too time-consuming and impractical (Bagarozzi, 1985). This points to a need to develop measures that evaluate multiple family levels (e.g., the Family Assessment Measure).

IMPLICATIONS FOR RESEARCHERS

As noted earlier, family research will advance most rapidly when there is a strong interplay among theory, measurement, and intervention (e.g., Cromwell, Olson, & Fournier, 1976; Larzelere & Klein, 1986; Schumm, 1982.) In addition, because the study of the family cuts across typical disciplinary boundaries, cross-disciplinary fertilization of family scholars will be essential. At minimum, family sociologists, family psychologists, family therapists, anthropologists, and biologists should be in dialogue.

As researchers study the family, careful attention should be paid to selecting and/or developing appropriate, psychometrically sound measures for the constructs under investigation. A useful protocol for the development of a psychometrically sound self-report instrument for family assessment may be found in Skinner (1987). In addition, because of the likelihood that different perspectives on the family will yield different results, investigators should think carefully about the need for both insider and outsider measures of the family and about assessing the family at multiple levels.

TECHNIQUES NOT REVIEWED IN THIS BOOK

Although the scope of this book has been limited to observational coding schemes, global rating scales, and self-report measures, other windows on family functioning are also available and may be valuable adjuncts to the measures reviewed here. These other measures may be grouped roughly into four categories: projective techniques, experimental tasks, structured interviews, and self-report measures of behavior.

Projective techniques provide opportunities for respondents to reveal aspects of their personalities and constructions of family relationships by presenting them with ambiguous stimuli or by asking them to create representations themselves. Examples of projectives used in family assessment include the Family Rorschach (Levy & Epstein, 1964), in which the family is brought together to respond to Rorschach inkblots as a group and their interaction is observed. Another kind of projective technique involves the use of family sculpture; family members are asked to create representations of the relationships in the family on paper (e.g., L. G. Bell, Eriksen, Cornwell, & Bell, 1984; Wedemeyer & Grotevant, 1982) or, within the context of a therapy session, physically place members of their family in the room to represent their feelings and thoughts about the relationships in the family (Constantine, 1978; Simon, 1972). Other relational mapping techniques, such as the genogram (McGoldrick & Gerson, 1986) and the ecomap (Holman, 1983), provide structured opportunities for individuals to convey perceptions of their family's functioning and their role in the family. A third projective technique is the sentence completion blank, which has been used by Coleman (1974) to assess adolescents' perceptions of relationships in their families. Finally, the Kinetic Family Drawing technique (Burns & Kaufman, 1970) has been used to elicit drawings of family members engaged in activity, which are in turn interpreted by a therapist. In general, projective techniques are most commonly used in clinical assessment as an adjunct to therapy. The psychometric qualities of these instruments typically preclude their use in research.

Two experimental tasks that have been used in family assessment include the Simulated Family Activity Measure (SIMFAM) (Straus & Tallman, 1971) and the Card Sort Procedure (Reiss, 1980, 1981). Both of these tasks place families in situations with ambiguous demands. In SIMFAM, family members play a shuffleboard-like game in which they are told that the object of the game is to learn the rules (Sprenkle & Olson, 1978). In the Card Sort Procedure, family members are seated in booths and are given decks of cards to sort in any way they wish. In both of these situations, the family is faced with a situation that has little direct relevance to daily life except the need to develop a strategy for making sense of the procedure. Both of these techniques have been used extensively in research.

Structured interviews have also been used in family assessment, especially as an aspect of clinical evaluation. A noteworthy example of a structured research interview for assessing relational development is the Family Relationships Interview of White and colleagues (White, Speisman, & Costos, 1983, 1984). The semistructured interview covers four areas: current interactions, resolution of differences of opinion, advice giving, and caretaking. Responses of young adults are coded with respect to one of three possible developmental levels of their relationships with each of their parents: self-focused, role-focused, or individuated–connected. This interview schedule, which has been used successfully in several research projects, provides evidence for an assessment device that is strongly based in theory, has creditable psychometric properties, and has relevance in the clinical setting as well.

Finally, strategies have recently been developed to collect self-report data on behavior in a systematic way. A renewed interest in the ecology of human and family development has stimulated the formation of methods for recording information about the behavior of family members both inside and outside the family. Examples of research applications of time use data include Montemayor's (1982) work relating parent–adolescent conflict to the proportion of time that adolescents spend by themselves, with their families, and with their peers; Huston's work on the time use of couples during the early years of marriage (Huston, Robins, Atkinson, & McHale, 1987); and Patterson's research and clinical use of the Parent Daily Report (Patterson, 1982).

CONCLUSIONS

Given the lack of consensus on theory or measurement in the family assessment field, we suggest that an understanding of the family would be best facilitated under the following conditions. First, a clear theoretical rationale linking theory and assessment strategy is needed (e.g., Reiss, 1983). Second, assessment of various levels of the family in which the individual is embedded is useful (Cromwell & Peterson, 1983; Peterson & Cromwell, 1983), provided that theory is used as a guide for interpreting the linkages among levels (Reiss, 1983). Third, the family studies field has matured sufficiently that psychometric integrity of measures is necessary. This means that measures should show evidence of appropriate types of reliability and validity. When multiple versions of measures have been developed, tested, and used in research, investigators should clearly report which versions were used and how they differed. Ease of administration and face validity cannot substitute for reliability and validity, especially when consequential decisions about children or families are made on the basis of the assessment (C. I. Carlson, 1987).

Section II
Observational Measures

2

INTRODUCTION TO
OBSERVATIONAL METHODS
IN FAMILY ASSESSMENT

The conceptual advances recently registered in the social sciences have spurred an increased interest in observational methods in the study of the family. Several factors have stimulated the use of observational techniques: the popularity of theories that emphasize the causal importance of family interaction in development; distrust of family members' ability to report accurately on the interactions in their family; research on the family as a context for the development of psychopathology as well as competence; acceptance of family systems theory by family therapist-researchers; the development of appropriate equipment for the collection and analysis of observational data (such as event recorders and large-memory computers); and the development of appropriate behavioral codes (B. C. Miller, Rollins, & Thomas, 1982).

In this section of the book, two contrasting types of observational data collection strategies will be discussed: in Chapter 3, family interaction coding schemes; in Chapter 4, rating scales of family functioning. Both techniques rely on observations made by individuals outside the family, but the levels of analysis at which observations are made differ substantially.

CODING SCHEMES

The trend toward increasingly widespread use of microanalytic observation codes in family research is understandable. Observational coding schemes preserve the precise actions of individuals in a group, the analysis of which is essential for understanding processes of interaction. Observational procedures lend themselves to flexibility in yielding quantitative indices of interaction and can generally be used reliably by nonprofessional observers (Cairns & Green, 1979). Furthermore, observational codes provide relatively unbiased responses (Hartmann, 1982a). Research aimed at delineating the lawful processes of family interaction traditionally places heavy emphasis on observation as a primary method of data collection (Patterson & Reid, 1984). Thus, as greater attention has been paid to interactional theories and research, many family interaction coding schemes have been created as research tools.

The foregoing factors have spurred the development of microanalytic observation coding schemes that capture the moment-to-moment contingencies of family members' behavior toward one another (Gottman, 1979; Jacob, 1975; Maccoby & Martin, 1983; Riskin & Faunce, 1972). Development of these schemes has required technological advances in the collection and reduction of data, now possible with the availability of videotapes and computers (Maccoby & Martin, 1983), as well as methodological advances in determining reliability and validity (Cairns, 1979).

Proponents of the microanalytic observational method argue for its superiority primarily on the basis of objectivity. The low correspondence between family members' subjective "insider" reality and objective "outsider" perspectives has been well documented (Olson, 1977). The increasing quantity of family interaction studies (e.g., Jacob, 1975) attests to the perceived value of observational work by family researchers. Unfortunately, theoretical conceptualizations regarding family interaction concern patterns, whereas family interaction research has examined, for the most part, rates of behavior (Gottman, 1979). Accordingly, a focus on frequencies of observable behavior, without attention to sequential descriptions of that behavior, appears inadequate for systems research. Family researchers are currently very interested in sequential data-analytic techniques that examine the relationships or contingencies among types of behavior, thereby permitting a focus on both process and relationship (Cousins & Power, 1986; Rogers, Millar, & Bavelas, 1985).

Although some family scholars are turning to sequential analytic techniques for the analysis of relational patterns, other investigators are beginning to note the shortcomings of such techniques. Specifically, Bakeman and Brown (1980) found that summary scores developed from microanalysis of mother–child interaction did not predict subsequent child characteristics as well as ratings of behavior did. Patterson (1982) found that moment-to-moment sequential contingencies did not reliably differentiate distressed from normal families, whereas base rates and duration of coercive interaction patterns did. Thus, whereas microanalytic observation techniques may be particularly suited to determining the moment-to-moment contingencies or sequences of behavior, a molar level of analysis may be essential to the description of stable relational patterns or dimensions of the family system (Cairns & Green, 1979). A further limitation of sequential analytic techniques is that they have been applied primarily to dyadic interactions and require a considerable number of data points for reliable evaluation even at this level of relationship. For family systems investigations, Rogers et al. (1985) have proposed that a minimum acceptable sequential analysis involves triadic interaction patterns and a three-event chain (a two-lag solution), thus requiring even more extensive data (Bakeman & Gottman, 1986). The labor-intensive nature of microanalytic observation procedures restricts their utility for both family clinicians and family researchers without sizable financial support.

One solution to the limitations posed by microanalytic observations of behavior is to change the level of analysis at which behavior is coded and analyzed. This approach appears to have considerable merit for family researchers in validating theoretical models of family interaction with relational behavior patterns. For example, Baldwin, Cole, and Baldwin (1982) combined the microanalytic level of behaviors of "helping one another" and "expressed approval," "hugging," "teasing," and "joking" into a molar behavioral construct of "warmth" to determine the parent interaction patterns predictive of children's school competence. Such a molar-level analysis, which groups similar behaviors, may in some cases enhance the reliability and validity of family interaction data.

Microanalytic observations of behavior, however—like their macroanalytic counterparts—are limited in their ability to capture qualities of whole relationships versus the behavior or characteristics of individuals within relationships. If the goal of family interaction assessment is to describe the global relational structure or characteristics of the whole family, then a rating scale may be the measure of choice.

RATING SCALES

Rating scales are similar to behavioral observation coding schemes in providing an objective, outsider view of the family, but they differ substantially in the level (molar versus molecular) of analysis. The distinctiveness of information elicited by rating procedures versus microanalytic observation procedures has been clarified by Cairns and Green (1979). Rating procedures involve a summary judgment on the part of an observer with regard to placement of an individual, dyad, or whole family on some psychological dimension. Although rating scales may differ from one another in psychometric properties, they have in common a reliance on the complex information-processing capabilities of the rater. Rating scales take advantage of the ability of human beings to process multiple sources of information and to abstract and integrate the relevant pieces in complex, unspecified ways to arrive at a summary judgment. Thus, rating scales appear particularly well suited for identifying relationship properties— that is, the summary indices of patterns of interpersonal events that occur in the family system (e.g., Huston & Robins, 1982). Moreover, unlike microanalytic techniques, for which behavioral interdependence across individuals poses a statistical dilemma, rating scales incorporate the interdependence of behavior in relationships into the rating process. Rating methods, therefore, provide an objective observation method that is well suited to the whole family or relational unit of analysis. The ease with which they can be constructed and used also makes them appropriate for both clinical and research settings.

Maccoby and Martin (1983) and Patterson and Reid (1984) have aptly noted that choosing the most meaningful level of analysis is one of the most challenging problems facing researchers who study the family. It is important for family clinicians and researchers to be keenly aware of the questions they are asking and to match the levels of their questions to the appropriate levels of data collection. Markman and Notarius (1987) point out the advantages of "cooperative interaction" between micro- and macro-level analyses. They note that microanalytic codes have the potential to reveal patterns of behavior that are too complex for human observers to detect. However, once detected, these patterns may be compatible with more global methods of coding. At the same time, global coding systems have the potential to generate hypotheses that can be tested at the microanalytic level. It seems to us that the field will advance more rapidly when multiple assessment strategies are used (both insider and outsider as well as macro and micro) and the information gained from all is integrated.

3

FAMILY INTERACTION
CODING SCHEMES

In this chapter, we will present summaries and critiques of 13 interaction coding systems used in the observation of families. The scope of our review is limited to measures involving the *verbal interaction of the family* with school-aged children and adolescents in at least a triadic situation (two parents and one child). Coding systems that focus on marital interaction or family interaction in therapy are not reviewed, as useful reviews are already available (Filsinger & Lewis, 1981; Gibb, 1961; Gilbert & Christensen, 1985; Pinsoff, 1981). Systems developed for coding parent–infant play or nonverbal behavior were deemed beyond the scope of this chapter, as their primary focus is not on verbal interaction. Finally, the majority of family interaction codes reviewed have been developed since 1970. Earlier coding systems have been included only if they are currently being used in either the original or a modified form. Thus, the focus of this review is family interaction coding systems designed to illuminate family patterns related to children's normal and pathological development.

In this chapter, the 13 coding systems will first be described, highlighting their theoretical origins and the constructs assessed by the codes. Then comparisons will be made of the coding systems' descriptions, administrative procedures, reliability and validity, and clinical and research utility. We will conclude with a general discussion and recommendations for use.

DESCRIPTIONS OF MEASURES

In this section, each interactive coding system is briefly described. The coding systems are roughly grouped into two sets, reflecting the primary purposes for which they were developed and have been used. The first nine coding systems have primarily been used to study the family as a context for the development or maintenance of psychopathology. The remaining four have primarily been used to study the family as a context for the development of individual differences in psychosocial development of children and adolescents. Within each group, however, important theoretical distinctions will be made.

As each coding system is discussed, the key constructs assessed by the code will be highlighted. In Table 3–1, the constructs have been arranged to reflect five dimensions that appear to differentiate most adequately among the family assessment systems: (1) *cognitive* constructs, which refer to patterns of interaction presumed to facilitate the cognitive development of family members; (2) *affective* constructs, which are indicators of the emotional climate of the family; (3) *interpersonal process* regulators, which are aspects of communication that regulate the flow of interaction within the family; (4) *structural* constructs, which reflect patterns of relationships within the family; and (5) *dominance* constructs, which reflect control, sanctions, or conflict within the family. This table illustrates the variability in coverage of the constructs addressed by family process coding systems.

The Family as a Context for the Development of Psychopathology

Each of the following nine coding systems was developed primarily to identify patterns of interaction in clinic populations. The study of differences in family interaction patterns between normal or unlabeled families and those with dysfunctional members (typically, schizophrenics or delinquents) has been motivated by the assumption that the discovery of differences might inform theories about the etiology of psychopathology as well as treatment efforts.

Family Interaction Code

The Family Interaction Code developed by Mishler and Waxler (Mishler & Waxler, 1968) is a microanalytic coding system designed to examine the interaction of families with a schizophrenic member. The coding system was developed to test the clinical observation that psychological communication may contribute to the etiology of schizophrenia and to identify new and unpredicted family interaction patterns. The coding system includes the Bales (1951) Interaction Process Analysis code, developed for small-group process research, and additional code categories of theoretical significance, derived from the clinical literature on schizophrenia. The Family Interaction Code is used to assess the affective constructs of *expressiveness* and *responsiveness*, the interpersonal process regulation construct of *speech disruption*, and the control and sanction construct of *strategies for attention and control*. Each complete sentence or idea is coded. The code was developed and used in one major study of communication in families with a schizophrenic member (Mishler & Waxler, 1968). In this study, family interaction was elicited in a 50-minute revealed differences task in which members were asked to come to a consensus on items about which they disagreed. The interaction was audiotaped and transcribed; coding required the use of both the tape and the transcript. This early code has been influential in the development of subsequent coding systems (e.g., D. C. Bell, Bell, & Cornwell, 1982).

Family Interaction Scales

The Riskin and Faunce (1969) Family Interaction Scales were developed from the family therapy theory of Jackson and Satir in order to provide an objective coding scheme for family interaction that would be superior to the impressionistic clinic observations used at that time. The purpose of the Family Interaction Scales is to contribute to the understanding of normal and pathological personality development by examining the family context in which the child's personality develops. The code includes six major dimensions: *relationship* and *intensity* (affective constructs), *clarity, topic continuity, commitment,* and *agree–disagree* (process regulation constructs). The coding system has been used in studies of both "healthy" and clinical families. Families are given 10 minutes in which to plan something that they could all do together; all family members are asked to participate in the planning. The interaction session is audiotaped; coding requires the use of both the tape and a verbatim transcript. Each speech of each family member is coded. In addition, interruptions are preserved, and the identities of the persons speaking and spoken to are recorded. The Family Interaction Scales have inspired the development of subsequent codes (D. C. Bell et al., 1982).

Family Conflict and Dominance Code

Several variations of the Family Conflict and Dominance Code (Henggeler & Tavormina, 1980; Hetherington, Stouwie, & Ridberg, 1971; Jacob, 1974) have been developed to assess conflict and dominance through microanalytic coding of family interaction. The coding systems are based on psychiatric theories (e.g., Farina & Dunham, 1963) concerning the role of maternal dominance and parental conflict in the etiology of schizophrenia. Indices of *conflict* typically include attempted interruptions, simultaneous speech, and disagreement; indices of *dominance* typically include successful interruptions, speaking first and last, and total talking time. In general, revealed or unrevealed differences tasks are used to elicit family interaction. Because variations of this coding system have been used by different researchers, specific details about the data collection and reduction processes also vary. In general, the interaction session is audiotaped. However, transcripts of the session are not always made or used as the basis for coding. This coding system has been used for a number of purposes, including comparison of family interaction styles in families with different types of delinquent adolescents and examination of changes in family interaction over time as a function of adolescent pubertal development (e.g., Steinberg, 1981).

Affective Style Measure

The Affective Style Measure (Doane, Goldstein, & Rodnick, 1981; Doane, West, Goldstein, Rodnick, & Jones, 1981) was developed, within the context of family systems theory, to predict the development of psychopathology in a

TABLE 3–1. Comparison of Family Interaction Coding Scheme Constructs

Coding Scheme	Cognitive	Affective	Interpersonal Process Regulation	Structural	Control and Sanction
Family as Context for Psychopathology					
Family Interaction Code		Expressiveness, responsiveness	Speech disruption		Strategies for attention and control
Family Interaction Scales		Relationship (support–attack), intensity	Clarity, topic continuity, commitment, agree–disagree		
Family Conflict and Dominance Codes					Dominance, conflict
Affective Style Measure		Style, support, criticism, guilt induction, intrusiveness			
Family Task				Transactional style, enmeshment, alliance, conflict, protectiveness	
Structural Analysis of Social Behavior		Affiliation	Focus	Interdependence	

Defensive and Supportive Communication Interaction System		Defensive, supportive			Aversive, prosocial
Family Interaction Coding System					
Parent–Adolescent Interaction Coding System					Positive, negative, neutral
Family as Context for Child Development					
Interaction Process Coding Scheme	Validation	Support			Power
Individuation Code				Self-assertion, separateness, mutuality, permeability	
Family Constraining and Enabling Coding System	Cognitive enablers and constrainers	Affective enablers and constrainers	Discourse change		
Developmental Environments Coding System	Stimulation, inhibition	Support, affective conflict	Mode, transactive–nontransactive, content		

sample of high-risk adolescents and to predict the course of a patient's illness and social functioning following release from a psychiatric hospital. The coding system is used to calculate the frequency of parental behaviors indicative of five affective constructs: *style, support, criticism, guilt induction,* and *intrusiveness.* Individual parents and marital dyads can then be classified as "benign," "inconsistent," or "negative." In the investigators' studies (Doane, Falloon, Goldstein, & Mintz, 1985; Doane, Goldstein, & Rodnick, 1981; Doane, West, et al., 1981), adolescents are observed in two dyadic situations with mother, two with father, and two triadic situations. In each 7-minute session, the participants discuss a problem that had previously been determined to be an issue for that particular family. The first dyadic situation with each parent and the first triadic situation are used for data analysis because they are the most emotionally charged. Speeches are coded from transcripts. Coded family interaction of clinic families has been used to predict adolescent diagnosis 5 years later (Doane, West, et al., 1981) and to predict relapse in schizophrenia (Doane et al., 1985) and in mania (Miklowitz, Goldstein, Neuchterlein, Snyder, & Doane, 1986).

Family Task

The Philadelphia Child Guidance Clinic Family Task is a procedure that involves five tasks for eliciting family interaction. The videotaped tasks include planning a menu, discussing a family argument, describing pleasing and displeasing qualities of other members, making up stories about family pictures, and putting together color-forms designs. The coding system applied to these tasks, developed by Rosman and Minuchin (Rosman, 1978), is based on structural family theory (Minuchin, 1974). Through the use of this coding system, five structural constructs are assessed: *transactional style, enmeshment, alliance, conflict,* and *protectiveness.* Each construct includes several subcategories of behavior that are coded every time a family member speaks. Additional details regarding the coding procedure are unpublished. The coding method has been used to compare the family functioning of psychosomatic and normal families, as evidenced by their family interaction patterns (Minuchin, Rosman, & Baker, 1978).

Structural Analysis of Social Behavior

The Structural Analysis of Social Behavior (SASB) (Benjamin, Giat, & Estroff, 1981) is a model for the classification of interpersonal transactions and includes a microanalytic coding process to classify social interactions and intrapsychic events in terms of three underlying dimensions: *focus* (a process regulation construct), *affiliation* (an affective construct), and *interdependence* (a structural construct). Focus refers to self, other, or introjection. Affiliation and interdependence both represent continuum ratings—very friendly to very unfriendly, very autonomous to very submissive. The model and coding system are designed to provide a scientific methodology for the diagnosis of psychosocial functioning and the investigation of psychotherapy process.

The SASB is theoretically derived from object relations theory, the personality theories of Murray (1938) and Sullivan (1953), and the interpersonal circumplex model of Leary (1957). It is considered to be compatible with structural and communication theories of family therapy. No specific task is essential to the use of SASB. However, because the coding process is microscopic and expensive, it is recommended for use with relatively brief (minimally, 10 minutes) but intense family process. The code is applicable to a range of units—for example, an individual, a coalition of individuals, and so on. The primary unit of analysis is a complete thought. The coding system's primary uses with regard to families have been to explicate the therapy process and to compare patterns of interpersonal relationships in normal and troubled families. The long-range goal of the SASB is to analyze the process of therapy scientifically and to reduce error in the prescription of patient interventions (Benjamin, 1987).

Defensive and Supportive Communication Interaction System

Alexander's (1973a, 1973b) Defensive and Supportive Communication Interaction System is theoretically derived from small-group research (Bales, 1951; Gibb, 1961) and family systems theory (Haley, 1971). It includes eight behavior types—four representing the affective construct of *defensiveness* (judgmental-dogmatism, control-strategy, indifference, superiority) and four representing the construct of *supportiveness* (genuine information seeking/giving, spontaneous problem solving, empathic understanding, and equality). In studies that use this coding system, the frequency and reciprocity of defensive and supportive communication in family interaction are scored as indicators of family adaptiveness. Approaches to coding include time sampling, examination of naturally occurring speech units, and examination of thought units. Family interaction data are obtained from two videotaped family discussions: a response to open-ended questions task, and a revealed differences task. The coding scheme has reliably discriminated between families of delinquent and nondelinquent adolescents (Alexander, 1973a, 1973b) as well as between more and less successful therapeutic interventions (Alexander, Barton, Schiavo, & Parson, 1976).

Family Interaction Coding System

The Family Interaction Coding System (FICS), developed by Patterson, Ray, Shaw, and Cobb (1969; Reid, 1978) is a microanalytic code designed to describe the aggressive behaviors of parents and children, their associated antecedents, and consequences within a field setting. The measure is based on social learning theory. It was developed to provide an assessment methodology that accurately measures changes in family interaction resulting from intervention and to provide data to support the development and validity of a theory of coercion and social aggression. The code consists of 29 categories, approximately half describing *aversive* behaviors and half describing *prosocial* behaviors. Examples of the aversive code categories include cry, humiliate, destructiveness, whine; examples of the prosocial categories are physical positive, compliance, talk, receive. In studies that use the code, data are collected in semistructured home settings prior to either lunch or dinner. Observations are conducted for a minimum of 70 minutes and are coded live in 5-minute blocks. The FICS has been used to identify sequences of interlocking contingencies of positive and negative behavior that differentiate families of nonclinical children from families of children identified as antisocial (Patterson et al., 1969).

Parent–Adolescent Interaction Coding System

The Parent–Adolescent Interaction Coding System (PAICS), developed by Robin and Fox (1979), is a microanalytic coding system grounded in social learning theory and based on the Marital Interaction Coding System (Weiss, Hops, & Patterson, 1973; Weiss & Summers, 1983). It is used to record verbal behaviors of parents and adolescents as they attempt to solve their problems. Each behavior unit is coded according to one of the following categories: *positive* behaviors (agree-assent, appraisal, consequential thinking, facilitation, humor, problem solution, specification of the problem); *negative* behaviors (command, complain, defensive behavior, interrupt, put down); or *neutral* behaviors (no response, problem description, talk). In studies that use the PAICS, prior to the family interactive session, both parents and the adolescent complete the Issues Checklist, in which they recall disagreements about 44 specific issues (such as curfew, chores, or smoking). The two topics that occur with greatest frequency and anger-intensity are used to elicit parent–adolescent communication. The family is audiotaped as it discusses these problems for 20 minutes. The PAICS has been used in a number of studies to evaluate changes in parent–adolescent communication following various kinds of family interventions (Robin, 1981; Robin & Canter, 1984; Robin & Weiss, 1980). A revised and simplified version of the PAICS is being developed.

The Family as a Context for Child Development

The following four coding systems were developed primarily to identify patterns of interaction in *normal* or *unlabeled* families. In general, these schemes have been developed to identify patterns of family process that predict individual differences in adolescent psychosocial development.

Interaction Process Coding Scheme

The Interaction Process Coding Scheme (IPCS), developed by Bell, Bell, and Cornwell (1982), is a microanalytic code for use with audiotaped family or marital interaction around a revealed differences task. The code, which has its roots in earlier codes of Mishler and Waxler (1968) and Riskin and Faunce (1969), is based on family systems theory, with secondary emphasis on family communication theory (Wynne, Ryckoff, Day, & Hirsch, 1958) and individuation theory (Bowen, 1976). Five major scales are coded from audiotapes and transcripts for each "speech unit": topic, orientation, focus, support, and acknowledgment. Before the interaction task in the home, each family member independently completes the Moos (1974) Family Environment Scale. Items on which dyads within the family disagree are used to generate interaction in a revealed differences task. The key constructs investigated have included *validation* (cognitive), *support* (affective). and *power* (reflecting control and sanctions). To date, the coding system has primarily been applied to a sample of intact families with adolescent daughters in order to investigate family processes associated with daughters' ego development (D. C. Bell & Bell, 1983).

Individuation Code

The Individuation Code of Condon, Cooper, and Grotevant (1984; Cooper & Grotevant, 1987; Grotevant & Cooper, 1985, 1986) provides a microanalysis of family verbal interaction that is designed to assess individuation in family relationships—that is, the interplay between individuality and connectedness within relationships in the family. The coding system is derived from family systems theory and from the psychological literature on the role of individuation in development and mental health. In addition, the code is based on work in speech and conversational analysis (e.g., Coulthard, 1977; Dore, 1979) that concentrates not on the grammatical form of each utterance, but on the interpersonal function of speech and on the way in which participants in conversation collaborate in order to sustain interaction. The Individuation Code is organized into two mutually exclusive and exhaustive categories (MOVE and RESPONSE) in order to acknowledge that all speech units represent both a response to previous conversation and a direction for subsequent discourse. Each speech unit is coded in both categories. A hierarchical organization is also imposed to resolve the problem of speech units that have more than one function. When factor analyzed, four independent factors indicative of the relationships in the family emerged from the 14 coded behavior categories. Two *(self-assertion* and *separateness)* are indicative of individuality, and two *(mutuality* and *permeability)* are indicative of connectedness.

The coding system is designed to analyze family discourse around a 20-minute plan-something-together task. All utterances (an utterance is defined as "an independent clause together with any dependent clauses") are coded from transcripts and audiotapes. To date, the code has been used to differentiate levels of adolescent identity exploration and role-taking, as predicted by family interaction variables at the levels of both the individual and the dyad (Cooper, Grotevant, & Condon, 1983; Grotevant & Cooper, 1985), and to examine links between adolescents' interactions within the family and with peers (Cooper, Grotevant, & Ayers-Lopez, 1987).

Family Constraining and Enabling Coding System

Hauser's Family Constraining and Enabling Coding System (Hauser, Powers, Jacobson, Schwartz, & Noam, 1982; Hauser, Powers, Noam, et al., 1984;

Hauser, Powers, et al., 1987) is a microanalytic system for coding family communication events and sequences. The coding system is based on the psychoanalytic work of Helm Steirlin, who was concerned with the ways in which family members inhibit adolescents who are attempting to individuate from the family. The code assesses two categories of *constraining* behavior (cognitive and affective), two categories of *enabling* behavior (cognitive and affective), and an interpersonal process construct *(discourse change)*. Each speech may be coded on these major categories as well as on the source and object (who to whom) of each speech. Family interaction has been assessed in a revealed differences task that follows the individual administration of the Kohlberg Moral Judgment Interview. Family members are asked to defend their positions and then come to a consensus. To date, Hauser's coding system has been used to characterize family interaction patterns that are predictive of adolescent ego development and of progressions or regressions in ego development (Hauser et al., 1982; Hauser, Powers, Noam, et al., 1984; Hauser, Powers, Schwartz, et al., 1980; Hauser, Powers, et al., 1987). In recent work, sequential analysis has been used to discriminate between psychiatric and nonpatient families along theoretically expected lines (Hauser et al., in press).

Developmental Environments Coding System

The Powers (1982) Developmental Environments Coding System (DECS) is similar to the foregoing Hauser code, in that both investigate patterns of communication presumed to stimulate (or enable) and inhibit (or constrain) development. Unlike Hauser's psychoanalytically derived system, however, Powers' coding system was derived from structural-developmental theory, as most clearly examplified by Piaget and Kohlberg.

The purpose of the code is to assess those family variables predicted to affect ego development of adolescents (Loevinger, 1976). The DECS codes 24 categories of family interaction that are indicative of two cognitive constructs *(stimulation* and *inhibition),* and two affective constructs *(support* and *affective conflict)* as well as codes for the interpersonal process regulators of *mode, transactive versus nontransactive,* and *content.* The coding system of Berkowitz and Gibbs (1979) for dyadic discussion of moral dilemmas was used as a model in the development of the DECS. Before the interaction session, both parents and the target adolescent respond individually to the Kohlberg Moral Judgment Interview. Family members are then brought together, their differences are revealed, and they are asked to reach a family consensus. To date, the primary application of this code has been to test hypotheses concerning the degree to which family interaction variables predict ego development of normal adolescents as well as adolescents undergoing psychiatric treatment (Powers, 1982; Powers, Hauser, Schwartz, Noam, & Jacobson, 1983) and to examine associations between family interaction and adolescents, and the use of defense mechanisms and adaptive coping processes (Powers et al., 1986; Powers, Jacobson, & Noam, 1987).

Discussion

Existing family interaction coding systems demonstrate considerable overlap in behavior coded at the level of the utterance. However, the theoretical diversity among the coding systems is noted when the behaviors are aggregated into constructs. Thus, there appear to be minimal interchangeability and overlap either between or within theoretical groupings at the construct level. Because of distinctive theoretical emphases, no one coding system includes constructs in all five dimensions.

The overarching context of research (clinical versus developmental) somewhat differentiates construct dimensions. For example, no clinically focused coding system includes cognitive variables, which are represented in three of the four systems that concern the family as a context for development. Of all the dimensions, the affective constructs appear to be represented more consistently in both clinical and developmental coding systems, possibly reflecting the historical importance attributed to the role of affect in the development of personality. The interpersonal process constructs follow a similar pattern. Coding systems that exclude affective variables (systems theory and social learning theory) reflect theoretical reactions to the weight given to affective variables in psychodynamic theory. Structural constructs are represented in coding systems that either are derived directly from or acknowledge the importance of family systems theory. Variables reflecting control and sanction span both clinical and developmental research contexts. Within developmental research, control and sanction categories are used to explicate parent–child interaction; whereas in clinical research, they are used to characterize the way that family members constrain the behavior of one another.

It should be noted that identical behaviors are sometimes represented with different constructs, on the basis of their theoretically derived function. For example, an acknowledging or supportive statement is coded as an indication of permeability (a structural construct) within the Individuation Code; whereas an identical statement would be coded as support (an affective construct) within the Interaction Process Coding Scheme, the Family Interaction Scales, and the Affective Style Measure. This difference in coding reflects the different emphases of systems and relational theories in contrast to individually oriented theories. In the Individuation Code, permeability is a reflection of a relational rather than an individual quality. Thus, because of the theoretical diversity represented in the family interaction codes, comparisons of research findings using the different coding systems must be made with caution.

PSYCHOMETRIC COMPARISONS OF THE CODING SYSTEMS

This section first compares the family interaction coding systems in terms of the techniques of data collection and reduction used and the level at which the interactions were coded. These considerations are typically linked to the code itself because the unit of analysis must be specified by each coding system. Next, the coding systems are contrasted in terms of their organization, the tasks used to elicit behavior, observation settings, duration of observation, and ease of use. Although interaction coding systems are not *inevitably* tied to specific data collection techniques, most interaction codes have been used in a small number of studies or by a small number of investigators, so that, in practice, the coding system and data collection technique are linked. It should be noted, however, that such links are not necessary.

Data Collection and Reduction

The coding systems were first compared with respect to the mechanics of data collection and reduction. Audiotaping was used most commonly in data collection (for 10 coding systems), followed by videotaping and live coding. The choice of some method of preserving a record of the interaction by 12 of the 13 coding systems reflected the complexity of the systems and the need to review interaction in depth, possibly a number of times, before completing the coding process. The advantages of videotaping include the ability to capture nonverbal behavior and to make accurate judgments of who is speaking to whom, especially when two or more family members have similar voices. The disadvantages, however, include the need for bulky, intrusive equipment and the difficulty of coding nonverbal behavior.

Most of the coding systems required the preparation of verbatim transcripts of the family's interaction, with the exception of the behavioral codes of Patterson and Robin, Alexander's Defensive and Supportive Communication code, and some users of the Conflict and Dominance Codes. In all cases except Patterson's FICS, a permanent record of the interaction was available on audio- or videotape for thorough analysis. Transcripts were essential for discourse-based codes in which behavior was analyzed in units such as an utterance or a speech. Determination of the boundaries of these units required a separate "unitizing" or "chunking" process before the actual coding could begin.

In addition to variations in the preparation of transcripts, studies in which the coding systems were used differed in terms of the source from which data were actually coded. Two systems coded only from tape (audio or video) (Alexander, Robin); three coded only from transcripts (Doane, Hauser, Powers); one coded live (Patterson); five coded from tape plus transcript. Although it has not been demonstrated empirically, it seems likely that coding from transcripts without the benefit of tapes could reduce the information available to the coder (e.g., tone of voice cues, such as sarcasm) and potentially lead to inaccuracies in coding, especially in the coding of affect. The studies using coding systems to assess affective constructs coded from actual speech rather than from written transcripts alone, with three exceptions (Hauser, Powers, Doane). Of course, it should be noted that subsequent researchers using these coding schemes could use both tapes and transcripts in coding.

The unit of coding also varied widely across coding systems. Four systems (Riskin and Faunce, Doane, Hauser, Powers) coded each "speech," typically defined as all of one person's conversation from the time he or she started to speak until someone else spoke. Thus, the actual duration of a speech could be very brief or quite lengthy. Three coding schemes (Mishler and Waxler; Bell, Bell, and Cornwell; Condon, Cooper, and Grotevant) used an approximation of the "utterance" as the unit of analysis. An utterance was typically defined as an independent clause and any dependent clauses connected to it; a complete sentence was the longest utterance coded. In the SASB, the "element," defined as a complete thought or a psychologically meaningful interaction, was coded; a given utterance might therefore have several elements. Four coding systems (Alexander, Patterson, Robin, and the Conflict and Dominance Codes) analyzed units of behavior. For example, in Robin's PAICS, a behavior unit is a verbalization that is homogeneous in content without regard to arbitrary syntactical properties. Thus, several very different means of unitizing are represented in this set of interaction codes. As of this date, methodological studies of family interaction have not addressed the impact of different styles of unitizing on analysis of the same data set. Such a study would seem very useful now.

Organization

Next, the codes were compared in terms of their organization. The number of behavior categories included in the codes varied widely. The structures of the codes were also very different. For example, in Patterson's system, each of six major scales was coded separately, and within each scale, the categories were mutually exclusive and exhaustive. In Alexander's system, however, categories were neither mutually exclusive nor exhaustive; specific behavior units could receive multiple codes. Other codes included conventions involving coding hierarchies (e.g., Bell, Bell and Cornwell; Condon, Cooper, and Grotevant; Hauser) for use when more than one code could logically be applied to a particular unit. Many of the organizational issues (such as coding hierarchies) appeared to be made on pragmatic and/or theoretical bases (see Table 3–1). Some were based on consideration of features of verbal interaction; for example, in the Individuation Code, each utterance was coded twice—once as it represents a "move" in the conversation, and once as it responds to preceding interaction.

Tasks Used to Elicit Interaction

The coding systems were next compared with respect to the tasks used to elicit family interaction, the setting in which interaction was observed, and the length of observation. Tasks used to elicit family interaction varied widely among studies using the 13 coding systems. They included revealed differences and unrevealed differences tasks, discussing actual family problems, plan-something-together tasks, naturalistically occurring behavior, describing qualities of other family members, making up stories about family pictures, and putting together color-forms designs. The choice of tasks typically reflected the different purposes of the investigators using the coding systems.

It is possible to place the coding systems on a continuum of the level of conflict that the tasks elicited. At one extreme of this continuum are those coding systems that called for the discussion of specific, emotionally charged family problems. All three of these coding systems were developed for use with clinical populations to elucidate and possibly intervene in problematic family interaction. The coding systems that employed revealed and unrevealed differences tasks typically did so to engage the family members in confrontation of their differences. However, this method was used both with clinical and normal families and was not designed to elicit the same intensity of family conflict as was the set of codes just described. Less conflictual behavior was elicited by those coding systems that used plan-something-together tasks. In the case of Individuation Code, the plan-a-vacation-together task was used to maximize participation of all family members by providing a topic of interest to which all members could contribute without making preexisting family roles salient.

The choice of task to elicit family interaction has the potential to influence strongly the interactional content and process. Therefore, it is important for developers of interaction coding systems to articulate clear theoretical or pragmatic reasons for their choice of task; and it is important for users of interaction coding systems to understand the potential impact of the choice of task on the content and process of the family's interaction.

Some studies attempting to assess the impact of task differences on family processes have found minimal differences across tasks, although the range of tasks investigated has not been as great as the range of tasks represented in the foregoing coding systems. Jacob and Davis (1973) compared family interaction in three tasks (plan-something-together, make up a consensus story for a TAT card, unrevealed differences task) in a sample of 10 family triads. Few reliable task differences emerged for the three indices studied: talking time, attempted interruptions, and successful interruptions. In a replication and extension, Zuckerman and Jacob (1979) examined interaction differences across three tasks (TAT story, Family Problem Questionnaire—hypothetical family issues, unrevealed differences task), this time with 30 family triads. Again, few reliable differences emerged for two indices: the ratio of successful to attempted interruptions (a measure of power) and the ratio of attempted interruptions to number of speeches (a measure of conflict). Task differences were found for the number of speeches, a measure of the amount of family activity. In both of these studies, the impact of task differences was felt to be minimal.

On the other hand, Henggeler, Borduin, Rodnick, and Tavormina (1979) compared family interaction in two unrevealed differences tasks, one focusing on instrumental/external family issues and the other focusing on expressive/ internal family issues. Dyadic measures of affect and dominance were not related to task content; however, strong task effects were observed for the conflict measure. Thus, it appears that measures of certain constructs may vary as a function of task content, whereas measures of other constructs may vary much less. Because of the breadth of the constructs assessed by the coding systems reviewed here as well as the variations in tasks, we feel that it is premature to conclude that different tasks would yield similar patterns of family interaction. Until the parameters of task differences are much more clearly understood, we believe that it is essential that investigators have clearly articulated reasons for their choice of tasks and that they be aware of the potential impact of that choice on family interaction. Studies observing families in multiple-task situations are seen as highly desirable.

Setting of Observation

The 13 family interaction coding systems also differed with respect to the setting in which the interaction took place—home, laboratory, clinic, or school. Choice of setting appeared related either to the hypothesis and sample under investigation or to the constraints of the chosen data collection technique. One might expect, for example, that the codes focusing on child-rearing expertise would utilize home observation in an effort to achieve greater approximation of typical or optimal parent behavior, whereas family pathology codes might benefit from a clinic or laboratory situation, which can be expected to increase the stress and thus provide a more stringent test of the coping of family members. In general, data to be analyzed with the family pathology coding systems were largely collected in clinic or laboratory settings. The coding systems of Patterson and Robin, based on social learning, represent exceptions to this rule and reflect the theoretical importance of environment for behavior within this tradition. The settings of the child development codes present a mixed picture. It is expected that the utilization of laboratory or clinic settings with those codes facilitates their administration.

Research supports the importance of setting to variations in family process. In a widely cited study, O'Rourke (1963) compared the interaction of 24 family triads in home and laboratory sessions. In both settings, families were presented with two problems of a hypothetical family and were asked to discuss alternative solutions. Interaction was coded in terms of a short form of the Bales Interaction Process Analysis: positive social-emotional behavior, negative social-emotional behavior, and instrumental behavior. As they moved from home to laboratory, fathers and adolescents became less positive and mothers became more positive. In addition, there was a general increase in instrumental and negative behaviors as the family moved from the familiar home setting to the unfamiliar laboratory. This study suggests that the setting in which behavior is observed may affect family process.

Users of the coding systems being reviewed here should be aware of the potential trade-offs involved in the observation of families in the home versus the more constrained setting of the laboratory, clinic, or school. For example, is the investigator willing to give up the familiarity of the home setting for the ability to videotape interaction in a laboratory? How will decisions about the location of family interaction influence family behavior? In sum, setting selection should be based primarily on theoretical concerns and secondarily on pragmatic considerations.

Duration of Observation

The coding systems also varied with respect to the length of family observation. Duration of observation ranged from 10 to 70 minutes for the coding systems under consideration, with most observations lasting from 20 to 30 minutes. Observations were not always coded in their entirety, however. For example, in the Family Interaction Scales of Riskin and Faunce, the first 80 speeches and the third block of 80 speeches were coded, reducing the amount of interaction analyzed to approximately 4 minutes. No empirically based rationale was presented for this decision. In Doane's Affective Style Measure, adolescents were observed in two dyadic situations with mother, two with father, and two triadic situations (for a total of 42 minutes). For purposes of analysis, the first dyadic situation with each parent and the first triadic situation were used (for a total of 21 minutes), because they were most emotionally charged. In the Individuation Code of Condon, Cooper, and Grotevant, the first 300 utterances of the 20-minute interaction were analyzed, because the authors had found that the frequencies of behaviors found in the first 300 utterances correlated substantially with the frequencies of behaviors for the entire transcript (Cooper, Grotevant, & Condon, 1982). An important issue concerning selection of a subsample of interaction to analyze involves the degree to which the subsample is representative of the entire interaction episode. Decisions of this type should be made on an empirical rather than an impressionistic basis. With the exception of Patterson's code, in none of the studies using the 13 coding systems were multiple samples of behavior taken over a short period of time or in multiple settings, although several of the interaction codes (e.g., Hauser, Powers) were designed for longitudinal studies in which behavior observations were separated by a year.

Ease of Use

To compare the family interaction coding systems on their ease of use, we specifically addressed the availability of norms and standardization, the availability and completeness of a coding manual, and the cost of training observers and coders.

   None of the family interactive codes has compiled adequate research data to provide norms for populations of interest. Patterson's Family Interaction Coding System has been used in the greatest number of research investigations. Mean behavior rates for the Patterson variables are available for clinic versus nonclinic children and their siblings and parents (Patterson et al., 1969). Clearly, the high cost of collecting and analyzing data with interactive systems discourages investigations with adequately representative samples that would permit norms to be established. In addition, the tendency to develop new coding systems to fit each investigator's theoretical focus rather than to replicate previous coding systems with new populations retards the integration of findings.

The availability and completeness of a coding manual is critical to the use of family interactive coding systems by a variety of researchers and, therefore, is a key to the development of the code's construct validity and utility. Eleven of the 13 family interaction coding systems had developed coding manuals. Specific information regarding the coding manuals is provided in Table 3–2.

There was considerable variability among the coding manuals in their clarity and coverage of topics. The majority of coding manuals provided clear explication of specific coding definitions, rules, examples, and sample transcripts. Exceptions to clarity occurred in particularly complex coding situations such as the Rosman and Minuchin Family Task, which utilized different codes for each of five interactive family tasks, and Benjamin's Structural Analysis of Social Behavior, which was based on complex theoretical premises requiring considerable inference. The most adequate manuals included descriptions of the theoretical basis of the code, scoring and data reduction guidelines, reliability and validity data, and information on coder training. Manuals that were part of a larger published work were reliably comprehensive. Approximately half of the available manuals did not provide adequate information to permit informed use of the code without obtaining information from a variety of sources—typically, journal articles.

Coder training is one of the costly aspects of family interaction methodology. Therefore, the 13 family interactive systems were compared on their requirements for coders. Information on coder training was available for 6 of the 13 codes. Coder reliability after training varied from 70% to 90%; the majority of studies reporting on coding indicated that ongoing reliability checks were customary. The majority of coders were post-BA-level personnel, which raises some concern regarding the expense of the coding process. However, few code authors indicated that such a level of education was essential. Coder training varied widely among the codes, with a minimum of 15 to 20 hours of training indicated (Family Interaction Coding System and Individuation Code) and a maximum of 160 hours reported for certain complex scales of Mishler and Waxler's Family Interaction Code. Duration of coder training varied with code complexity, level of inference required, number of simultaneous coding decisions, and code stimulus (written transcript versus live or videotape coding).

GENERALIZATION OF THE CODING SYSTEMS: ISSUES OF RELIABILITY AND VALIDITY

The value of any observation code is ultimately limited by its reliability and validity. Most recently, these issues have been discussed as an aspect of gen-

TABLE 3–2. Mechanics of Data Collection and Reduction in Family Interaction Tasks

Coding Scheme	Availability[a]	Theoretical Rationale	Administration Instructions	Coding Instructions	Coding Examples	Sample Transcripts	Scoring	Coder Training	Data Reduction Method	Reliability	Validity
Family Interaction Code	1	***	***	***	***	***	***	***	***	***	***
Family Interaction Scales	2	*	***	***	***	***	***	*	*	***	*
Family Task	2	*	***	**	***	*	**	*?	*	*	*
Structural Analysis of Social Behavior	2	**	***	***	***	*	***	***	***	***	*
Defensive and Supportive Communication Interaction System	2	**	***	***	***	*	***	*	*	*	*
Family Interaction Coding System	1	***	***	***	***	***	***	***	***	***	***

Coding System	Availability[a]									
Parent–Adolescent Interaction Coding System	2	*	*	***	***	*	*	*	*	*
Interaction Process Coding Scheme	2	**	***	***	***	*	***	***	***	*
Individuation Code	1	***	***	***	***	***	***	***	***	***
Family Constraining and Enabling Coding System	2	*	*	***	*	*	***	*	*	*
Developmental Environments Coding System	1	***	***	***	***	***	***	***	***	***

Note: Two interaction coding schemes did not have manuals available: Family Conflict and Dominance Codes and Affective Style Measure.
[a] Availability: 1—from publisher, 2—from author.
*Not covered in manual **Covered but material not clearly explicated ***Comprehensive coverage

eralizability theory (Cronbach, Gleser, Nanda, & Rajaratnam, 1972), which focuses on the adequacy of the coding system—to be representative and non-reactive and to discriminate (Gilbert & Christensen, 1985). Cronbach's theory of generalizability enables the researcher to make a detailed conceptual analysis, through analysis of variance procedures, of the many and various components that contribute to the reliability and subsequent validity of observational data (Hartmann, 1982b). Reliability as evidenced, for example, by coder/observer accuracy—comparison of coder with a criterion (Hartmann, 1982b), interrater reliability (Pinsoff, 1981), and reliability of unitizing as well as coding (Pinsoff, 1981)—has been noted as critical to the reliability of systems. However, in family process studies (Patterson, 1982, is an exception), reliability has emphasized one variance component: consistency of codings between two or more individuals. As noted in more comprehensive discussions of these issues, the generalizability of observational coding systems, particularly the determination of their reliability, is a substantive methodological issue that requires a careful matching of the coding system's application in research to appropriate reliability methodology (see Gilbert & Christensen, 1985, Hartmann, 1982b, Pinsoff, 1981, for additional discussion of these complex issues). While acknowledging the importance of matching coding systems with reliability methods, this section compares the 13 observation coding systems in terms of their reliability on one variable, interrater reliability, as the most commonly assessed reliability estimate. Highlights of reliability and validity findings for each of the observation systems are presented in Table 3–3.

Reliability

Three statistical indices have been most commonly used to estimate interrater reliability: percentage agreement, Cohen's kappa, and correlation. Percentage agreement and Cohen's kappa are recommended for categorical scores (response frequency, duration, and so on). Cohen's kappa, unlike percentage agreement, corrects for chance agreement by coders; therefore it usually provides a more conservative estimate.

Clear standards have not been established regarding appropriate reliability values for observation systems (Hartmann, 1982b). In fact, Pinsoff (1981) argues that the establishment of arbitrary levels of acceptable reliability is inappropriate, because reliability levels are relative to the validity demands placed on the task. Adequate reliability is attenuated by the number of code categories, the complexity of the coding systems, and the difficulty of the experimental task.

Other researchers (e.g., Hartmann, 1982b) have suggested ranges for acceptable reliability. The recommended reliability range is 70% to 90% for percentage agreement; .60 to .75 is acceptable for Cohen's kappa, with statistical significance considered adequate by some investigators; and .60 is considered necessary for correlation (Hartmann, 1982b). In addition, reliability estimates

TABLE 3–3. Reliability and Validity Information for Coding Schemes

Coding Scheme	Number of Codes	Interrater Reliability	Validity
Family Interaction Code (Mishler & Waxler)	22	Codes: 64–97%; kappa = .59–.87 Composites: 81–100%	*Criterion:* Normal and schizophrenic families were differentiated on 5 composite indices.
Family Interaction Scales (Riskin & Faunce)	8	80–95% (over time)	*Criterion:* Differentiated 5 family groups (4 clinical), $n = 44$. Ranking derived from observed variables correlated significantly with clinical ranking, $n = 12$. *Construct:* Codes combined to reflect family systems theory significantly correlated with clinical ranking.
Family Conflict and Dominance Codes (Hetherington, Stouwie, & Ridberg)	11	94–100%	*Criterion:* Differentiated 4 delinquent groups. *Construct:* Did not correlate with questionnaires.
(Jacob)	3	96% (informal)	*Criterion:* Composite correlated with age and social class.
(Henggeler & Tavormina)	8	$r = .73–.95$	*Criterion:* No consistent race/class differences.
Affective Style Measure (Doane)	5 (3 composite)	kappa = .78 ($p < .001$)	*Criterion:* Marital and cross-situational parent classifications predicted young adult pathology 5 years later and schizophrenic relapse.
Family Task (Rosman & Minuchin)	5 composite, 3–14 specific	None reported	*Construct:* Presumably differentiates among psychosomatic family types; however, claim unsupported by data.
Structural Analysis of Social Behavior (Benjamin)	3 composite	kappa = .45–.91 (process), .62–.94 (content)	*Criterion:* Code validity not formally established; SASB dimensionality validated.
Defensive and Supportive Communication Interaction System (Alexander)	8 (2 composite)	81–94% (over time)	*Criterion:* Differentiated delinquent and nondelinquent adolescent families. *Construct:* Subcategories intercorrelated; composite categories negatively correlated.
Family Interaction Coding System (Reid & Patterson)	29	30–96%; $r = .59–1.00$	*Criterion:* Differentiated normal and antisocial child families. Families with social aggressors differentiated from hyperactives and stealers. *Construct:* Correlated with alternative measures of family coercion, the Parent Daily Report.

(continued)

TABLE 3–3. CONTINUED

Coding Scheme	Number of Codes	Interrater Reliability	Validity
Parent–Adolescent Interaction Coding System (Robin)	15	51–81%; (mean, 64%); $r = .73–.92$	*Criterion:* Differentiated family therapy, communication training, and no treatment groups as well as distressed and nondistressed mother–son dyads. *Construct:* Correlated with global ratings.
Interaction Process Coding Scheme (Bell, Bell, & Cornwell)	5 composite (average of 7 codes per composite)	71–97%	*Criterion:* Coding system differentiated between dual-career and husband-employed families
Individuation Code (Condon, Cooper, & Grotevant)	4 composite, 14 codes	52–100% (11 > 75%)	*Criterion:* Individuality and connectedness in family communication predictive of identity exploration and individuation in interaction with peer. *Construct:* Factor analysis yielded four independent factors, $n = 444$.
Family Constraining and Enabling Coding System (Hauser)	15 (3 composite)	81–99%; kappa = 43 ($p < .05$) to .93 ($p < .001$)	*Criterion:* Differentiated families with children at two levels of ego development, $n = 2$. Differentiated family process in low versus high-ego-development adolescent, $n = 3$. Ego development predictably correlated with family process, $n = 61$. *Construct:* Viewed as supporting Loevinger's ego development theory.
Developmental Environments Coding System (Powers)	8 major codes	84–98%; kappa = .63–.73; $r = .85–.98$	*Criterion:* Family interaction correlated with adolescent ego development.

should be based on assessments that occur covertly and periodically throughout the study; chance-corrected statistics should be used, or the chance-level agreement for the statistics should be reported for each variable that is the focus of analysis, rather than only for the average of all variables (Gilbert & Christensen, 1985; Hartmann, 1982b; Pinsoff, 1981).

A comparison of reliability statistics used by the 13 family interaction systems reveals that the majority (10) estimate reliability using the percentage agreement index appropriate to categorical data. Of these 10, 6 reported reliability within the recommended range. Lower reliability appeared to reflect lack of consistency in coding one or two specific behaviors rather than overall inconsistency, because mean percentage agreements fell within the acceptable range. Several investigators (Mishler and Waxler, Hauser, and Powers) calculated Cohen's kappa estimates of reliability in addition to percentage agreements; others (Benjamin, Doane) relied solely on Cohen's kappa. All reported kappas met acceptable criterion levels. Three coding systems reported correlational indices of reliability, all of which fell within acceptable levels. Choice of the correlational method of reliability was warranted for the Family Conflict and Dominance Codes, because the data being compared were response totals rather than interval-by-interval agreement.

In general, the family interaction codes report respectable levels of reliability. However, few studies conformed to all of the recommended procedures for reporting reliability. In particular, greater attention to establishing reliability repeatedly over the course of the study and increasing use of chance-corrected statistics appears warranted.

Validity

Although several types of validity are applicable to observation systems, the most frequently considered types are content, construct, and criterion-related. *Content validity* is present when a judgment is made that the variables included within a coding system reasonably represent the domain that the investigator wishes to study. Establishment of content validity is usually a first step in code development; however, it is generally not considered sufficient by itself to determine the value of a coding system. *Construct validity* is crucial when an observation system has been derived deductively from theoretical considerations. It is typically established by obtaining positive correlations of the observation scores with other measures of the same construct (convergent validity) and negative or nonsignificant correlations with measures of different constructs (discriminant validity). *Criterion-related validity* is established by relating scores for variables or constructs to external criterion scores that are relevant to the purpose of the coding system. The criterion may be studied at the same point in time (concurrent validity), or the variable or construct may be used to predict a later outcome (predictive validity). Criterion-related validity is sufficient when coding systems are derived inductively from observed covariations (Cone, 1982). It is recognized, of course, that validation is a process that occurs through empirical investigation over time.

Attention to construct validation of the family interactive systems has been limited. The coding systems of Riskin and Faunce, Patterson, and Robin found interactive process scores to correlate with alternative measures of the same constructs, such as rankings or daily reports. A comparison of scores across multiple measures written by the same investigator does not provide as stringent a test of validity as is desirable. The one system (Hetherington's version of the Family Conflict and Dominance Code) that compared observation scores with scores on a standardized measure of the same construct did not obtain a significant relationship.

In comparing the family interaction systems, 12 of 15 (variations of the Family Conflict and Dominance Code are considered independently) provided at least one investigation demonstrating evidence of criterion-related validity. In general, composite scores derived from most of the coding systems differentiated family types of interest. However, specific variables within coding systems provided little criterion-related validity support. As has been previously determined for individually focused, behavioral observation systems, criterion-related validity appears to be more easily established with summed or composite scores derived from molecular behaviors.

Although promising validation efforts have been made on several coding systems, the high cost of data collection and analysis discourages rapid advancement. The validation of available coding systems is also hindered by the tendency for each investigator to create a new code to address his or her specific research questions. Finally, a significantly overlooked research area is the within-method comparison of existing family interaction coding systems.

CONCLUSIONS

Despite the similar purposes of many of the coding systems reviewed in this chapter, it should be abundantly clear that they differ from one another in a number of substantive ways: in the theoretical foundations underlying code constructs, in the tasks and setting in which interaction is elicited, in the means of data collection and reduction, in the units of coding and analysis, in the ease of use of coding manuals and documentation, and in the evidence accrued to date in support of the coding system's reliability and validity. Each of the decisions required by an investigator in the choice and use of a coding system has a potential impact on how the data are collected, reduced, and aggregated. It should be assumed that these differences are not inconsequential until critical comparative studies of the coding systems are undertaken.

The 13 family interaction coding systems reviewed here reflect a broad array of theoretical perspectives. Each theoretical viewpoint is appropriate for certain research questions but is not so useful for others. It is therefore imperative that researchers consider theoretical issues when selecting a coding system. Within theoretical perspectives, studies have not yet compared the extent to which different coding systems sample the same dimensions. We view comparative studies of family interaction codes both within and across theories as important directions for future research. Weinrott, Jones, and Boler (1981) provide an example of research investigating the correspondence among coding systems. Until further comparative studies are completed, investigators must rely upon psychometric data, such as the data presented in this review, to guide their choice of coding system.

Psychometric evidence in support of some of these coding systems is beginning to mount, but most of the systems have been used in only one or a few studies. This appears to be due, in part, to the time-consuming and expensive nature of most of the data collection strategies. It is imperative that much more extensive use of these measures be made before we have ample evidence for their usefulness. To date, the largest body of evidence available is for the Family Interaction Coding System (Patterson et al., 1969), reflecting the maturity of Patterson's family research program. The lack of psychometric studies for other measures does not indicate that these measures are less valid, but simply means that their validity has not been adequately established.

As existing coding systems become more fully utilized, researchers not only may provide evidence of adequate psychometric quality, but also may identify the most salient aspects of social interaction captured by the coding system for making particular predictions. Such ''short forms'' might enhance the usefulness of lengthy and complex coding systems in research without jeopardizing their validity. A parallel situation exists regarding the clinical utility of family interaction codes. Currently, the microscopic analysis of behavior does not lend itself readily to the clinical setting. Again, however, once a body of supporting evidence has been established for particular coding systems, it might be possible for clinical versions of the codes to be developed in order to capture ''critical events'' in treatment that would be theoretically and practically meaningful.

Given the variations noted within the coding systems reviewed in this chapter, it is incumbent on the researcher to make the most informed decision possible when choosing data collection and reduction techniques in family interaction research. It is hoped that this comparison of the coding systems will stimulate potential users to articulate their research questions clearly and to choose a coding system that is consistent with their goals. We concur with Hartup (1978, p. 40) that ''there is no substitute for rational selectivity in avoiding the tyranny of one's own data.''

4

RATING SCALES OF
FAMILY FUNCTIONING

The purpose of this chapter is to offer family clinicians and researchers a critical comparative analysis of eight family rating scales to assist them in making decisions regarding the quality and utility of the scales. To enhance comparability, the scope of this review is limited to rating scales that involve the whole family unit. Rating methods that focus only on marital or parent–child dyadic relationships are not included. Rating scales reported only in dissertations were also omitted. One identified rating scale was not evaluated at the request of its author.

This chapter begins with a brief discussion of psychometric issues regarding the use of rating scales and a presentation of the criteria used for evaluating them. Then the eight rating scales are described and individually evaluated according to the specified criteria. A comparative analysis of the rating methods follows. The chapter concludes with an integrative discussion, recommendations for use, and issues to be addressed in the future development of family rating measures.

ISSUES IN RATING SCALE MEASUREMENT

Issues concerning both psychometric quality and rater competence constrain the reliability and validity of rating scales. One pattern of rating errors reflects the stylistic or personality tendencies of the rater. These errors include the error of central tendency, the leniency/severity effect, and the contrast effect. The *error of central tendency* reflects the propensity of the rater to assign ratings in the middle of a scale rather than at the extremes. The *leniency/severity effect* results from the reluctance or propensity of a rater to assign either overly unfavorable or overly generous ratings to a family. The leniency error may be interrelated with the *contrast effect,* whereby families are rated in the opposite direction to the rater's own family or family of origin.

A second pattern of rater errors reflects errors in the cognitive processes by which raters evaluate families. These include the logical error, the proximity error, and the halo effect. The *logical error* occurs when the rater constructs logical relationships between items such that they are rated similarly. Logical errors are exacerbated by the *proximity error,* which occurs when two items placed together on the rating scale receive similar ratings. A final type of error to which raters are vulnerable is the *halo effect.* This error occurs when raters construct a global impression about the family that is carried across specific differentiated items or qualities. In other words, the raters fail to discriminate among potentially independent aspects of a family's behavior (Saal, Downey, & Lahey, 1980).

Rating errors reduce the reliability and validity of ratings in a variety of ways. Several of the errors (e.g., central tendency) restrict the range of scores, whereas other errors (e.g., the halo effect) create spurious correlations among the items. Both types of errors can be expected to cause data problems, particularly for correlational or predictive research designs. The high cost associated with rating errors underscores the importance of training raters thoroughly and assessing their reliability. Whereas reliability is typically assessed with percentage agreement statistics, the use of generalizability theory, which permits the differentiation of rater error from scale error, would appear to be important. The reader is referred to Hartmann (1982b) for further discussion of this method of reliability.

The psychometric quality of rating scales can be enhanced in several ways (Saal et al, 1980). First, rating scale quality is enhanced when the dimension to be measured reflects a single construct indexed by overt behavior that occurs within a specified time frame. Broad, abstract dimensions that require a high level of inference typically result in low reliability and validity. When global ratings of family functioning are used, it is essential to identify the significant elements. Second, rating scale dimensions must reflect behavior that is likely to occur in the family's stream of behavior during the period of observation. Third, the dimensions most suitable for the rating method are the stable, enduring characteristics of families.

The availability of clearly defined anchor points and equal psychological distance between anchor points also increases the likelihood that ratings will be both reliable and valid. Reliability is further increased with an adequate number of anchor points or steps. Nunnally (1978) has suggested that five scale steps represent the minimum acceptable level and that reliability increases substantially with seven scale points.

Psychometric quality enhances the potential quality of the rating—a key concern because the rating method depends on the complex information-processing capabilities of the rater. In contrast to the observer in behavioral observation coding schemes, who need only be an accurate recorder, the rater is assumed to be a competent family theorist, methodologist, observer, and psychometrician. Specifically, the following assumptions have been identified regarding rating methods (Cairns & Green, 1979): (1) raters share with the scale author, and with other raters, a theoretical concept of the quality or attribute to be rated; (2) raters share a concept of which behaviors reflect that quality or attribute; (3) raters are able to detect information relevant to the attribute in the stream of behavior; (4) raters share the same underlying psychometric "scale" (e.g., normal distribution), on which the attribute will be judged; and (5) raters have sufficient knowledge about the comparison or reference group to place observed behavior on a distribution. Because of these assumptions, rater quality and training assume heightened importance for this method of family assessment.

Users of rating scales reviewed in this chapter should realize that most of the studies using the scales have employed raters who have extensive clinical training and experience in addition to training on the instrument. The necessity of such background should be noted by the user of the rating scale but will not be the primary focus of subsequent discussion.

EVALUATION CRITERIA

When the relative strengths and limitations of the family rating scale method of family assessment have been discussed, two sets of issues have emerged: those that reflect rating scale properties and those that concern rater competence and training. The quality of each of these categories directly affects the reliability and validity of a particular scale. The key issues within each of these areas may be summarized as follows:

Properties of Scales
1. Dimensions are clearly defined.
2. Dimensions reflect enduring, stable characteristics.
3. Dimensions reflect overt, observable behavioral constructs.
4. Dimensions reflect a single or unitary construct rather than multiple or mixed constructs.
5. Dimensions reflect behaviors that are likely to occur in the observation setting.
6. Dimensions are constructed on a uniform and explicit standard of reference.
7. Dimensions have an adequate number of discrimination points.

Rater Competence and Training
1. Rater level of training/experience is specified.
2. Manual is available and adequately comprehensive for training.

Psychometric Validity and Reliability
1. Normative data are available.
2. Interrater reliability rater errors have been examined.
3. Validity studies have been conducted.

These criteria will be considered as the family rating scales are individually and comparatively evaluated in the remainder of the chapter.

DESCRIPTIONS AND EVALUATIONS OF SCALES

Beavers-Timberlawn Family Evaluation Scale (BT)

The BT is a 14-item rating scale designed to assess family health. Its primary purpose is for descriptive classification and family research; a secondary purpose is to influence treatment. Each item represents a construct derived from the Beavers System Model of Family Functioning (Beavers, 1982; Lewis, Beavers, Gossett, & Phillips, 1976). The model is based on a clinical interpretation of general systems theory, which holds the view that key family challenges are separation and individuation and that individual functioning and family functioning are interrelated.

The BT consists of six major scales: Family Structure (subscales are Overt Power, Parental Coalition, and Closeness); Mythology; Goal-Directed Negotiation; Autonomy (subscales are Clarity of Expression, Responsibility, Invasiveness, and Permeability); Family Affect (subscales are Range of Feelings, Mood and Tone, Unresolvable Conflict, and Empathy); and Global Health/Pathology Rating. These variables are rated on scales ranging from 1 to 5, with nine half-point differentiations. Individual subscale scores are averaged, and this score is compared with the Global subscale score as an "ecological check." It is unclear from the manual what the rater is to do if the "ecological check" is invalid. A scoring guide provides conversion scores that permit placement of a family on the Beavers Model classification scheme.

The BT has significantly differentiated healthy families from those containing psychiatric patients (Lewis et al., 1976). In the most recent psychometric studies of the BT, interrater reliabilities ranging from .58 to .77 for the subscales and .79 for the Global scale have been found (Hulgus, 1985). Preliminary data indicate that all but two of the BT subscales (Mythology and Invasiveness) can be reliably rated, but only when the raters are highly experienced family therapists (Green, Kolevzon, & Vosler, 1985; Hulgus, 1985).

A strength of the BT is its clear theoretical foundation. The BT provides adequate differentiations for dimensions and clear descriptions for three of the five scale points. Limitations of the BT construction are reflected in the degree to which dimensions reflect covert processes and, therefore, are highly susceptible to subjective ratings with low reliability. Another concern with this measure is that several scales combine more than one construct (e.g., power and flexibility are combined within the Overt Power subscale; expression of thought is integrated with expression of feeling in the Clarity of Expression subscale). Raters also face the challenge of placing the dimensions on a family systems health/pathology continuum rather than on a more standard linear continuum. Though consistent with the theoretical foundation from which the rating scale is derived, this scale construction property underscores the necessity of highly qualified, clinically trained raters.

Beavers-Timberlawn Centripetal/Centrifugal
Family Style Scale (CP/CF)

The CP/CF is a seven-item rating scale intended to evaluate the family's "manner of being together" or style of systemic interaction without regard to health or pathology. When used in conjunction with the BT, the family may be located on a "map" of the Beavers System Model. Subscales include Social Presentation, Verbal Expression of Closeness, Positive Expression of Feelings, Parental/Adult Conflict, Parental Control—Clinging, and Parent Control—Aggressive. An impressionistic Global scale is also included.

Subscale ratings are made on 5-point scales ranging from centripetal at one end to centrifugal at the other. Descriptions are provided for three of the five anchor points on each dimension. The scores from the individual subscales are added, averaged, and compared with the Global subscales, as in the BT. The average CP/CF score is then mapped, along with BT scores, on the Beavers System Model.

The CP/CF scales have differentiated types of families with midrange competence. In preliminary studies, interrater reliability has ranged from .33 to .63; reliabilities for the Dependency, Scapegoating, and Physical Spacing subscales were not reported (Hulgus, 1985). The Parental Control—Clinging and Parental Control—Aggressive subscales demonstrated inadequate reliability (.33 and .39, respectively). Low reliability could be due to low frequency of occurrence of these events, lack of clarity in the dimension descriptions, or inadequate training of raters.

In summary, the primary strength of the CP/CF is its theoretical fit with the Beavers Model of Family Competence and its complementarity with the BT. Currently, the scale suffers from inadequate subscale reliability and limited psychometric assessment of its properties.

McMaster Clinical Rating Scale

The McMaster Clinical Rating Scale (CRS) (Epstein, Baldwin, & Bishop, 1982) evaluates family functioning to determine the need for professional intervention. The McMaster Model of Family Functioning (MMFF) (Epstein, Bishop, & Levin, 1978) is based on systems theory, which assumes that the parts of the family are interrelated and that the whole does not equal the sum of the parts. Therefore, the McMaster CRS rates whole-family functioning rather than individual dysfunction. Within the model, family "health" is equated with "normality." The dimensions of family functioning measured by the CRS (problem solving, communication, roles, affective involvement, affective responsiveness, behavior control) are hypothesized to have the most impact on the emotional and physical health of family members. The CRS also evaluates Overall Family Functioning. Each dimension is rated on a 7-point scale with three defined anchor points: severely disturbed (1), nonclinical (5), and superior

(7). Ratings of 1 through 4 indicate family dysfunction and the need for intervention. Although scale dimensions arc uniformly constructed along a logical continuum, anchor points are not individually defined. Raters may differ in their ability to differentiate among scale points. A further threat to rater competence is that the multidimensionality of each scale requires a high level of inference by raters.

Despite these difficulties, preliminary data indicate that the CRS has demonstrated good interrater reliability (range, $r = .57$ to .91). It has also shown acceptable criterion validity, when compared with the objective McMaster Family Assessment Device, on all dimensions except Problem Solving (Little-Bert, personal communication, 1984).

Family Assessment Measure
Clinical Rating Scale (FAM-CRS)

The FAM-CRS (Skinner & Steinhauer, 1986) evaluates family functioning according to the Process Model of Family Functioning (Steinhauer, Santa-Barbara, & Skinner, 1984). The Process Model of Family Functioning is similar to its antecedent model, the McMaster Model of Family Functioning, but greater emphasis is placed on the interaction of the individual family and family with social environment systems. Thus, the FAM-CRS contains items that evaluate family dyadic relationships as well as values and norms reflective of the extrafamilial social press. The dimensions assessed by the FAM-CRS include Task Accomplishment, Role Performance, Communication, Involvement (including dyadic relationships), Control and Values and Norms. Each dimension is rated on a 5-point scale, with all anchor points defined (e.g., Major Strength [1] = almost always appropriate and likely to remain a strength under stress; Major Weakness [5] = a severe problem area, likely to worsen family functioning if not changed, destructive in individuals).

Strengths of the FAM-CRS include its theoretical derivation, dimensional consistency with the self-report FAM, well-defined anchor points, and the assessment of dyadic relationships within at least one dimension. Because it has been developed recently, scoring procedures are currently unavailable, and empirical validation studies of the scale have not yet been conducted. Familiarity with the Process Model of Family Functioning is necessary for valid use of the rating scale.

Global Family Interaction Scales (FIS-II)

The FIS-II rating scale (Riskin, 1982) is a global, macroanalytic form of the original FIS, a microanalytic family interaction measure (Riskin & Faunce, 1972). The goal of the rating scale is to identify family interaction patterns that contribute to the understanding of the personality development of family members. Thus, the scale is intended primarily for descriptive research.

The FIS-II rates each of 17 dimensions of family interaction on a 5-point scale rating from "very much," or "high," to "very little," or "low." Thus, differentiations reflect a uniform standard of reference. Ratings are based on the whole-family unit. Dimensions include Clarity, Topic Continuity, Appropriate Topic Change, Commitment, Request for Commitment, Information Exchange, Agreement, Disagreement, Support, Attack, Intensity, Humor, Interruptions, Laughter, Who Speaks, Intrusiveness, and Mind Reading. Most of the dimensions reflect observable behaviors.

The reliability of the FIS-II was assessed by Kendall's coefficient of concordance (Riskin, 1982). Based on 18 raters and two families, reliability was deemed adequate (probability of ratings occurring by chance ordering was less than .10) for 12 of the 17 subscales. Low reliability could reflect limited observer training, inadequate clarity of dimensions, low frequency of occurrence, or high within-family variability of events.

In a longitudinal study comparing several nonclinical families, the FIS-II has differentiated families significantly on nine dimensions (Riskin, 1982). Results supported the content validity of at least several dimensions of the measure regarding family style and led Riskin to hypothesize a range in which normal functioning may be observed on the scale dimensions. However, further investigation of these hypotheses has not been undertaken as yet (J. Riskin, personal communication, 1986).

The strength of the FIS-II appears to be the simplicity of the code and the ease with which it can be mastered. Several shortcomings are evident, however. First, the measure is limited by the lack of a strong empirical or theoretical basis for the selection of rating scale dimensions. Its utility must therefore await considerable empirical investigation, which has not, to date, been forthcoming. Second, the dimensions of the FIS-II are directly derived from a microanalytic procedure in which behaviors of individuals are coded. Thus, they tend to reflect individual behaviors rather than whole-family system qualities. Within-family variability on dimensions evaluated by the FIS-II are likely to reduce the reliability and validity of the rating scale. Further empirical work with the FIS-II will be necessary to establish its validity as an effective whole-family system measure.

Clinical Rating Scale
for the Circumplex Model of Marital and Family Systems

The Clinical Rating Scale for the Circumplex Model (Olson & Killorin, 1985) permits a clinician to make global ratings of marital and family systems on the basis of a semistructured family interview. Although the substance of the interview is not prescribed, the scale's authors recommend an interview that asks the family members to engage in a discussion with one another about how they handle general family issues such as time, space, and discipline. "Asking the family to describe what a typical week is like and how they handle their daily routines, decision making, and conflict is often illuminating'' (Olson & Kil-lorin, 1985, p. 2). Following the interview, the clinician rates the family on subscales for three major dimensions: Cohesion, Adaptability, and Communication. Anchor points for all dimensions are clearly specified in a table supplied with the scales. Six subscales contributing to the Cohesion score (Emotional Bonding, Family Involvement, Marital Relationship, Parent–Child Coalitions, Internal Boundaries, External Boundaries) are each measured on scales of 1 (disengaged) to 8 (enmeshed); five subscales contributing to the Adaptability score (Leadership, Discipline, Negotiation, Roles, Rules) are each measured on scales of 1 (rigid) to 8 (chaotic); and six subscales contributing to the Communication score (Continuity Tracking, Respect and Regard, Clarity, Freedom of Expression, Listener's Skills, Speaker's Skills) are each measured on scales of 1 (low) to 6 (high). The psychological distances between scale points seem to be roughly equal.

On the basis of the Cohesion and Adaptability ratings, families may be placed on the Circumplex Model grid, which was derived directly from Olson's theory of family systems functioning (e.g., Olson, Sprenkle, & Russell, 1979; Olson, Russell, & Sprenkle, 1983). Although the scale has not been used widely in research, Olson (personal communication, 1985) found that, using five raters in a sample of 45 families, the average interrater correlation was .88 for Cohesion, .84 for Adaptability, and .92 for Communication. In addition, the level of agreement within one scale point on the global ratings was found to be 91% for Cohesion, 89% for Adaptability, and 94% for Communication. Validity studies are currently under way. The major strengths of this instrument seem to be its flexibility for use in a clinical setting with both families and couples and its clear ties to the Circumplex Model. Its major weaknesses include unknown validity and failure to integrate the ratings on the Communication dimension into the Circumplex Model. An additional consideration in the use of this instrument is the current debate over the curvilinearity of the dimension of family adaptability (Beavers & Voeller, 1983; Lee, 1988).

Global Coding Scheme

The Global Coding Scheme (L. G. Bell, Cornwell, & Bell, 1985) is intended for macroanalysis of family interaction in a research context using a battery of three audiotaped tasks: revealed differences based on items from the Moos Family Environment Scale (for the marital couple); a similar revealed differences task for the mother–father–adolescent triad; and interactions surrounding the creation of a family paper sculpture by the mother, father, and adolescent. The coding scheme is based on family systems theory. The scales themselves were modeled on the Beavers-Timberlawn Family Evaluation Scale and the Family Behavioral Snapshot (see L. G. Bell et al., 1985). The total scale includes 55 rated items and also provides several opportunities for written descriptions by the observer. Individual items are typically rated on 5- to 6-point scales from "almost always" to "almost never" or on a scale relevant to the item (e.g., "very vague" to "very clear"). Within each section, various items are combined to form composite scales. Seven such composite scales have been developed: Interpersonal Boundary, Comfort with Differences, Ability to Resolve Differences, Covert Conflict, Warmth and Support, Depression, and Influence of Children. Since a detailed theoretical framework is not set out in the manual, it is difficult to say whether the items comprehensively sample the domains considered important. Interrater reliability (correlations) for two coders assessing nine families ranged from .44 to .81 (median, $r = .73$); single-item reliability correlations for 15 items ranged from .51 to .90.

To date, several items and scales have shown themselves to be useful as predictors of theoretically relevant outcomes. For example, ratings on Accurate Interpersonal Perception, Comfort with Differences, and Positive Receptive Attitude were predictive in theoretically meaningful ways of Differentiated Self-Awareness and Positive Self-Regard in adolescent females (D. C. Bell & Bell, 1983). The emotional closeness among family members was also predictive of the degree to which adolescents' friendship choices were reciprocated (L. G. Bell et al., 1985). The primary strengths of these scales lie in their theoretical foundation and promising validity evidence. The primary weaknesses concern the high degree of inference involved, the extensive clinical training of the coders who have worked with the scales so far, and the unspecified breadth of the theoretical domain that the scales were intended to assess.

Family Interaction Q-Sort (FIQ)

The FIQ (Gjerde, Block, & Block, 1983) provides a macroscopic assessment of parent–child and parent–parent relationships in dyadic and triadic situations. The 33 items that make up this research technique were not chosen on the basis of any single theory, although they were chosen to represent a variety of family relationship issues. Six tasks are used to elicit behavior: three dyadic tasks (phenomenology of emotions, consequences test, Lowenfield Mosaic test) and three triadic tasks (description of ideal person, strategies, Venn diagrams). Q-sorts for dyadic relationships are completed after judges view videotapes of family interaction. The 33 items are sorted into a forced-choice distribution of nine categories, ranging from "most uncharacteristic" to "most characteristic." The variable clusters that emerged from factor analysis included disregard, ambivalence, affiliation, withdrawal, and control. To date, the FIQ has been used primarily in the Block longitudinal study of personality development being conducted at the University of California at Berkeley. The measure has been found to discriminate successfully between mother–child and father–child interaction patterns in families characterized by high parental disagreement on child-rearing issues (Morrison, Gjerde, & Block, 1983a, 1983b). In addition, the measure has been used to predict the development of adolescent depression at age 14 from FIQ assessments made between the ages of 3 and 13 (Gjerde,

1985). It has also been used to distinguish in predictable ways between mother–son and mother–daughter relationships in single-parent families (J. Block, Block, & Gjerde, in press). A strength of this technique is that behavior is assessed in a variety of tasks. Some items are anchored very clearly in behavioral terms, whereas others require more subjective summary judgments. The technique's weakness lies in its lack of an explicit theoretical foundation; hence, the comprehensiveness of item coverage of the scale is impossible to assess. To date, the FIQ methodology has been used successfully in several research endeavors and promises to be useful in future work.

COMPARATIVE EVALUATIONS OF SCALES

A comparative evaluation of existing family rating scales across key dimensions appears in Table 4–1. Dimensions selected for comparative evaluation reflect the psychometric quality of the measure and thus influence its reliability and validity. Most family rating scales are based theoretically on family systems theory and therefore are congruent with an evaluation focus on whole-family functioning. Although theoretical foundations are similar, the primary function of existing rating scales varies and includes screening for treatment, classification, and descriptive-normative research. The psychometric concerns discussed next are important for all of these functions.

Clearly Defined Dimensions

The clarity of the dimensions to be rated varied considerably among and within measures. Two specific problems were noted most commonly. First, some scale items required simultaneous ratings of more than one quality. For example, on the BT, the Responsibility scale includes consideration of the degree to which family members voice responsibility for their own actions with the degree to which they blame others. A similar problem was noted with an item on the Bell Global Coding Scheme: "In general members take responsibility for their own actions, feelings, and thoughts, and do not take responsibility for the actions, feelings, or thoughts of others." A second problem involved dimensions that did not appear to fall along a logical continuum. For example, the progression rated on the Overt Power item of the BT goes from "chaos" to "marked dominance" to "moderate dominance" to "led" to "egalitarian."

Overt Behaviors

The reliability of rating scales depends on the extent to which observable behaviors are rated. Items within scales varied with respect to the degree to which they assessed overt behaviors. Problematic items included, for example, the BT's Mythology scale: "Every family has a mythology; that is, a concept of how it functions as a group. Rate the degree to which this family's mythology

TABLE 4–1. Comparative Evaluation of Rating Scale Properties

Scale	Theory	Assessment Function[a]	Clearly Defined Constructs	Overt Behaviors	Stable Characteristics	Frequency of Event	Uniform Logical Standard of Reference	Adequate Number of Scale Steps	Manual	Reliability	Validity
BT	Family systems	1,2,3,4	**	**	**	**	**	***	**	**	***
CP/CF	Family systems	1,2 3,4	**	***	***	**	***	**	**	**	**
CRS for the Circumplex Model	Circumplex Model	1,2,3,4	***	***	***	**	***	***	**	***	*
McMaster CRS	Family systems	1,3,4	**	**	**	**	**	***	**	***	**
FAM-CRS	Family systems	1,3,4	***	**	***	**	***	**	*	*	*
FIS-II	Interactional	4	**	***	*	***	***	**	*	**	*
FIQ	None	4	**	**	*	**	***	***	***	**	***
Global Coding Scheme	Family systems	4	***	**	**	**	*	***	***	**	***

[a]1 = influence treatment; 2 = classification; 3 = intervention evaluation; 4 = normative descriptive research.
* Absent or inadequate; ** Present but mixed/minimum requirements met; *** Present and adequate

seems congruent with reality.'' The Gjerde FIQ required assessment of a subtle, poorly defined type of behavior: ''A tends to be aware of and to be comfortable with B's sexuality.'' The Bell Global Coding Scheme included the item ''The task seemed scary and they tended to pull back from it,'' and the FAM-CRS included the item ''Family members internalize a sense of responsibility and self-discipline.'' Inclusion of such high-inference items would appear to tax the observational abilities of the best raters and would likely lead to low reliability on such items.

Characteristics Observed

Ratings are designed to capture global characteristics or patterns in family behavior; thus, dimensions should reflect observable, repetitive, and patterned behavior. Most of the rating scales presented a mixed picture with regard to this criterion. Low ratings were given to the Gjerde FIQ for the situational specificity of its items, and to the FIS-II for its failure to integrate micro-level overt behaviors into theoretically meaningful global family patterns or characteristics. These measures would probably be less useful to a clinician than the others, since they would not as effectively provide summary conclusions about the family's functioning. In contrast, the low inference demanded by the FIQ and FIS-II enhance their utility in research, which is their expressed purpose.

Frequency of Events

Within rating scales, dimensions varied in terms of the degree to which they reflected events expected to occur with reasonable frequency in a family interaction. Although an advantage of rating scales over behavioral observation techniques is that low-frequency events that are highly salient may be given appropriate weight in the inferences drawn by the rater, some items may be difficult to rate because of insufficient information. For example, both the McMaster CRS and the FAM-CRS assess role performance, a category for which evidence may not occur in the stream of behavior without directive questioning.

Standards of Reference

With several noteworthy exceptions (e.g., FAM-CRS, BT, CP/CF, FIS-II), clear anchor points were not consistently provided across measures, and manuals did not typically provide sufficient examples for training of raters. It is likely that clinicians would bring a different frame of reference to these rating scales than would researchers who are studying normal family processes. For example, the 5 scale points for rating ''clear vs. unclear speech'' on Riskin's FIS-II may have very different meanings for a clinician and a researcher. Although this problem would not prevent the establishment of adequate interrater reliability within a particular research or clinical team, comparability across research teams or clinicians working independently would be questionable. One strategy that would obviate this problem would include the development of "criterion tapes" that could be shared (with corresponding ratings and rationales) among clinicians and researchers. Another model for ensuring similarity of ratings across investigators includes scoring workshops used for training with such measures as Ainsworth's "strange situation," Loevinger's measure of ego development, and Kohlberg's Moral Judgement Interview. To the best of our knowledge, the workshop method has been used only informally by the Beavers-Timberlawn group.

Number of Scale Steps

All scales had at least 5 scale steps, the minimum necessary for reliability according to Nunnally (1978). The CP/CF, FIS-II, and FAM-CRS scales had 5; all other scales had more, with the FIQ and the BT having 9 scale differentiations. Since reliability is not significantly enhanced beyond 7 steps, additional differentiation would appear cumbersome and may reduce interrater reliability.

Manuals

The availability of a clear, detailed training manual is essential to ensure comparability of ratings across professionals using the rating scales. Few of the scales had detailed manuals, and no manuals were available for the FAM-CRS or the FIS-II. Only the Bell and Gjerde manuals provided full behavioral descriptions of differentiations among scale points. None of the manuals contained detailed information about rater training, despite the critical role played by the rater in this type of family assessment methodology.

Reliability

All scales except the FAM-CRS, for which data have not been collected, demonstrated minimally acceptable reliability, although some individual scales had unacceptable reliability. The most consistently high reliability was reported with the McMaster and Olson scales.

Validity

Validity evidence for most of the measures reviewed is promising but incomplete. Several of the rating scales were developed quite recently, and few if any validity studies have been conducted. Insufficient studies on which to base a judgment of validity were noted for the Olson and Killorin rating scale, the Skinner and Steinhauer FAM-CRS, and the Riskin FIS-II. Most of the individuals involved with the development of these measures have ongoing programs of research in which further validity evidence will be developed.

DISCUSSION

The comparative evaluation of the eight rating scales for family assessment has brought into focus several issues that must be addressed by family scholars involved in scale construction and use. The psychometric quality of existing family rating scales appears mixed. Areas in which family rating scales can be improved include the use of clearly defined anchor points on single dimensions that reflect observable, stable behavioral patterns; the development of comprehensive manuals and rater training procedures; and the conduct of reliability and validity studies. Thus, the state of the art of the family rating scale methodology might be considered "good enough" to "promising," but not "excellent."

The issues involved in the use of rating methods in family assessment extend beyond psychometric concerns, however, and mirror unresolved methodological dilemmas of the field. The operationalization of family systems theory continues to provide a source of methodological challenges. Existing family rating scales appear most compatible with the systemic principle that the whole is greater than the sum of the parts and, therefore, that the whole should be the appropriate unit of assessment and change. Although consistency with this principle is appropriate in many cases, it poses serious limitations to the researcher's ability to obtain a comprehensive view of family functioning. In particular, data on family hierarchy or structure, as well as within-family variability, cannot be obtained. Family researchers have noted the importance and the somewhat neglected stature of both hierarchy and individual variability in family methodology (Gurman & Kniskern, 1981b; Oliveri & Reiss, 1982).

A pervasive problem with family rating scales is the difficulty of assessing a quality of the whole family when a rating might differ for certain individuals or dyads within the family. For example, the degree of emotional bonding (Olson & Killorin, 1985) might be very high for three of five family members and very low for the other two. How is the family to be rated? When marked within-family variability is noted, some raters may base their judgments on the most salient or vocal family members. Others may base ratings on some "average" level for the family, which may not reflect the actual behavior of any specific individual or dyad within the family. Identifying rater biases in this regard is critically important for both researchers and clinicians using family rating scales and heightens the value of explicit training and rater evaluation procedures.

In contrast to the whole-family perspective of the rating scales, the Gjerde FIQ, the Bell Global Coding Scheme, and the FAM-CRS permit dyadic judgments. This appears to enhance the accuracy of the rating procedure. However, the inclusion of the assessment of hierarchical or dyadic relationships raises an additional concern; that is, how does one "score" or weight subsystem evaluations vis-à-vis whole-system scores? Clearly, wholeness and hierarchy, milieu, and variability are important to both researchers and clinicans. Researchers who are interested in family cohesion, for example, would benefit from knowing where in the family the levels of cohesion differ. Clinicians might plan interventions to shift dysfunctional dyadic levels of closeness to optimize the identified patient's development.

It would appear that solutions to the problem of measuring whole versus interdependent but variable parts can best be determined from empirical investigation. Studies that examine the correspondence of ratings across hierarchical levels of family functioning on the same dimension would appear essential before assuming that the whole can be measured validly. This appears particularly salient for some dimensions—such as closeness, communication, and control—and for theories that emphasize the individual–family interface (e.g., the Process Model of Family Functioning). In summary, family scholars who develop rating scales are encouraged to consider a multilevel methodology and to validate empirically the differential utility of a whole versus variable-parts rating across salient dimensions of family functioning.

Global ratings are also problematic to the degree that they summarize a variety of impressions in a single score. This summarizing may yield a misleading score (albeit a highly reliable one), because it does not take into consideration the full range of the family's behavior during the period of observation. This consideration is a concern for all scales reviewed in this chapter.

Observers must also decide whether judgments are to be based on the frequency or salience of events or on a combination of the two. With microanalytic family interaction codes (see Chapter 3 for review), summary judgments are typically derived from the frequencies of specified events or sequences of events, even though certain highly salient events may have occurred with low frequency. With rating scales, observers have the flexibility to weight both frequency and salience in making judgments. Although this should be an advantage, such weighting requires careful training and extensive experience in order to make reliable and valid judgments. This factor is an important consideration for all rating scales reviewed here, with the possible exception of the Family Interaction Q-Sort, in which items are placed relative to one another in a fixed distribution.

Several advantages of Q-sort methodology suggest that further instrument development in this area could be beneficial (Waters & Deane, 1985): Observers can be kept unaware of the constructs they are evaluating; observers do not need to have internalized norms for each behavior they are rating; response biases are reduced because items are sorted into a fixed distribution; and rating on a variety of items makes possible the development of a variety of scales and a variety of criterion sorts against which the family can be compared. Q-sorts can also be repeated on dyadic relational or individual levels, thus permitting a more complete assessment of the complexity of the system.

Another concern raised by this review of scales is the appropriateness of family classification on dimensions or in typologies. Some have argued that typological classification is premature, given the level of knowledge regarding family functioning (Epstein et al., 1982), and that as the number of empirical studies increases, the time will be more appropriate for the construction of classification schemes. Others (e.g., Olson), argue for the clinical utility of typologies. This debate is reflected in the rating scales reviewed, which include both dimensional and categorical construction. It would appear that the solution to this problem requires further empirical study of the validity of family typologies derived from ratings.

In summary, the rating method of measurement, and the specific family rating scales reviewed in this chapter, demonstrate both strengths and limitations for use by family scholars in research and clinical practice. Family rating scales vary in their capacity to accomplish measurement functions reliably and validly because of differences in the clarity and observability of their dimensions or subscales and the competence and training of raters required to make the ratings. Although replete with methodological challenges, family rating scales may still be the family assessment method of choice. When evaluated against one set of criteria proposed for the selection of family measures for clinical use, rating scales appear uniquely sound (Margolin & Fernandez, 1983). Ratings give perspective on the intensity of the problem, assist in targeting areas of intervention, are cost-effective, and are not intrusive to the family. The research utility of existing family rating scales is far less clear. Although ratings have demonstrated predictive validity in areas such as developmental psychology, their usefulness remains uncertain in family psychology. The unique challenges posed by the systems framework appear simultaneously to support the use of this methodology as a means of capturing patterns of behavior in families and to underscore the necessity of construction based on empirical data to reconcile the unique whole–part interdependencies.

Section III
Self-Report Measures

5

INTRODUCTION TO SELF-REPORT MEASURES IN FAMILY ASSESSMENT

The self-report method is perhaps the most commonly employed clinical and research measurement strategy for the study of human relationships (Cromwell, Olson, & Fournier, 1976). Questionnaires have been used primarily to assess whole-family functioning, including family stress and coping, marital relationships, and parent–child relationships. More recently, assessment of sibling relationships has emerged.

Self-report measures are standardized questionnaires that provide information about individual family members' subjective reality or experience, including their perceptions of self and other family members, attitudes regarding family (e.g., roles, values), and satisfaction with family relationships (Huston & Robins, 1982). Information obtained with self-report measures, although completed by an individual family member, may assess the individual, dyadic, nuclear family, or extended family levels.

Self-report methods have numerous advantages. It requires considerably less training to administer and score questionnaires than observational methods. Thus, self-report methods are often the necessary family assessment choice of clinicians and researchers. Using the subject as informant is also necessary when reliable observational data are difficult to obtain, such as in the assessment of behavior across time and situations or the assessment of behavior not typically displayed in public (Maccoby & Martin, 1983). Finally, self-report methods provide an "insider" view of family relationships (Olson, 1977), and the subjective reality of relationship partners has been demonstrated to be interrelated with their behavioral interaction patterns (Gottman, 1979).

Despite the strengths of self-report questionnaires for family assessment, this methodology has historically received considerable criticism (Maccoby & Martin, 1983). Concerns regarding self-report methodology include: (1) the sensitivity of informants to their own behavior; (2) individual response differences in subjective anchor points; and (3) the inaccuracy of retrospective reports by informants (Maccoby & Martin, 1983). These criticisms limited the development of self-report measures of family functioning in the 1960s. However, the recent cognitive trend in psychology, which emphasizes the relationship between cognitive processes and behavior, has validated, in part, the measurement of family members' subjective reality regarding their family relationships. Therefore, family self-report methods are currently used primarily for assessment of the attitudes, beliefs, and perceptions—that is, the subjective reality—of family members. These questionnaires most commonly focus on concurrent rather than retrospective information about family interaction (Maccoby & Martin, 1983); however, with increased interest in the transgenerational transmission of psychopathology (e.g., Bowen, 1966; Sroufe & Fleeson, 1986), retrospective measurement of parent–child relationships in the family of origin has reemerged. In contrast with earlier use of these data, however, the subjective bias inherent in these retrospective data is now acknowledged and considered to be theoretically relevant.

Numerous methodological advances in psychometrics have also increased interest in the use of self-report methods of family assessment. For example, the use of statistical methods for determining reliability and validity, as well as investigation of mechanisms by which error can be reduced in the construction of questionnaires, has greatly enhanced the trust that can be placed in this type of data. As with other methods of measurement, self-report measures must possess adequate reliability, validity, and normative data in order to be useful. Furthermore, the instruments must bear consistent and meaningful relationships to the constructs they were designed to measure.

The value of family self-report measures is ultimately limited by their established reliability and validity. Validity is the degree to which evidence accumulated from a variety of sources supports the inferences that are made about families on the basis of members' test scores. Thus, as noted in *Standards for Educational and Psychological Testing* (1985), it is the inferences regarding specific uses of the test, not the test itself, that are validated. Test validation should include the gathering of evidence across all three categories of validity—*content-related, criterion-related,* and *contruct-related. Content validity* is present when a judgment is made that the items included in the subscales of a self-report measure reasonably represent the domain. Establishment of content validity is usually a first step in test development; however, it is generally not considered sufficient by itself to determine the value of a measure. *Construct validity* is the extent to which the measure, or subscales of the measure, correlate positively with other measures of the same construct (convergent validity) and do not correlate with measures of constructs hypothesized to be distinct (discriminant validity). *Criterion-related validity* is established by relating scores for variables or constructs to external criterion scores that are relevant to the purpose of the self-report measure. The criterion may be studied at the same point in time (concurrent validity), or the measure may be used to predict a later outcome (predictive validity).

Reliability, which constrains validity, is the degree to which test scores are free of error. Since methods of establishing reliability vary, it is imperative that the sources of error most salient to the use of the measure be evaluated. The statistical indices most commonly used to estimate reliability of self-report measures are the coefficient alpha, based on the internal consistency of the test, and the test–retest correlation, based on multiple administrations of the test. The coefficient alpha is considered to be a good estimate of reliability, as the major source of test measurement error is the sampling of content (Nunnally, 1978). The split-half method of reliability is considered appropriate for measuring the variability of traits when alternative test forms are unavailable, as is the case with most self-report family measures; however, it can be employed only with tests of adequate length (20 items per half) and should not be considered a measure of stability. The retest method of reliability is the key statistic in determining the long-range stability of a test; thus, it is important for family measures that are designed to assess enduring family relationship traits or characteristics. However, the retest method over short time intervals (e.g., 2 weeks) has serious flaws as a method of estimating reliability. Thus, if the coefficient alpha is low for a measure, a short-term high retest correlation should not be taken as evidence of adequate reliability (Nunnally, 1978).

Acceptable levels of reliability vary, depending on the purpose of the instrument. Reliability coefficients of .50 to .60 are considered modest but acceptable for some situations. Reliability coefficients greater than .80 are considered unnecessary for purposes of research. However, in clinical settings, where significant decisions depend on test scores, reliability coefficients of .90 are considered the minimum, and a reliability coefficient of .95 is considered the optimal standard (Nunnally, 1978).

Normative data are essential to provide meaning for scores from self-report measures, especially when they are used for purposes of clinical prediction. Norms provide a basis for interpreting the test performance of a person or group in relation to a defined population (*Standards,* 1985). Because the collection of an adequate normative sample is recognized to be costly, evaluation of the adequacy of test norms varies, depending on the purpose of the test. Measures that are designed for research purposes and that are in the test development phase are not expected to have representative norms. Rather, clearly defined descriptive statistics regarding the various populations of research interest are imperative. In contrast, measures that are designed for clinical use or for classification purposes demand an adequate normative sample, usually based on probability sampling techniques across geographic, socioeconomic, and cultural groups.

A number of response set, or attitudinal, influences on the accuracy of self-reports have been identified and should be considered in constructing, evaluating, and using self-report measures. *Social desirability*—or "faking good" to appear in a positive light—is the most common and most troublesome source of inaccurate responding. Strategies aimed at reducing the effect of social desirability include (1) using responses to a social desirability scale to partial out the effects of social desirability statistically, (2) constructing socially neutral items, (3) using rapport and test instructions to convince the respondent that accurate responses are to his or her advantage, (4) including scales or keys within the instrument to detect faking, and (5) using a forced-choice format, in which two items are equated for social desirability.

Malingering—or "faking bad"—is a possible source of error in some situations. The problem of *acquiescence*—a tendency to give all "yes" or "true" answers or all "no" or "false" answers—is easily remedied by equating the number of "yes" or "no" responses that are keyed positively. A less common response set is *deviation*—a respondent's tendency to give unusual or uncommon responses. In research, such factors as perceptions of the experimenter's expectations and the desire to please or frustrate the experimenter are other possible sources of inaccurate responding to self-report measures.

Self-report measures are also subject to semantic problems and the effect of situational factors. An item may have different meanings to different respondents, and it may have different meanings to the same respondent at different times and in different situations (Nunnally, 1978). Clearly worded items and adequate reliability and validity take on added importance in view of these issues.

In the assessment of family systems, it is important to remember that self-report measures are measures of one individual's perceptions of the system (e.g., Fisher, 1982; Huston & Robins, 1982). The extent to which an individual respondent can provide useful information about systems variables is an important consideration in the use of self-report measures for family research. Self-report measures are appropriate when knowledge of individual family members' attitudes or comparisons of different family members' points of view are of interest (B. C. Miller et al., 1982; Olson, 1977).

In summary, issues related to the use of self-report measures for family assessment include the need for adequate reliability, validity, and normative data, as well as consideration of the effect of response sets upon the accuracy of data obtained. The key issues within each of these areas may be summarized as follows:

Properties of the Measures
1. Response format is clear and adequate in range.
2. Item length is reasonable.
3. Item content reflects differentiation of individual, dyadic, or subsystem behavior from whole-family behavior when appropriate.
4. Item verb tense clearly indicates the time frame of reference.
5. Item content is nonreactive and is keyed in both positive and negative directions to reduce social desirability.
6. Anchor points are clearly defined.
7. Reading level is appropriate.
8. Items are adequate to capture the constructs intended.

Administration and Scoring
1. A manual is available.
2. Cut-off scores and/or profile forms are available when appropriate for the instrument's purpose.
3. Directions for administration are clear, and administration is simple.
4. Directions for scoring are clear, and scoring is simple.

5. Scoring is consistent across the measure.
6. Social desirability is controlled.

Psychometric Validity and Reliability
1. Normative data are available.
2. Internal consistency and test–retest reliability have been established.
3. Validity studies have been conducted.

In the following chapters, self-report measures of family relational functioning will be discussed and evaluated individually and comparatively, using the foregoing criteria. Chapter content is biased toward self-report measures of whole-family functioning—reflecting the strong pull from family systems theorists toward assessing at the level of the whole family. To assist the comparative analysis, whole-family measures have been divided into two categories: measures of general family functioning (Chapter 6) and measures of family stress and coping (Chapter 7). Although consideration of whole-family measures is primary in this book, the choice of the appropriate level of analysis is acknowledged as one of the key issues in family research (Carlson & Grotevant, 1987a, 1987b; Maccoby & Martin, 1983). Each level of analysis (e.g., the individual, parent–child dyads, the marital dyad, sibling dyads, the whole family) adds unique explanatory power to an understanding of family phenomena that is not captured by one superordinate measurement (Cowan, 1987). The family systems tenet that the whole is greater than the sum of its parts implies that subsystems are embedded within one another; thus, assessment is appropriate at each potential level (Carlson & Grotevant, 1987a, 1987b). To facilitate multilevel family assessment with self-report methods, self-report measures of the parent–child relationship are reviewed in Chapter 8. For assessment of the marital dyad, see Filsinger (1983a, 1983b, Filsinger & Lewis, 1981).

6

SELF-REPORT MEASURES OF WHOLE-FAMILY FUNCTIONING

with Margaret Koranek

Self-report questionnaires were the predominant methodology in studies of the family through the 1970s (Galligan, 1982). The reliance on self-report measures reflected not only convenience but also the prevalence of the positivistic orientation of science, which implied that ideas could be measured and that these ideas or constructs were, in fact, representative of the real world (Galligan, 1982). However, the reliability and validity of self-report methods was seriously challenged within the field of psychology, resulting in considerable investigation of the psychometric properties of questionnaires, such as response style and response set, and more circumscribed use (see Maccoby & Martin, 1983). This method has also been criticized within the field of family studies, particularly as a method for measuring interactive reality (Galligan, 1982). Despite the criticism, however, self-report questionnaires, particularly as measures of a respondent's subjective reality, are again regarded as having broad research and diagnostic significance. Furthermore, in the past 20 years, the growing popularity of family systems theory has resulted in the development of a new set of self-report questionnaires, designed to capture qualities of the family system.

In this chapter, we will present summaries and critiques of 17 self-report measures of family relationships. Each measure will be described, highlighting its theoretical origins, the constructs assessed, and preliminary evidence of its utility. Measures will be critically evaluated and comparatively analyzed according to the criteria specified in Chapter 5. The chapter will conclude with an integrative discussion, guidelines for use, and issues to be addressed in the future development and refinement of self-report measures of family relationships.

DESCRIPTIONS AND EVALUATIONS OF MEASURES

Family Assessment Measure (FAM-III)

The FAM-III (Skinner, Steinhauer, & Santa-Barbara, 1984) is a measure of family strengths and weaknesses that is appropriate for completion by preadolescent, adolescent, and adult family members. The FAM-III is based theoretically on the Process Model of Family Functioning, an elaboration of the McMaster Model of Family Functioning (Steinhauer, Santa-Barbara, & Skinner, 1984), and thus bears some resemblance to the McMaster Family Assessment Device (see FAD discussion). The FAM-III is unique in that it provides a multilevel (within-family) assessment of family functioning across seven dimensions: *Task Accomplishment, Role Performance, Communication, Affective Expression, Affective Involvement, Control, and Values and Norms.* Items reflecting each dimension, all with a 4-point Likert-type response format, appear in each of the three FAM-III scales: a 50-item General Scale, which measures overall level of family health; a 42-item Dyadic-Relationships Scale, which is completed separately for different dyadic relationships and examines how each member views the specific dyadic relationship; and a 42-item Self-Rating Scale, which allows each person to rate his or her own functioning within the family. The FAM-III was standardized on 475 families (28% problem families) (Skinner, Steinhauer, & Santa-Barbara, 1983). Preliminary psychometric studies of the FAM-III support the reliability and validity of the overall ratings of the three scales but find variability in the internal consistency of the dimensions within the scales, particularly in the Self-Rating Scale.

The FAM-III, acknowledged by its authors to be in the development phase, represents a unique contribution to the family assessment field in providing a measure of the multiple levels (individual, dyadic, whole) of the family system.

Family Functioning in Adolescence Questionnaire (FFAQ)

The FFAQ (Roelofse & Middleton, 1985) was developed to assess the adolescent's perception of the psychosocial health of the family during the stage of having adolescent children. It focuses on six dimensions of the family system as they bear on the developmental tasks and identity formation of the adolescent: Structure, Affect, Communication, Behavior Control, Value Transmission, and External Systems. The instrument is based on family systems theory, family development theory, and Erikson's identity formation theory. It consists of 42 items, each of which is responded to on a 4-point Likert scale ranging from "almost always true" to "hardly ever true." Reliability estimates for the FFAQ are .90 for the full scale and .40 to .79 for the subscales. Scale intercorrelations are very high, suggesting that the instrument may be assessing one overall dimension rather than six distinguishable subscales. Factor analysis of the items yielded a single factor with eigenvalue exceeding 1.0. One criterion-related validity study has been conducted. In summary, the FFAQ shows promise as a single-dimension measure but is still largely untested.

Family Evaluation Form (FEF)

The theoretical base of the FEF (Emery, Weintraub, & Neale, 1980) is best described as eclectic. Items were derived empirically and from relevant theoretical constructs in the literature in order to provide an easily obtained yet comprehensive measure of family functioning to be used by researchers. The revised form of the instrument consists of 128 items, with a 7-point rating scale response format. Scales included in the 1984 version are Family Centeredness, Conflict and Tension, Open Communication, Emotional Closeness, Community Involvement, Children's Relations, Children's Adjustment, Parenting—Nurturance, Parenting—Independence Training, Parenting—Effective Discipline, Parenting—Strict/Punitive Discipline, Parenting—Negative Style, Husband/Wife Dominance, Marital Satisfaction, Homemaker Role, Worker Role, Financial Problems, and Extrafamilial Support. Norms are available for a small sample of suburban New York families. The original version of the instrument exhibited moderate to high internal consistency and test–retest reliability, with little evidence of validity. The only psychometric data available on the 1984 revised version of the FEF are alpha coefficients, which range from .61 to .88.

The FEF lacks clear scoring instructions, a broadly based normative sample, adequate evidence of validity, and an empirical basis for its numerous scales. Work in progress (including more normative work and work on test–retest reliability and construct validation) with the revised version of the Family Evaluation Form should add to our knowledge of the instrument's usefulness.

McMaster Family Assessment Device (FAD), Version 3

The FAD (Epstein, Baldwin, & Bishop, 1983) is a 60-item, Likert-scale screening instrument that distinguishes between healthy and unhealthy family functioning on seven clinically relevant dimensions, which form the scales: Problem Solving, Communication, Roles, Affective Responsiveness, Affective Involvement, Behavior Control, and General Functioning. It is appropriate for use with adolescent and adult family members. The FAD is based on the McMaster Model of Family Functioning (Epstein et al., 1978), a model compatible with family systems theory, which assumes that family health is related to the accomplishment of essential tasks. Means and standard deviations (Epstein et al., 1983) and health–pathology cut-off scores (I. V. Miller, Epstein, Bishop, & Keitner, 1985) for the FAD have been determined; however, adequate normative data have not as yet been collected. Although additional reliability and validity studies are essential, preliminary psychometric evidence suggests that the FAD is internally consistent (e.g., alphas range from .72 to .92), reliable over short periods, unrelated to measures of social desirability, and successful in discriminating clinical from nonclinical groups (Epstein et al., 1983; I. V. Miller et al., 1985).

Family Process Scales (FPS), Form E

The purpose of the FPS (Barbarin & Gilbert, 1979) is to assess the interdependence of family members, dynamic homeostasis in the family, and the family's ability to provide an environment that fosters healthy psychological development and promotes a sense of well-being in its members. The scale, which is based on family systems theory, includes 50 items, each of which is responded to on a 5-point Likert scale ranging from "strongly agree" to "strongly disagree." Five factor-analytically derived scales (10 items each) are included: Enmeshment, Mutuality, Flexibility, Support, and Satisfaction. Cronbach alpha reliability coefficients for the five scales range from .74 to .96, and tests for concurrent validity indicate moderate correlations between FPS scale scores and those of similar constructs on other measures (Barbarin & Tirado, 1985). The Enmeshment scale successfully discriminated between families whose interactions seemed to influence maintenance of weight loss and families whose interactions did not (Barbarin & Tirado, 1985).

The FPS has undergone several revisions to increase its psychometric quality. In its current version, it is simple to administer, appears useful in both clinical and research settings, and is subject primarily to limitations common to all self-report family assessment measures.

Self-Report Family Inventory (SFI)

The SFI (Beavers, Hampson, & Hulgus, 1985) was designed to translate family systems constructs from the Beavers Model of Family Functioning into a self-report format. It consists of 36 items, each of which is responded to on a 5-point scale from "Yes: Fits our family very well" to "No: Does not fit our family." The constructs assessed are Family Health/Competence, Conflict, Family Communication, Family Cohesion, Directive Leadership, and Expressiveness. According to the authors, the measure is most beneficially used in conjunction with the Beavers-Timberlawn Family Evaluation Scale (Lewis et al., 1976) and the Centripetal/Centrifugal Family Evaluation Scale (Kelsey-Smith & Beavers, 1981) in a multimethod, multilevel family systems evaluation. The SFI demonstrates good internal consistency reliability (range, .84 to .88) and mixed test–retest reliability (Hulgus, unpublished data, 1986). Tests of concurrent validity yield differential patterns of correlations across the scales (Hulgus, unpublished data, 1986).

In summary, the SFI is a potentially useful instrument that permits multimethod family assessment within the Beavers theoretical model. However, the process of instrument validation remains in the early stages, and the SFI may require further refinement before a final version is ready for use. Specifically, the independence or distinctiveness of the scales has not as yet been established.

Colorado Self-Report Measure of Family Functioning

The purpose of the Colorado Self-Report Measure of Family Functioning (Bloom, 1985) is to provide a description of whole-family functioning along 15 dimensions that cover three general headings: relationship dimensions, personal growth or value dimensions, and system maintenance dimensions. The measure is based on constructs in family systems and family development theories. The instrument includes 75 items, each of which is responded to on a 4-point scale, from "very true for my family" to "very untrue for my family." The 15 subscales include Cohesion, Expressiveness, Conflict, Intellectual-Cultural Orientation, Active-Recreational Orientation, Religious Emphasis, Organization, Family Sociability, External Locus of Control, Family Idealization, Disengagement, Democratic Family Style, Laissez-Faire Family Style, Authoritarian Family Style, and Enmeshment. Internal consistency has been demonstrated to be adequate (Bloom, 1985). A factor analysis yielded 13 factors with eigenvalues exceeding 1.0 and closely matching the anticipated theoretical constructs. Criterion-related validity was established in one study.

Although this relatively new measure is still largely untested, the careful attention paid to theoretical and psychometric issues during its development suggests that it has the potential to be a very valuable clinical and research tool. Its primary limitation lies in its current form as a retrospective measure.

Family Environment Scale (FES)

The FES (Moos & Moos, 1986) is a 90-item, true–false questionnaire designed to provide researchers and clinicians with a systematic assessment of the social environment or climate of the family unit. The measure is theoretically based in social ecological psychology and general systems theories. The FES comprises 10 subscales that assess three underlying dimensions: Interpersonal Relationship (subscales: Cohesion, Expressiveness, Conflict); Personal Growth (subscales: Independence, Achievement Orientation, Intellectual-Cultural Orientation, Active-Recreational Orientation, and Moral-Religious Emphasis); and System Maintenance (subscales: Organization and Control). Three forms of the FES are available: the Real Form (Form R) evaluates the current environment; the Ideal Form (Form I) assesses the desired environment; and the Expectations Form (Form E) measures perceptions of a new environment.

The FES Form R demonstrates adequate reliability (range for alphas, .61 to .78) and has been standardized and normed on a sample of 1,125 normal and 500 distressed families (Moos & Moos, 1986). Although several investigations have challenged the factor structure of the FES (Fowler, 1981, 1982; Nelson, 1984), the validity of the measure has been established in more than 200 studies (Moos, Clayton & Max, 1979; Moos & Spinrad, 1984). The primary limitation of the FES centers on the generalizability of the measure across populations. Like most family assessment measures, the FES provides information only about whole-family functioning. Despite its limitations, however, the FES is the most widely used and validated self-report measure of family functioning; thus, it is frequently the standard for determining the criterion validity of newly developed measures.

Children's Version of the FES (CVFES)

The CVFES (Pino, Simons, & Slawinowski, 1984) is a 30-item pictorial, multiple-choice measure designed to assess children's (ages 5 to 12) perceptions of their family's social climate. The CVFES is conceptually equivalent to the FES, with identical dimensions and subscales (see FES discussion). The CVFES represents an important potential contribution to the family assessment field, both as an extension downward in age of the widely used FES and as a means of systematic family assessment with children for whom most instruments are inappropriate. Although it has been commercially published, the psychometric properties of the CVFES have received only limited investigation to date, and the conceptual equivalence of the measure with the FES has not been examined. Furthermore, the utility of the CVFES across the developmental range for which it is intended must be established. Finally, although some content validity has been established, it is our opinion that the pictorial stimuli in the CVFES are ambiguous and may increase the likelihood of response error.

Index of Family Relations (IFR)

The Index of Family Relations, part of the Clinical Measurement Package (Hudson, 1982), was developed for repeated use with a client to monitor and evaluate progress in therapy. The instrument was designed to measure the magnitude of a problem in family members' relationships as seen by the respondent, and it can be viewed as a measure of intrafamilial stress. Although the scale can be used in a variety of settings, its initial use was in single-subject, repeated measures designs to monitor and guide treatment. The scale includes 25 items, each of which is responded to on a 5-point scale ranging from "rarely or none of the time" to "most or all of the time." The IFR was designed to be a unidimensional scale and therefore does not include subscales. Internal consistency estimates exceed .90. Hudson feels that test–retest reliability is "of dubious value" because the instrument's purpose is to assess change in the clinical setting. The construct and criterion validity of the IFR have been established in several studies (Hudson, 1982; Hudson, Acklin, & Bartosh, 1980).

In summary, the IFR is a short, easily administered self-report measure of the severity of family relationship problems. Although the measure demonstrates adequate reliability and validity, IFR items are quite transparent and anchor points are vague, thus increasing the potential response error. As intended, the measure appears to be more useful for a clinical than a research setting.

Conflict Tactics Scale (CTS)

The purpose of the CTS is to measure the use of reasoning, verbal aggression, and violence as modes of dealing with conflict in dyadic relationship within a family (Straus, 1979). The scale is based on sociological conflict theory and the work of Murray Straus and his colleagues on family violence. The CTS is composed of three subscales: the Reasoning subscale, which taps the use of such tactics as rational discussion to resolve disputes; the Verbal Aggression subscale, which refers to the use of verbal and nonverbal acts as a means of symbolically hurting the other; and the Violence subscale, which is designed to measure the use of physical force against the other. The instrument is available in two forms: Form A, the original self-report instrument, or Form N, which was designed to be administered as an interview and which places greater emphasis on violent tactics. National norms are available for use with Form N. The Verbal Aggression and Violence subscales have shown adequate to high intensity consistency reliabilities, but internal consistency for the Reasoning scale has been low. Extensive evidence for construct-related validity and some evidence for criterion-related validity has been presented for the scale. The CTS is versatile and easy to use, has demonstrated usefulness in research about family violence, and has good potential for use in a clinical setting as well.

Family Relationship Questionnaire (FRQ)

The FRQ (Henggeler & Tavormina, 1980) was developed for use with families that vary in cultural composition and socioeconomic status, including families with low literacy rates, and was designed to measure each family member's perception of the affect, conflict, and dominance within family dyads. The instrument is based on scales developed by Hetherington and Frankie (cited in Henggeler, Borduin, & Mann, 1987), which were derived from psychiatric theories concerning the role of family interaction in the etiology of schizophrenia. The FRQ consists of 11 Likert-type items, with 5-point response formats. At present, no norms are available for the instrument. The FRQ has exhibited test–retest reliability ranging from .67 to .70 over short time intervals, and several studies support the criterion-related validity of specific dimensions of the FRQ. No studies to date have provided validity support for the dominance dimension or for the FRQ as a whole. The FRQ has potential for use in family research because of its simplicity, which lends itself to use with diverse types of families. However, the usefulness of the measure is limited by weak documentation regarding administration and scoring, lack of normative data, and lack of psychometric support, particularly evidence of validity.

Inventory of Family Feelings (IFF)

The Inventory of Family Feelings (Lowman, 1980) is a 38-item, 3-point Likert-type scale in which each family member indicates agreement with items in terms of his or her feelings at that moment toward every other member. The purpose of the IFF is to determine the affective structure of the family, partic-ularly the strength of positive family affect. The IFF is theoretically based in the Multilevel Model of Family Functioning (Lowman, 1981), a model that is compatible with family systems theory but focuses on the integration of the behavioral, cognitive, and affective components of individual and family func-tioning. The IFF measures the affective component of the model. The validity of a single affective dimension has been substantiated empirically in a factor analysis of the IFF (Lowman, 1980). Along the single affective dimension, a variety of scores can be derived from the IFF that permit evaluation of dyadic, as well as whole-family, affective relationships. The IFF is designed for family members who can read at the fifth-grade level. However, the use of double negatives in the items may raise the comprehension level.

The IFF has demonstrated excellent reliability with a college sample (Low-man, 1980). Validity support has also been strong, with the IFF correlating positively with a marital adjustment measure and with clinical ratings (Fineberg & Lowman, 1975) as well as significantly differentiating clinical from nonclin-ical families (Lowman, 1980).

In summary, the IFF provides a valid and reliable assessment of a single key dimension of family functioning: family affect. The IFF is limited primarily by the lack of normative data, the lack of a manual, and the lack of systematic evaluation of its suitability for the lower age limits of the test.

Family Adaptability and Cohesion Evaluation Scales III (FACES III)

FACES III (Olson, Portner, & Lavee, 1985) was designed to measure family cohesion and adaptability as well as perceived and ideal family functioning within the context of the Circumplex Model of Family Functioning (Olson et al., 1979). Family members complete the 20-item scale twice, once indicating the present perception of their family and once indicating how they would like their ideal family to be. Each item is responded to on a 5-point Likert scale ranging from "almost never" to "almost always." From scores on the Cohe-sion and Adaptability scales, family members may be placed on a circumplex grid, which allows their perception of family functioning to be classified into one of 16 types. Internal consistency reliabilities were .77 for Cohesion and .62 for Adaptability; test–retest correlations were in the .80's. Construct validation of the scales has demonstrated that Cohesion and Adaptability are orthogonal, as assumed in the Circumplex Model; when factor-analyzed, the Cohesion and Adaptability items load on the appropriate factors (Olson et al., 1985).

In summary, FACES III provides a simple and reliable assessment of current and ideal family functioning as perceived by family members, consistent with Olson's Circumplex Model. As with other measures derived from specific family functioning theories, the utility of FACES-III may be limited by the universal acceptance of its theoretical foundation. In addition, FACES-III may be deceptively simple in its effort to assess complex family-level variables with 20 items.

Personal Authority in the Family System Questionnaire (PAFS-Q)

The PAFS-Q, based on intergenerational family theory (Bowen, 1978; Williamson, 1981, 1982a, 1982b; Williamson & Bray, in press), was designed to assess an individual's perception of important relationships in the three-generation family system. The PAFS-Q has eight scales: Spousal Intimacy, Spousal Fusion/Individuation, Nuclear Family Triangulation, Intergenerational Triangulation, Intergenerational Intimacy, Intergenerational Intimidation, Intergenerational Fusion/Individuation, and Personal Authority. Nuclear Family Triangulation is not included in the versions for persons without children (versions B and C). The PAFS-Q has internal consistency coefficients ranging from .73 to .97, adequate test–retest reliability, dimensions generally supported by factor analysis, and promising evidence of validity. Norms calculated from several samples are available. This instrument, which seems to be the only measure of intergenerational family functioning available, should be especially useful to practitioners and researchers who are interested in intergenerational family functioning.

Family APGAR

The Family APGAR (Smilkstein, 1978) is a screening instrument based on family systems theory and stress and coping theory; it is designed to give family physicians an overview of family functioning as perceived by the patient. The five-item instrument consists of one question designed to measure each of the following components of family functioning: Adaptation, or family problem solving; Partnership, or sharing of responsibility and decision making; Growth; Affection; and Resolve, or commitment to share time, space, and material resources with other family members. Two response formats are available: a three-choice format (almost always, some of the time, hardly ever), which is recommended for clinical use, and a five-choice format (never, hardly ever, some of the time, almost always, always), which is recommended for research. The instrument has demonstrated good criterion-related and construct validity, good test–retest reliability (.83), and low to moderate internal consistency reliability. Norms are available for small samples of graduate students and clinic and psychiatric outpatients and for a large sample of 10- to 13-year-old Taiwanese children. The Family APGAR will probably be most useful as a screening instrument for physicians or for others who need to make quick assessments of family functioning and as a rough and global assessment of family functioning for research.

Structural Family Interaction Scale (SFIS-R Form A)

The most recent revision of the SFIS—SFIS-R Form A (Perosa, 1986)—is a 76-item, 4-point Likert-type questionnaire that assesses family functioning in accordance with structural family therapy theory (Minuchin, 1974). The SFIS-R Form A contains eight subscales, derived from factor analysis: Spouse Conflict, Parent Coalition/Cross-Generational Triads, Father–Child Cohesion/Estrangement, Mother–Child Cohesion/Estrangement, Enmeshment/Disengagement, Family Conflict Avoidance/Expression, Flexibility/Rigidity, and Overprotection/Autonomy. The SFIS-R Form A represents a recent revision of the SFIS (Perosa, Hansen, & Perosa, 1981) that was undertaken to strengthen the measure's psychometric properties. Alpha reliabilities for the eight scales ranged from .76 to .93; test–retest reliabilities exceeded .80 for every scale. Validity studies are under way. The SFIS represents the only objective family assessment measure to be developed solely from structural family theory; therefore, it represents a significant potential contribution to the field. Current utilization is limited, however, by multiple revisions and the lack of psychometric investigation of the updated version.

COMPARATIVE EVALUATIONS OF MEASURES

Theoretical and Conceptual Comparisons

To facilitate comparisons among the 17 measures, their subscales were grouped into one of five categories. The categories were rationally derived for this project, although they are based on (but are different from) groupings proposed by Fisher (1976). The five categories are structure, process, affect, orientation, and other. *Structure* refers to how the family is organized and concerns the roles and patterns that provide a framework within which the family functions. *Process* refers to actions and activities within the family, including control, regulatory, and communication functions. *Affect* refers to the expression of emotion within the family. *Orientation* refers to the family's attitudes about itself, especially in terms of its relations with the outside world. Subscales that could not reasonably be included in one of these four categories were included in the *other* category.

The categorized listing of subscales (see Table 6–1) attests to the theoretical

TABLE 6–1. Conceptual Groupings of Subscales of the Whole-Family Assessment Measures

Measure; Author(s); Theory	Structure	Process	Affect	Orientation	Other
Family Assessment Measure; Skinner, Steinhauer, & Santa-Barbara; Process Model of Family Functioning	Role Performance	Task Accomplishment, Communication, Control	Affective Expression, Affective Involvement	Values and Norms	
Family Functioning in Adolescence Questionnaire; Roelofse & Middleton; family systems theory, family developmental theory, Erikson's identity formation theory	Structure	Behavior Control, Communication, Value Transmission	Affect	External Systems	
Family Evaluation Form; Emery, Weintraub, & Neale; eclectic theory	Family Centeredness, Husband/Wife Dominance, Homemaker Role, Worker Role	Conflict, Parenting–training, Independence–training, Parenting—Effective Discipline, Parenting—Strict Discipline, Parenting—Negative Style, Open Communication	Parenting—Nurturance, Marital Satisfaction	Emotional Closeness, Community Involvement, Extrafamilial Support	Children's Relations, Children's Adjustment, Financial Problems
McMaster Family Assessment Device; Epstein, Baldwin, & Bishop; McMaster Model of Family Functioning	Roles	Problem Solving, Communication, Behavior Control	Affective Responsiveness, Affective Involvement		General Functioning

(continued)

Family Process Scales; Barbarin & Gilbert; family systems theory	Enmeshment	Flexibility	Mutuality Support Satisfaction		Family Health
Self-Report Family Inventory; Beavers, Hampson, & Hulgus; Beavers Systems Model	Cohesion	Conflict Directive Leadership	Expressiveness		
Colorado Self-Report Measure of Family Functioning; Bloom; Structural family systems theory	Cohesion Enmeshment Disengagement	Conflict Democratic Family Style Laissez-Faire Family Style Authoritarian Family Style Expressiveness		Intellectual-Cultural Orientation Active-Recreational Orientation Religious Emphasis Family Sociability External Locus of Control Family Idealization Organization	
Family Environment Scale; Moos & Moos; Social-ecological theory, family systems theory	Cohesion Organization	Expressiveness Conflict Independence Control		Achievement Orientation Intellectual-Cultural Orientation Active-Recreational Orientation Moral-Religious Emphasis	

TABLE 6–1. CONTINUED

Measure; Author(s); Theory	Structure	Process	Affect	Orientation	Other
Children's Version of the Family Environment Scale; Pino, Simons, & Slawinowski; Social-ecological-psychological theory, family systems theory		*Same as Family Environment Scale*			
Index of Family Relations; Hudson; atheoretical					Intrafamilial Stress
Conflict Tactics Scale; Straus; Sociological conflict theory		Reasoning Verbal Aggression Violence			
Family Relationship Questionnaire; Henggeler & Tavormina; Psychiatric theory concerning schizophrenia		Conflict	Affect		
Inventory of Family Feelings; Lowman; Multilevel Model of Family Functioning			Affect		
Family Adaptability and Cohesion Evaluation Scales III; Olson, Portner, & Lavee; Circumplex Model of Family Functioning	Cohesion	Adaptability			

Measure; author; theory	Subscales		
Personal Authority in the Family System Questionnaire; Bray, Williamson, & Malone; intergenerational family systems theory	Spousal Fusion/Individuation Intergenerational Fusion/Individuation Nuclear Family Triangulation Intergenerational Triangulation	Spousal Intimacy Intergenerational Intimacy	Intergenerational Intimidation Personal Authority
Family APGAR; Smilkstein; family systems theory		Adaptation Partnership Growth Affection Resolve	
Structural Family Interaction Scale; Perosa; structural family therapy theory	Parental Coalition Enmeshment Overprotection Mother–Child Cohesion Father–Child Cohesion	Spousal Conflict Family Conflict Avoidance Flexibility	

and conceptual heterogeneity of self-report measures of whole-family relational functioning. In developing Table 6–1, it became clear that subscales are not always labeled consistently with their content. In the table, subscales were placed with the domains that corresponded with the content of the items used, rather than simply with the scale name. A noteworthy example concerns the meaning of *expressiveness*. In the Self-Report Family Inventory, the items assessing expressiveness concern family members' hugging and touching one another and feeling close to one another. In this case, therefore, expressiveness was considered within the domain of affect. In the Colorado Self-Report Measure of Family Functioning, *expressiveness* was used to refer to family members' willingness to discuss problems and say what was on their minds. Thus, the Expressiveness subscale was categorized in terms of process rather than affect. The lack of correspondence in meaning of constructs across measures reflects the lack of concensus within the family study field regarding the meaning and operationalization of theoretical variables. The diverse meanings of similarly labeled constructs presents considerable difficulty to researchers and clinicians in communication, diagnosis, and comparative analysis of research.

Although variations of family systems theory form the basis for many of the measures, others are based on idiosyncratic or eclectic models; one measure appears to be atheoretical. Although it is difficult to group the instruments according to theoretical derivation, they may be grouped in terms of degree of comprehensiveness. There appear to be three such groupings: (1) comprehensive measures that assess structure, process, affect, and orientation; (2) broad measures that assess three of the four areas; and (3) specialized measures, which assess only one or two areas. Three of the measures (Family Assessment Measure, Family Functioning in Adolescence Questionnaire, and Family Evaluation Form) appear to be comprehensive, in that they assess all four areas. Even so, they assess different constructs within each area. Six measures (McMaster Family Assessment Device, Family Process Scales, Self-Report Family Inventory, Colorado Self-Report Measure of Family Functioning, Family Environment Scale, and Children's Version of the Family Environment Scale) are broad, in that they consider three of the four areas of family functioning. The remaining eight measures appear to be specialized, focusing on only one or two of the assessment domains.

Physical and Administrative Comparisons

The family relationship self-report measures were evaluated according to the criteria discussed in Chapter 5. Table 6–2 summarizes the physical and administrative characteristics that differentiate the measures. The most variability among measures was noted in the areas of response format, response set, and availability of norms and manuals. Unique strengths or weaknesses associated with each instrument are provided in the "Notes" column of the table.

Norms are essential for determining the applicability of a test to different

TABLE 6–2. Physical and Administrative Characteristics of the Whole-Family Assessment Measures

Measure	Norms	Manual	Response Format	Obvious Response Set Problems	Notes
Family Assessment Measure	Yes	Yes	4-choice	None noted	Includes a Social Desirability and Denial Defensiveness scale within the General Functioning scale
Family Functioning in Adolescence Questionnaire	Limited	Yes	4-choice	None noted	Scoring recognizes curvilinear relationships
Family Evaluation Form	Limited	No	7-choice	None noted	No scoring directions available
McMaster Family Assessment Device	Limited	No	4-choice	None noted	Unrelated to social desirability (Miller et al., 1985)
Family Process Scales	Profile scores	No	5-choice	None noted	
Self-Report Family Inventory	Limited	None	5-choice	None noted	Instructions available from authors
Colorado Self-Report Measure of Family Functioning	Limited	None	4-choice	None noted	
Family Environment Scale	Yes	Yes	True/False	None noted	
Children's Version of the Family Environment Scale	Limited	Yes	3-choice	None noted	Cartoons ambiguous; more guidance in administration needed
Index of Family Relations	Cutoff scores only	Yes	5-choice	Social desirability	Vague anchor points
Conflict Tactics Scale	Yes (Form N)	No	6-choice (Form A), 7-choice	Social desirability	Scoring directions must be gathered from several sources

(continued)

TABLE 6–2. CONTINUED

Family Relationship Questionnaire	None	No	5-choice	None noted	No scoring directions available; purports to measure to dyadic relationship but some items reflect whole-family functioning
Inventory of Family Feelings	Limited	No	3-choice	None noted	Lengthy instructions; double negatives increase reading difficulty
Family Adaptability and Cohesion Evaluation Scales III	Yes	Yes	5-choice	Acquiescence problems	Items keyed in one direction
Personal Authority in the Family System Questionnaire	Limited	Yes	5-choice	None noted	Unequal item weighting; scoring time-consuming; items lengthy, possibly hard to understand
Family APGAR	Limited	Yes	3-choice (clinical), 5-choice (research)	Acquiescence problems	Limited to five questions; items keyed in one direction
Structural Family Interaction Scale	None	No	4-choice	None noted	No instructions for administration; item format lacks clarity

groups and are especially necessary when a measure is used for clinical diagnosis or intervention. Normative data for family self-report measures are limited. Four of the measures report adequate normative data and standardization samples; others report data from limited samples or report only profile or cutting scores. No normative data are reported for two of the measures: the Family Relationship Questionnaire and the Structural Family Interaction Scale.

A manual is a convenient source of standardized administration and scoring instructions, interpretation guidelines, theoretical premises, and normative and psychometric data. Manuals are available for 8 of the 17 instruments. Information typically contained in a test manual can be gleaned from the references for most of the measures that do not have manuals; however, this is haphazard and time-consuming and risks utilization of outdated information. Three measures (Family Evaluation Form, Family Relationship Questionnaire, Structural Family Interaction Scale) lack adequate scoring and/or administration information.

The reliability of a measure increases as a function of the number of response choices per item up to the point at which multiple choices confuse the respondent. The increase in reliability has been found to level off at about seven response choices (Nunnally, 1978). Response formats of the self-report measures range from two to seven choices, with most of the instruments falling in the four- or five-choice range. One instrument, the Index of Family Relations, has problems with vague anchor points in the response format.

As discussed earlier, a variety of response set problems have the potential for introducing systematic error into scores on self-report measures. For the majority of the measures, such problems were not obvious. However, researchers and clinicians should be aware that response set is a potential problem with any self-report measure. Of the measures reviewed, the Family APGAR and FACES-III are susceptible to acquiescence problems because the items are all keyed in one direction. The author of the Index of Family Relations (Hudson, 1982) provides administrative instructions to offset possible social desirability effects. Although social desirability difficulties were expected with the Conflict Tactics Scale because of social sanctions against family violence, evidence for minimal social desirability effects has been presented (Schumm, Martin, Bollman, & Jurich, 1982; Straus, 1979; Straus, Gelles, & Steinmetz, 1980).

In summary, additional normative studies are needed for most of the family functioning self-report instruments. Furthermore, manuals—essential to scoring, administration, and interpretation—are available for one half of the measures. Most measures offer adequate response formats; however, the potential response set problems of self-report measures of family functioning have seldom been examined.

Reliability and Validity

Highlights of the reliability and validity findings for each of the family relationship self-report measures are presented in Table 6–3. A comparison of re-

TABLE 6–3. Comparative Reliability and Validity of the Family Relationship Self-Report Measures

| Measure | Purpose[a] | Reliability | | Validity | |
		Test–Retest	Internal Consistency	Criterion-Related	Construct-Related
Family Assessment Measure	1,3,4	Unknown	Alphas: across scales = .89–.93 (adults), .86–.94 (children); subscales—General = .67–.87 Dyadic = .64–.82 Self = .25–.63	Various subscales differentiated problem families (specifically, Role Performance and Involvement) (Skinner et al., 1983); anorexic from normal differentiated (Garfinkel et al., 1983)	Subscales negatively correlate with defensiveness ($r = -.28$ to $-.48$) and social desirability ($r = -.35$ to $-.53$) (Skinner, in press)
Family Functioning in Adolescence Questionnaire	1	Unknown	Alphas:: .90 (whole measure), .40–.79 (subscales)	Correlated with Erikson Psychosocial Inventory ($r = .46$); correlated with problem solving in the family (Roelofse & Middleton, 1985)	Factor analysis yields a single factor that accounts for 54% of the variance (Roelofse & Middleton, 1985)
Family Evaluation Form	1	2 wk: .94–.40 subscale range (1980 version)	Alphas: .41–.89 (1980), .61–.88 (1984 revision)	Significant correlations between mothers' and fathers' scores for all but one subscale; significant differences among family income groups (Emery et al., 1980)	Unknown
McMaster Family Assessment Device	1	1 wk: .66–.76 subscale range	Alphas: .72–.92; scale intercorrelations: .37–.76; partial correlations approach zero when General Functioning held constant	Discriminant analysis of FAD scores predicted clinical (64%) and nonclinical (67%) groups; predicts 28% of variance of the Locke-Wallace Marital Satisfaction Scale; Predictive: FAD more power-	Correlations between the FAD and FUI fit theoretical hypotheses; Low correlation with social desirability; high correspondence with clinical ratings for six of seven scales (Miller et al., 1985)

Measure		Test–retest	Internal consistency	Validity	
Family Process Scales	1,2,3,4	Unknown	Alphas: .74–.96	...ful predictor of morale in geriatric sample than Locke-Wallace (Epstein et al., 1983) Enmeshment scale differentiated families with successful and unsuccessful weight loss maintenance (Barbarin & Tirado, 1985)	Significant correlations of the FPS scales with conceptually similar scales on the FACES, FEB, and Deger-McCullough Happiness-Contentment measure obtained (Barbarin, submitted)
Self-Report Family Inventory	1,2	1–3 mo: .30–.87 for factors	Alphas: .84–.88 for factors	Factors differentiated clinically rated high from low functioning families (Hulgus, 1986)	Convergence of the SFI scales with conceptually similar scales on the UCFES, FACES II, FACES I, FES, and FAD obtained; SFI scores uncorrelated with social desirability, but SFI correlated significantly with State–Trait Anxiety Inventory, undermining the discriminant validity of the measure (Hulgus, 1986)
Colorado Self-Report Measure of Family Functioning	1	Unknown	Alphas: .59–.86	Significant differences obtained on 12 of 15 scales in divorced vs. intact adolescent families (Bloom, 1985)	Factor analyses yielded 13 factors that closely matched the anticipated constructs (Bloom, 1985)
Family Environment Scale	1,3,4	2 mo: .68–.86; 12 mo: .52–.89	Alphas: .61–.78	Differentiated normal and clinical families in over 200 studies (Moos et al., 1979, 1984, 1986); predictive: predicted alcoholic treatment	Subscale correlations not consistently greater than between dimensions; subscale intercorrelations range from 0.1 to .45; constructed with factor

(continued)

TABLE 6–3. CONTINUED

Measure	Purpose[a]	Reliability		Validity	
		Test–Retest	Internal Consistency	Criterion-Related	Construct-Related
				gains and relapses (Moos & Moos, 1984); predicted attrition from treatment and treatment outcome (Moos & Moos, 1986)	analysis, but the factor structure does not replicate consistently (Fowler, 1982; Robertson & Hyde, 1982; Nelson, 1984); multiple studies support the convergent and discriminative construct validity of FES subscales with conceptually similar/dissimilar measures (Moos & Moos, 1986)
Children's Version of the Family Environment Scale	3	4 wk: .80	Unknown	Unknown	Unknown
Index of Family Relations	2,4	Unknown; considered irrelevant	Alphas: .91, .98, .97	Differentiated therapy clients with/without family problems. $r = .92$ between groups and IFR score (Hudson, Acklin, & Bartosh, 1980); related to college students' report of family problems ($r = .56$) (Hudson et al., 1980)	Items correlate with scores on other measures, as predicted (Hudson, 1982)
Conflict Tactics Scale	1	Unknown	Alphas (Form N): Verbal Aggression, .77–.88; Violence, .62–.88; Reasoning,	Parent and child reports: Reasoning, –.12–.19; Verbal Aggression, .43–.51; Violence, .33–.64 (Strauss,	Numerous correlations between CTS scores and other variables, consistent with theory; factor analysis supported

Instrument		Reliability (test–retest)	Reliability (internal)	Validity	Structure
			.50–.76; Interitem (Form A) $r = .44$–.91	1979; Strauss et al., 1980); significant parent–adolescent correlations (Schumm et al., 1982)	Form A structure; Form N factor analysis yielded four factors (Strauss, 1979)
Family Relationship Questionnaire	1	1–2 wks: .67 (Hengeler et al. in press); .70 (Hengeler & Tavormina, 1980)	Unknown	Affect scale differentiated adolescent offender status (Hengeler et al., 1984); Conflict scale (mother–son) differentiated violent, nonviolent, and control adolescents (Hengeler et al., 1985)	Unknown
Inventory of Family Feelings	1,2,3,	2 wk: .96	Split-half = .98	Correlated with Marital Adjustment scores (Lowman, 1980); correlated with therapist ratings ($r = .49$) (Fineberg & Lowman, 1975); significantly related to degree of individual pathology; differentiated families with a pathological member; significantly differentiated maritally distressed couples (Lowman, 1980)	Unknown
Family Adaptability and Cohesion Evaluation Scales III	1,3,4	4 wk: Cohesion = .83; Adaptability = .80	Alphas: Cohesion = .77; Adaptability = .62	Unknown	Subscales uncorrelated, consistent with theory; factor analysis yielded appropriate item loading (Olson, 1986); item total correlations high ($r = .42$–.74) Olson et al., 1985)

(continued)

TABLE 6–3. (*continued*)

| Measure | Purpose[a] | Reliability | | Validity | | |
		Test–Retest	Internal Consistency	Criterion–Related	Construct–Related
Personal Authority in the Family System Questionnaire	1,3,4	2 wk: .55–.95; 2 mo: .56–.80	Alphas: range across multiple studies = .73–.97	Correlated in expected direction with measures of psychological well-being and the SFIS; differentiated clinical from nonclinical college students (Bray et al., undated; Bray & Harvey, undated)	Factor analysis confirmed conceptual scales with exception of item overlag on two scales; factor analysis has been replicated (Bray & Harvey, undated); results of studies have supported the theoretical model from which the PFAS-Q was derived (Harvey & Bray, 1986; Harvey, Curry, & Bray, 1986)
Family APGAR	2	2 wk: .83	Interitem r = .24–.67; Split-half r = .93 (Good et al., 1979); interitem r = .46–.74 (5-choice); alphas: 5-choice = .86; 3-choice = .80 (Smith et al., 1982)	Total scores differentiated clinic (physical health) from nonclinic families, maladjusted from well-adjusted adolescents, adopted from biological children, intact from separated families (Smilkstein et al., 1982); predictive: predicted postpartum complications in high-risk mothers (Smilkstein et al., 1984)	Correlated .80 with FFI (Pless & Satterwhite, 1973); inter-spouse r = .67; correlation with therapist ratings r = .64 (Good et al., 1979)
Structural Family Interaction Scale	1,3	Greater than .80 for all scales	Alphas: .76–.93	Differentiated nonclinic families from families with a learning-disabled child (Perosa & Perosa, 1982) (initial version)	Factor analyses of the SFIS-R Form A yielded eight scales (Perosa, 1986)

[a] 1 = research; 2 = screening; 3 = diagnosis; 4 = evaluation of treatment.

liability statistics used by the 17 family self-report measures reveals that the majority (14) estimate reliability using the coefficient alpha. A substantial number (10) also provide test–retest data, and 5 use this method appropriately to determine long-term stability (range = 1–12 months). Split-half reliability estimates were available for two measures (Inventory of Family Feelings, Family APGAR).

A comparison of the adequacy of reliability of the family relationship self-report measures, using the alpha coefficients across measures, yields generally positive but also mixed findings. Two measures (Index of Family Relations, Inventory of Family Feelings) demonstrate adequate reliability (alpha > .90) for use in significant clinical decision making. Several additional measures (Self-Report Family Inventory, Family APGAR) evidence good reliability for clinical use and excellent reliability for research purposes (alpha > .80). The reliability of the majority of measures varies considerably across subscales. The Family Assessment Measure, Family Functioning in Adolescence Questionnaire, Family Evaluation Form, McMaster Family Assessment Device, Family Process Scales, Conflict Tactics Scale, and Personal Authority in the Family System Questionnaire, for example, all yield reliability coefficient ranges that vary from .60 to .95. Often reliability is excellent (alpha > .90) across subscales but not for individual scales. Thus, use of these measures for clinical decision making deserves caution. For purposes of research or screening, however, the majority of family self-report measures demonstrate adequate reliability. Several measures evidence inadequate reliability on some or all subscales and, thus, would benefit from additional test revision prior to use in research or clinical practice; these are the Structural Family Interaction Scale, the Colorado Self-Report Measure of Family Functioning, and the Self scale of the Family Assessment Measure.

The stability of the family relationship self-report measures presents a mixed and complex picture. Test–retest reliability studies have not been completed on a number of measures (seven), and of those that have such indices, the majority reflect short-term stability (1–2 weeks). Furthermore, stability coefficients are quite variable within and across measures. Evidence of the long-term stability of measured traits is provided only with the Family Environment Scale. It can be argued that many of the constructs measured by family self-report measures would not be expected to be stable over time and that determinations of long-term test–retest stability may be unnecessary or even inappropriate. Furthermore, measures may include some subscales that are expected to be unstable and others that purport to measure stable family characteristics. This suggests that test developers must present a clear statement of the purpose of their measure and its theoretical premises, especially with respect to predicted stability.

In summary, the internal consistency of the family relationship self-report measures is promising. The majority yield reliability coefficients that are more than adequate for research purposes. Reliance on any single family self-report measure for clinical diagnosis would appear inappropriate at this time. However, this circumstance is deemed unlikely, given the emphasis within clinical practice on assessment of multiple systems with multiple methods (Cromwell & Peterson, 1983). Regarding short-term stability, it would appear that the split-half method has been underutilized; however, this may reflect the typical multiple-subscale composition of family self-report measures, with subscales containing fewer than 20 items. The mixed stability of measures does suggest that additional clarification of constructs being measured, as well as their expected stability, is warranted.

As discussed in Chapter 5, several types of validity are applicable to self-report measures. The focus of this discussion will be a comparative analysis of the construct validity and criterion-related validity. Since the family assessment field is relatively young, and since a measure's validity is established over time, evidence for the validity of all measures (the Family Environment Scale may represent the exception) can be considered preliminary at this time. It should also be noted that evidence for validity does not necessarily generalize to populations outside those used in the validation studies.

Regarding the construct validity of family relationship self-report measures, eight measures provide evidence of their convergent validity with conceptually similar measures or subscales of measures. Four measures provide evidence of discriminant validity; however, for at least one measure, the Self-Report Family Inventory (SFI), results do not support the discrimination of the measure. The positive correlation of the SFI with anxiety suggests that this is a potentially confounding construct that deserves discriminant validity studies with other measures.

Several measures (five) have been factor-analyzed to support the integrity of their subscales or constructs. Results of the factor analyses generally support the construct structure of the measures; however, only the Family Environment Scale has attempted to replicate the factor analysis, and this has proved unsuccessful. In summary, the construct validation of existing family self-report measures is in a rudimentary stage. For some measures, no construct validity studies have been completed. Measures with evidence of construct validity have placed greater emphasis on convergent rather than discriminant validity of constructs. Attention to discriminant construct validity appears particularly warranted.

In comparing the criterion-related validity evidence of the family relationship self-report measures, 13 of 17 provide at least one investigation, the majority provide several supportive studies, and one (Family Environment Scale) has more than 200 studies demonstrating the criterion-related validity of the instrument. In some cases (Family Assessment Measure and Family Relationship Questionnaire), subscales, but not the whole scale, relate to an external criterion. In general, total scores differentiated some form of clinical from normal families. Three measures (Family Environment Scale, McMaster Family Assessment Device, Family APGAR), provide evidence of predictive validity. In summary, as with the construct validity of these measures, criterion-related validation is promising but very preliminary. Little attention has been given to the discriminative criterion-related validity of individual measures for various clinical subsamples; rather, clinical comparison groups represent a heterogenous population. In addition, a significantly overlooked research area is the within-method comparison of existing measures with similar measurement goals.

CONCLUSIONS: CONSIDERATIONS FOR RESEARCHERS AND CLINICIANS

Seven issues have emerged from this review as important considerations for individuals who wish to use self-report measures for assessing whole-family relational functioning. The first involves the psychometric quality of available measures. At present, the internal consistency of the majority of measures reviewed is promising; however, the stability of most measures is not established. Validation of most family self-report measures is in a preliminary stage, with studies of discriminative concurrent and predictive validity particularly lacking. Only four measures currently provide adequate normative data to permit population comparisons. On an optimistic note, the authors of existing measures appear to be actively engaged in continuing test validation and revision. At present, however, researchers and clinicians must be judicious in their use of measures.

The second issue involves the comprehensiveness of assessment. Even though all 17 measures discussed in this review purport to measure family relational functioning, the scope of assessment varies widely across the measures. Only 3 of the 17 measures actually assess all four dimensions of family structure, process, affect, and orientation. Ultimately, of course, selection of a measure should be based on the particular research or diagnostic question and theoretical perspective. These considerations then need to be matched with the degree of comprehensiveness required for the specific study.

Third, this review points to the importance of looking behind the names of scales to their item content. Several inconsistencies were noted in the issues assessed by scales that have the same name. Given this problem, it is no wonder that studies of concurrent and construct validity yield only modest correlations across measures. Researchers would be well advised to examine the specific item content of scales and factors in selecting a measure of a particular construct. In addition, from both content and construct validity points of view, it is important to ensure that the items fully measure the complexity implied in the constructs.

Fourth, although a multilevel assessment of the family may be desirable (see discussion in Chapter 5), at present it is impossible, as existing self-report measures are limited to adolescent and adult respondents. The lack of child self-report measures may reflect the predominance of an adult orientation in mental health treatment and family studies. Moreover, the cognitive limitations of elementary school–aged children may be expected to constrain their capacity to provide valid and reliable subjective evaluations of their family. However, the developmental capacities of younger children with regard to objective family assessment measures have not, as yet, been investigated.

Fifth, just as different levels of assessment within the family may yield different results, different types of assessment techniques are likely to yield different results, even if they focus on the same construct. Many of the constructs assessed by the measures reviewed in this article focus on *relationship properties*—qualities of relationships that arise out of recurring interpersonal interactions or subjective experiences (Huston & Robins, 1982). Although Huston and Robins (1982) argue persuasively that relationship properties should be assessed at the event level, many measures attempt to assess relationship properties at an inappropriately global level. For example, family cohesion is a relationship property that is explicitly measured in a number of the measures reviewed here. In most cases, it is assessed by questions that require that the respondent make summary judgments based on a long history of interactions. Threats to validity with such measures include inadequate sampling of interpersonal events and memory distortions that affect recall of events. Consequently, the correspondence between such measures and outsiders' views (such as those captured in interaction codes or clinical ratings) should not necessarily be high. For example, the meaning of specific behaviors to the participants in interaction can be strongly influenced by context (Sroufe & Rutter, 1984). Outside coders or raters may not have access to the frame of reference within which the participants are interpreting behavior (Coyne, 1987).

Finally, the theoretical diversity noted among the 17 measures reviewed here strikingly points out the lack of theoretical consensus among family researchers. The foci of the measures are quite different, and even measures of the same construct may differ in emphasis. Regarding research using whole-family system self-report measures, it seems, at this point, that energy should be devoted to theory development and that such work should involve multidisciplinary teams of family scholars that would include, at minimum, family sociologists, developmental psychologists, and clinicians. Increased theoretical sophistication should benefit the field of measurement in direct ways. For clinicians, it would appear imperative that selected self-report measures of family relationship quality be consistent with their theoretical perspective of etiology and treatment.

7

SELF-REPORT MEASURES OF
FAMILY STRESS AND COPING

with Rhonda Hauser

Stress is a concept that is widely used and assessed in a variety of disciplines, including biology, medicine, psychology, and sociology. Stress has been associated with both short-term and chronic psychiatric disorder and physical illness (Rutter, 1983). Thus, stress is a familiar concept that is of interest to researchers, clinicians, and laypersons. Despite its widespread use, however, the concept of stress is poorly defined and seems to apply equally to a form of stimulus (a stressor), a force requiring adaptation (strain), a mental state (distress), and a form of physiological response (Rutter, 1983). Although definitional issues divide researchers, the central questions regarding stress remain consistent: (1) Which life events may predispose to dysfunction? (2) Are certain stressors associated with certain types of dysfunction? (3) What are the underlying processes or mechanisms? Given our culture's concern with stress-related topics, as well as the viewpoint that one's milieu can either buffer or exacerbate stress, family scholars, as expected, have turned their attention to the role of the family in individual stress and coping (see McCubbin & Figley, 1983).

From developmental and family systems perspectives, stress is viewed as a normal part of the developmental process of individuals and families (Carter & McGoldrick, 1980; McCubbin & Figley, 1983). As individuals make developmental changes, it is anticipated that other family members and the family system must adapt. Similarly, family members and systems must adapt to external stressors, such as the loss of employment. The response of an individual or family to stressful events is considered "coping." Of increasing research and clinical interest is the phenomenon of resilience of individual family members or family units in the face of inordinate stressors (Rutter, 1983).

The earliest family-based conceptual model of families and stress, which emerged from the field of sociology, was Hill's (1949, 1958) ABCX family crisis model. In this model, A (the stressor event) was hypothesized to interact with B (family's crisis-meeting resources) and with C (family's definition of the crisis) to produce the magnitude of X (the crisis). This model and other models of stress from the fields of medicine, physiology, and psychology (Lazarus, 1966; Mikhail, 1981; Selye, 1974) have recently been integrated by

McCubbin and Patterson (1983) into the Double ABCX model. In contrast to the original ABCX model, which emphasizes precrisis variables, the Double ABCX model expands the original model and adds postcrisis variables. In the expansion of the original model, three levels of analysis are employed in the Double ABCX model: the individual, the family, and the community. Identified postcrisis variables include family pile-up of demands, family adaptive resources, and family definition and meaning. This multilevel analysis of pre- and postcrisis adjustment and adaptation is called the family adjustment and adaptation response (FAAR) (McCubbin & Patterson, 1983). These models of stress and coping, as well as others, have formed the basis for the development of techniques for measuring the stress and coping capacity of families.

In this chapter, nine whole-family system self-report measures of stress and coping are discussed and evaluated. As in the previous chapter, each measure will be described, critically evaluated, and comparatively analyzed according to the criteria specified in Chapter 5. The chapter will conclude with an integrative discussion and recommendations for future development of family measures of stress and coping.

DESCRIPTIONS AND EVALUATIONS OF MEASURES

Family Crisis Oriented Personal Scales (F-COPES)

The F-COPES (Olson et al., 1982) is a measure of the problem-solving attitudes and behaviors that families use when responding to difficulties. The F-COPES is based on the sociological research tradition of family stress (i.e., Hill's ABCX model and McCubbin and Patterson's Double ABCX model). The measure integrates individual coping strategies with intrafamilial process and the role of the community in the management of family stress. Five conceptual subscales have been derived from factor analysis of the F-COPES: Acquiring Social Support, Reframing, Seeking Spiritual Support, Mobilizing Family to Acquire and Accept Help, and Passive Appraisal. The questionnaire's 29 items are ranked on a 5-point Likert scale ranging from "strongly disagree" (1) to "strongly agree" (5). Subscale and total score norms are available for both adults and adolescents by sex (Olson et al., 1982). All 29 items are keyed in a positive direction, thus social desirability response bias is a possibility. The scale has demonstrated adequate reliability, with a test–retest reliability coefficient for the total scale of .81 and internal consistency correlations .86 and .87, respectively, across two samples (Olson et al., 1982). Advantages of the F-COPES include ease of administration and scoring, availability of norms, and a theoretical base. Further psychometric support, particularly construct and criterion-related validity data, will assist in determining the utility of this measure for clinicians and researchers.

Family Function Questionnaire (FFQ)

The FFQ (Sawa, 1986a; 1986b) was designed for use by health care professionals to examine a family's coping difficulties. Derived from the McMaster Model of Family Functioning (see Chapter 6), the FFQ consists of 49 items in two parts, with an additional open-ended section for gaining information about individual family members. Part I contains 26 questions with a yes/no response format. The 23 questions in Part II include a variety of response formats, including listing, a 5-point rating scale, and specified choices. The dimensions of the FFQ are Connectedness, Life Cycles, Internal Family Function, and Health and Coping. The questionnaire is designed to be completed independently by each family member. Although age of children is not specified, the length and reading level required would probably exclude children younger than 12. No norms are currently available for the FFQ, although descriptive data on a clinical sample have been collected. The Family Function Questionnaire is still in the development stage, with a scoring system and the collection of psychometric data currently in progress. Considerable psychometric evaluation of this measure will be necessary to determine its clinical and research utility.

Family Functioning Index (FFI)

The FFI (Pless & Satterwhite, 1973) is a 15-item questionnaire designed to assess the relationship of family functioning and psychological adjustment of children with chronic illness. Although described by the authors as theoretically eclectic, the FFI seems to be derived, in part, from sociological family role theory. A factor analysis yielded six factors: Marital Satisfaction, Frequency of Disagreements, Happiness, Communications, Weekends Together, and Problem Solving. The FFI items are responded to with a variety of response formats. Parallel forms for the husband and wife are available, but formal norms have not been published. Psychometric evidence suggests that the instrument is stable over time, with 5-year test–retest correlations of .83 for total score (Satterwhite, Zweig, Iker, & Pless, 1976); however, internal consistency data are unpublished. Validity support for the FFI is mixed. The FFI correlated highly (.80) with the Family APGAR, a measure of similar constructs. As a discriminator of psychosocial adjustment of children, however, studies report contradictory findings (Heller, Rafman, Zvagulis, & Pless, 1985; Pless & Satterwhite, 1975). The Family Functioning Index may have potential for use as a screening instrument by physicians; however, further psychometric evaluation is needed. A modification of the FFI, the Family Life Questionnaire (FLQ) by Seeman, Tittler, and Friedman (1985) may prove to be more useful. The FLQ has demonstrated moderate internal consistency (alpha = .69) and adequate stability ($r = .79$) at six weeks (Seeman et al., 1985).

Family Inventory of Life Events and Changes (FILE)

The FILE (Olson et al., 1982) was designed to assess the normative and non-normative stressors and intrafamilial strains experienced by members of the family during the course of one year. Based on the Double ABCX model of family systems and family stress theory, the FILE is a 71-item questionnaire in which the respondents are instructed to check whether or not each item has occurred in the past year. The measure consists of nine subscales: Intra-Family Strains, Marital Strains, Pregnancy and Childbearing Strains, Finance and Business Strains, Work–Family Transitions and Strains, Illness and Family Care Strains, Losses, Transitions "In" and "Out," and Legal Strains. Norms are available for a sample of 980 couples, ranging from young married couples to retired couples. The overall scale reliability of the FILE is adequate (alpha = .81); however, the reliability of the individual subscales was low and variable (.30 to .73), leading the authors to suggest that the total score be used rather than the less reliable subscale scores (Olson et al., 1982). Test–retest reliability over a 4- to 5-week period ranged from .64 to .84 (total scale = .80). Validity data on the FILE are very limited. Although the Family Inventory of Life Events and Changes is conceptually appealing, its clinical and research utility await further evaluation.

Family Relationships Index (FRI)

The FRI (Holahan & Moos, 1981) was designed to assess the quality of support found in social relationships within the family environment. The instrument consists of the items from three subscales of the Family Environment Scale (FES): Cohesion, Expressiveness, and Conflict. Twenty-seven true/false items make up the questionnaire, with the items being viewed as a unitary dimension of family support. Although no normative data are available specifically for the FRI, considerable normative data for its parent measure, the Family Environment Scale, would apply to the FRI. The internal consistency (Cronbach alpha) of the FRI is .89. The validity of the measure is supported by several studies that found family social support to be related to resistance to stress and psychological adjustment of family members (Holahan & Moos, 1981, 1982, 1986). The Family Relationships Index is a theoretically grounded measure of family support that demonstrates usefulness for both research and clinical settings.

Family Routines Inventory

The Family Routines Inventory (Boyce, Jensen, James, & Peacock, 1983) is theoretically based on the social-epidemiological model that postulates that stressful life changes contribute to disease susceptibility and that social support—specifically, family routines—buffer stress by providing a sense of stability and permanence during times of major life changes. The instrument is a

28-item inventory designed to measure a family's endorsement of and adherence to positive family routines. Items are rated on two response formats, with frequencies of behavior rated on a 4-point Likert scale ranging from "always" to "almost never" and perceived importance items rated on a 3-point scale ranging from "very important" to "not at all important." Ten domains are tapped by the Family Routines Inventory: Workday Routines, Weekend and Leisure Time, Children's Routines, Parent(s) Routines, Bedtime, Meals, Extended Family, Leaving and Homecoming, Disciplinary Routines, and Chores. All of the measure's items are keyed in a positive direction; thus, the possibility of socially desirable responses is present. Normative data are not available. Initial studies indicate that the Family Routines Inventory is stable over time, with a 30-day test–retest coefficient of .79. Internal consistency data are not published. Data comparing the Family Routines Inventory with theoretically similar measures support the measure's construct validity (Jensen, James, Boyce, & Hartnett, 1983). The predictive validity of the Family Routines Inventory was demonstrated in a study of mothers of infants (Sprunger, Boyce, & Gaines, 1985). Although further psychometric validation is needed—particularly exploration of internal consistency and additional validity studies—preliminary research supports the usefulness of the Family Routines Inventory in research as a measure of the role of family routines in buffering stress. The clinical utility of this measure has yet to be substantiated.

Family Strengths

The Family Strengths measure (Olson et al., 1982) is designed to measure a family's sense of pride and competency on the basis of the resources available to the family. The Family Strengths measure is based on sociological family theories concerning family resources and is theoretically consistent with family systems theory. The questionnaire consists of 12 items, each of which is responded to on a 5-point Likert scale ranging from "strongly disagree" (1) to "strongly agree" (5). The instrument includes two dimensions: Pride (including pride, loyalty, trust, and respect) and Accord (tapping a family's sense of competency). National norms are available for a sample of 1,140 Lutheran couples and 412 adolescents. The transparent purpose of the Family Strengths measure and its item content makes it very susceptible to social desirability response bias. The instrument demonstrates good internal reliability (Cronbach alphas = .87–.88 for Pride, .72–.73 for Accord, .83 for total score; Olson et al., 1982) and moderate stability (Pearson correlations) over a 4-week interval ($r = .73$ for Pride, .79 for Accord, .58 for total score). Little evidence of validity is available. Simple test construction and ease of use are advantages of the Family Strengths measure. Its limitations center on the content and construct validity of the measure and its susceptibility to social desirability, issues that await further research in order to assess the clinical and research utility of the measure.

Feetham Family Functioning Survey (FFFS)

The FFFS (revised) (Roberts & Feetham, 1982) is a 27-item inventory, based on ecological theory, that is designed to measure three areas of family relationship functioning: (1) relationships between the family and the social environment; (2) relationships between the family and subsystems; and (3) relationships between the family and each individual. The measure is useful for assessing the functioning of families that are experiencing various developmental events (e.g., birth of a child, illness of family member). More recently, the measure has been interpreted as a measure of social support as well as a measure of change in family functioning. Though moderately easy to use, the FFFS has a complicated response format. Each item is rated three times, on a 7-point Likert scale ranging from "little" (1) to "much" (7), in response to three different questions that assess current existence, desired existence, and importance of the item in the family. The resulting three dimensions of the FFFS are *degree of need fulfillment, discrepancy between achieved and expected levels of need fulfillment, and importance.* Factor analysis has supported the dimensional structure of the FFFS (Roberts & Feetham, 1982). Psychometric data are available only for the original 21-item version of the FFFS. These data indicate that the FFFS possesses moderate internal consistency, with subscale alphas ranging from .66 to .84, and is stable over short periods of time, with a 2-week test–retest correlation of .85 (Roberts and Feetham, 1982). The FFFS correlates with tests of similar constructs, thus supporting the construct validity of the measure (Roberts & Feetham, 1982). No normative data for the FFFS are available. There are limited descriptive data for a sample of mothers of children with myelodysplasia, and Feetham's work in progress contains data for normal children. Given the lack of psychometric investigation of the revised version of the FFFS, additional research is necessary before the usefulness of the measure can be determined.

Procidano Perceived Social Support Questionnaire— Family (PSS-Fa)

The PSS-Fa (Procidano & Heller, 1983) is a 20-item measure of perceived family support. Derived from community psychology theory, the PSS-Fa measures the extent to which an individual perceives that his or her needs for support, information, and feedback are fulfilled by the family. The items are responded to in a three-choice response format whereby the respondent answers "Yes," "No," or "Don't know." The PSS-Fa consists of a single scale, Family Support. Currently, no normative data are available. The PSS-Fa was found to be internally consistent, with an alpha coefficient of .90 (Procidano & Heller, 1983). No test–retest reliability data are available for the final version of this measure. Construct validity was evidenced by the significant relationships found between the PSS-Fa and theoretically relevant subscales of the MMPI.

Although social desirability presented a threat to validity, when controlled, partial correlations still remained significant. Although psychometric investigation of the PSS-Fa is limited and is currently based entirely on a college sample, preliminary work suggests the potential usefulness of the PSS-Fa as a measure of perceived family support that is applicable to both clinical and research settings.

COMPARATIVE EVALUATIONS OF MEASURES

Theoretical and Conceptual Comparisons

As seen in Table 7–1, most of the stress and coping measures were derived theoretically from either sociological family theory or family systems theory. Although several measures were based on additional theories (e.g., community psychology, ecological psychology) or eclectic models (e.g., the Family Functioning Index), the underlying theoretical emphasis of all the measures is consistent with the family stress literature, which recognizes the family as a dynamic unit and acknowledges the relationship among the variables of adaptive functioning, coping strategies, and sources of social support in the family. This framework assumes that a breakdown in family functioning occurs as a result of the presence of family stressors, the use of inappropriate coping strategies, and misperceptions or misallocations of family resources and support.

To facilitate comparison among the nine stress and coping measures, their subscales were grouped into one of four categories. The categories, though rationally derived for comparative purposes, were based on the Double ABCX model of family adaptation by McCubbin and Patterson (1983). The categories include stressors, coping strategies, mediating family perceptions, and other resources. *Stressors* are family life events that, when accumulated past an optimal level, can reduce the quality of family adaptation. *Coping strategies* are the processes and resources utilized by families to adapt to stress resulting from the accumulation of stressful family life events. *Mediating family perceptions* are attributions assigned by family members to social support systems available to the family. Subscales that could not be reasonable included in one of these categories were included under *other resources*.

The categorized listing of subscales (see Table 7–1) attests to the conceptual diversity of the family stress and coping measures. As we have found consistently in our review of family measures, subscales are not always labeled consistently with their content. In Table 7–1, subscales of the stress and coping measures were categorized according to the *content* of their constructs, rather than the construct label. An example of the content–label discrepancy is provided by Communications, which is often conceptualized as a coping process utilized by families in response to stress. In the Family Functioning Index, however, the items that assess the subscale Communications refer to a family member's perception of the ease of verbal communication with other family

TABLE 7–1. Conceptual Groupings of Subscales of the Stress and Coping Measures

Measure; Author(s); Theoretical Base	Stressors	Coping Strategies	Mediating Family Perceptions	Other Resources
Family Crisis Oriented Personal Scales; McCubbin, Larsen, & Olson; sociological theory based on family stress literature		Acquiring Social Support Reframing Seeking Spiritual Support Acquire and Accept Help Passive Appraisal		
Family Function Questionnaire; Sawa: Family systems theory, specifically the McMaster Model of Family Functioning	Life Cycles	Health and Coping	Connectedness Internal Family Functioning	
Family Functioning Index; Pless & Satterwhite-Stevenson; eclectic theory derived from sociological family role theory		Problem Solving Communication	Disagreements Weekends Together Marital Satisfaction Happiness	
Family Inventory of Life Events and Changes; McCubbin, Patterson, & Wilson; family systems theory and family stress theory	Losses Transitions "In" and "Out" of Family Pregnancy and Childbearing Strains Illness and Family "Care" Strains Marital Strains Intrafamily strains Financial and Business Strains Work–family Transitions and Strains Legal Strains			

Family Relationships Index; Holahan & Moos; ecological psychology theory		Family Support
Family Routines Inventory; Boyce, Jensen, James, & Peacock; social-epidemiological model	Workday Routines Weekend and Leisure Time Children's Routines Parent(s) Routines Bedtime Meals Extended Family Leaving and Homecoming Disciplinary Routines Chores	
Family Strengths: Olson, Larson, & McCubbin; sociological family theories		Pride Accord
Feetham Family Functioning Survey; Roberts & Feetham; family ecological theory, family systems theory		Need Fulfillment Importance
Procidano Perceived Social Support Questionnaire—Family; Procidano & Heller; prevention/community psychology		Family support

members. In this case, Communications was categorized as a mediating family perceptions construct rather than a coping strategies construct. The relative infancy of this field of family study may contribute to the confusing operationalization of theoretical variables. As noted in other chapters, the diverse meanings of similarly labeled constructs presents considerable difficulty to researchers and clinicians in communication, diagnosis, and comparative analysis of research.

As shown on Table 7–1, no measure (with the exception of the Family Function Questionnaire) contains a comprehensive set of subscales; that is, the subscales within each measure fall into only one or, at the most, two of the stress and coping categories. This suggests that existing stress and coping measures focus assessment on one aspect of the family stress and coping model, rather than seeking to provide a comprehensive measurement of family stress and coping. At present, a comprehensive assessment of family stress and coping would appear to necessitate the utilization of more than one measure, each tapping a particular category of proposed family adaptation models. The need to use multiple measures to assess family stress and coping increases the complexity of the interpretive task of clinicians and researchers, in that the interrelations among measures must also be considered.

As noted, most of the measures focus on the assessment of one aspect of family stress and coping. When variations within categories are examined, implicit conceptual groupings appear. For example, the subscales placed in the stressors category can be further grouped into intrafamilial stressors (e.g., marital strains, illness and family care strains), extrafamilial stressors (e.g., work–family transition and strains, financial and business strains). The subscales placed in the mediating family perceptions category can be grouped into perceived family support (e.g., connectedness, happiness), perceived marital support (e.g., disagreements, weekends together), and perceived satisfction (e.g., need fulfillment).

A view within and across categories suggests that family stress and coping, as reflected in existing theoretical models (e.g., the Double ABCX model) is a complex process involving multiple family levels, multiple areas of focus, and multiple constructs within areas. Although no single measure reviewed here provides a comprehensive evaluation of family stress and coping, an examination of constructs within and across categories provides a useful model for future development of comprehensive family stress and coping measures.

Physical and Administrative Comparisons

The family stress and coping measures were evaluated according to the criteria discussed in Chapter 5. The physical and administrative characteristics that differentiate the measures are summarized in Table 7–2. The most variability among measures was noted in response format, response set, and availability of norms and manuals. Unique strengths and weaknesses associated with each instrument are provided in the ''Notes'' column of the table.

Regarding the availability of norms, only the measures developed by Olson et al. (1982) (F-COPES, FILE, and Family Strengths) have normative data; and the generalizability of their normative sample, which was primarily Lutheran and middle-class, is uncertain. It is likely that norms for the Family Relationships Index could be determined, as it is derived from the Family Environment Scale, which has extensive psychometric documentation (see Chapter 6 for a reveiw of the FES). The majority of the family stress and coping measures, however, have no normative data available, thus limiting their current usefulness, particularly for clinical purposes. Since most of these measures have been developed recently and continue to undergo psychometric evaluation and revision, the lack of normative data is not surprising. However, at present, caution is appropriate in the use of family stress and coping measures because of the lack of adequate norms.

A manual serves as a source for standardized administration and scoring instructions, interpretation guidelines, theoretical premises, and normative and psychometric data. Manuals are available for four of the nine measures. The lack of manuals creates interpretive problems. For example, no scoring procedures are available for the Family Function Questionnaire; scoring procedures are confusing for the Family Functioning Index; and although a manual is available for the FILE, it contains no interpretive guidelines for the scores. In sum, the careful development of manuals is essential for the appropriate use of family stress and coping measures.

Perhaps the most variability in the stress and coping measures occurs in their response formats. Response formats of the measures range from two-choice to seven-choice, in addition to specified choice and open-ended listings. The response formats vary not only across measures, but often within measures as well. Three measures (Family Function Questionnaire, Family Functioning Index, Family Routines Inventory) have at least two response formats. Because of the lack of uniformity in response format, scoring procedures can become confusing.

As with all self-report measures, response set bias can be a potential problem. Of the measures reviewed, the Family Routines Inventory appears susceptible to acquiescence problems because the items are all keyed in a positive direction. For four of the nine measures, social desirability was noted as a possible limitation on the basis of the transparent purpose of the questionnaire and the expected reactivity of item content.

In summary, a comparative analysis of the physical and administrative features of the stress and coping measures reveals the need for additional work on all measures. Normative studies are needed for most of the measures. The development of interpretive manuals should help remedy the problem of nonexistent or confusing scoring procedures. The potential problem of social desirability as a response set problem deserves examination and/or control. Since a

TABLE 7–2. Physical and Administrative Characteristics of the Stress and Coping Measures

Measure	Norms	Manual	Response Format	Response Set Problems	Notes
Family Crisis Oriented Personal Scales	Yes	Yes	5-choice	Possible social desirability	Variation in anchor points may occur across family members; passive appraisal scale needs further clarification
Family Function Questionnaire	No	None	Part I, 2-choice; Part II, 5-choice, specified choice, listing	None noted	No available scoring procedures
Family Functioning Index	No	None	2-choice; 5-choice	None noted	Measure unsuitable for single-parent families due to marital adjustment items; confusing scoring procedures
Family Inventory of Life Events and Changes	Yes	Yes	2-choice	None noted	No interpretive guidelines for scores; lack of weights for FILE items

Measure					
Family Relationships Index	None available for this dimension of the FES	Yes	2-choice	None noted	This measure composed of a subset of items from the Family Environment Scale (Moos, 1974)
Family Routines Inventory	No	None	4-choice; 3-choice	Possible social desirability	All items keyed in a positive direction
Family Strengths	Yes	Yes	5-choice	Likely social desirability	
Feetham Family Functioning Survey	No	None	7-choice	Possible social desirability	Instrument not suitable for subjects with less than high school education; assesses whole-family functioning, but items refer to one person's perception of family life
Procidano Perceived Social Support Questionnaire— Family	No	None	3-choice	None noted	Measure may have limited generalizability beyond college-age sample

number of these family stress and coping measures remain in the developmental stage, it is hoped that many of the physical and administrative concerns will be addressed.

Reliability and Validity

The reliability and validity data for the family stress and coping measures appear in Table 7–3. A comparison of the reliability statistics used by the measures reveals that internal consistency (Cronbach alphas) and stability (test–retest) data are available for six of nine measures. A comparison of the adequacy of reliability of the family stress and coping measures yields moderate to good internal consistency coefficients, with total scale coefficients generally superior to subscale coefficients. Assuming that a reliability coefficient of .90 is desirable for clinical use (Nunnally, 1978), the Family Relationship Index and the Procidano Perceived Social Support Questionnaire are noteworthy. Both the F-COPES and the FILE approach acceptable reliability estimates for clinical use. The remaining measures either lack internal consistency data or require additional psychometric revision to obtain adequate internal consistency for both clinical and research purposes.

A comparison of the stability of the six family stress and coping measures for which data were available finds generally high (range = .79–.85) test–retest correlations for total measure scores. It should be noted that test–retest duration varied considerably, from 2 weeks to 5 years. Given the nature of stress and coping measures, which evaluate crisis and change, their stability is unexpectedly high and may, in fact, argue against their suitability as measures that are sensitive to change (e.g., Family Functioning Index).

In summary, either internal consistency or stability data are lacking for five of the nine family stress and coping measures reviewed, which to some extent reflects the developmental phase of the field. Most of the evaluated measures appear to possess good total measure internal consistency and stability; however, caution is appropriate in the use of measures for clinical purposes until further psychometric evaluation is conducted.

As discussed in Chapter 5, several types of validity are applicable to family stress and coping measures. The focus of this discussion, as in other chapters, will be on the comparative analysis of criterion-related and construct validity. Since the family stress and coping field is relatively young, and since a measure's validity is established over time, evidence for the validity of all measures at this time can be considered preliminary. It should also be noted that evidence for validity does not necessarily generalize to populations outside those used in the validation studies.

Regarding the construct validity of family stress and coping measures, three measures (Family Functioning Index, Feetham Family Functioning Survey, Procidano Perceived Social Support Questionnaire) provide evidence of convergent or divergent construct validity with conceptually similar or dissimilar measures or subscales. Two measures (F-COPES and Feetham Family Func-

TABLE 7–3. Comparative Reliability and Validity of the Stress and Coping Measures

Measure	Purpose[a]	Reliability		Validity	
		Test–Retest	Internal Consistency	Criterion-Related	Construct-Related
Family Crisis Oriented Personal Scales	1,3	4 wk: .61–.95 (5 scales): .81 (total scale)	Alphas: .86 (sample 1, whole measure); .87 (sample 2, whole measure); .62–.84 (subscales)	Unknown	Factor analysis yields five factors, each having eigenvalues greater than 1.0
Family Function Questionnaire	1,3	Unknown (in progress)	Unknown (in progress)	Unknown (in progress)	Unknown (in progress)
Family Functioning Index	1,2	6 wk: .79 (modification of index into 5-point Likert scale; Seeman, Tittler, & Friedman, 1985); 5 yr: .83 (total scores); .04–.71 (individual items) (Satterwhite, Zweig, Iker, & Pless, 1976)	Alpha: .69 (whole scale—modified)	Low FFI scores positively related to psychosocial adjustment scores; significant differences between random samples and counseling-seeking samples (Pless & Satterwhite, 1975); no relationship found between FFI and Achenbach Child Behavior Checklist (Heller, Rafman, Zvagulis, & Pless, 1985)	FFI scores positively correlated with ratings of family functioning; FFI socres of parents with a chronically ill child positively related to family functioning ratings (Pless & Satterwhite, 1973); FFI positively correlated with Family APGAR scores (Good et al., 1979)

(continued)

TABLE 7-3. CONTINUED

		Reliability		Validity	
Measure	Purpose[a]	Test–Retest	Internal Consistency	Criterion-Related	Construct-Related
Family Inventory of Life Events and Changes	1,2	4–5 wk: .64–.84 (subscales); .80 (whole scale)	Alphas: .81 (whole scale); .30–.73 (subscales)	Correlations with Moos Family Environment Scale ranged from −.41 to .42, and −.24 to .23 on the total scale score; FES conflict was positively related to total life changes; FES Cohesion negatively correlated with total life changes (Olson et al., 1982)	Due to variance in the frequency of occurrence of items, the items were grouped conceptually rather than empirically (Olson et al., 1982)
Family Function Questionnaire	1,3	Unknown	Unknown	Unknown	Unknown
Family Relationships Index	1,3	Unknown	Alpha: .89	Multiple studies have used the FRI in the role of family support in resistance to stress (Holahan, 1981, 1982, 1983, 1985, 1986); decreases in support in family and work environments related to increases in psychological maladjustment over a 1-year period (Holahan & Moos, 1981)	Unknown

Measure	[a]	Test-retest reliability	Internal consistency	Validity	Construct validity
Feetham Family Functioning Survey	1	2 wk: .85 (Roberts, 1979)	Alphas: .66–84 (dimensions)	Unknown	Negative correlation between FFFS and Pless & Satterwhite's Family Functioning Index; factor analysis yielded three factors; all but 3 items loaded onto the factors with eigenvalues of at least .43 (Roberts & Feetham, 1982)
Family Routines	1	30 day: .79 (Jensen, James, Boyce, & Hartnett, 1983)	Unknown	Family rhythmicity predicted mothers' sense of competence as parents (Sprunger, Boyce, & Gaines, 1985)	Positive correlations between FRI and family satisfaction and FES subscales of Cohesion, Organization, and Control; FRI scores negatively related to the FES subscale Conflict (Jensen et al., 1983)
Procidano Perceived Social Support Questionnaire— Family	1	Unknown	Alpha: .90	Unknown	Significant negative correlations between PSS-Fa and MMPI subscales of D, Pt, and Sc; PSS-Fa positively related to MMPI subscale K (Procidano & Keller, 1983)

[a] 1 = research; 2 = screening; 3 = diagnosis; 4 = evaluation of treatment

tioning Survey) have been factor-analyzed, with results generally supporting the integrity of their subscales or constructs. Support for the integrity of the single-scale Procidano measure and the Family Relationships Index is provided by the aforementioned internal consistency data. For four measures, construct validity studies are in progress or have not yet been completed. Continued attention to construct validity of existing measures appears warranted.

Criterion-related validity data are available for four of the nine family stress and coping measures. For three measures that assess family functioning, total scores were related to psychological adjustment of family members; the fourth, a measure of life events, was found to relate to perceived family functioning. Although generally supportive of validity, one measure, the Family Functioning Index, yields equivocal criterion-related findings.

In summary, continued efforts to determine the criterion-related and construct validity of existing family stress and coping measures remain critical. Existing studies are limited, and numerous measures lack any evaluation of criterion-related validity at this time. Thus, the value of these measures, for the most part, remains uncertain.

DISCUSSION

The concepts of family stress and coping have become important components of family theory and research in the 1980s, as both theories and methods have become more sophisticated (McCubbin & Boss, 1980). As this field moves toward greater maturity, several issues warrant further attention.

The domain of family stress and coping is in need of further theoretical development, just as we have noted in earlier chapters in regard to other research areas. Even when theories such as McCubbin and Patterson's (1982) Double ABCX model and Reiss's (1981) family paradigm model are available, assessment measures do not treat the theoretical components comprehensively. In general, the theoretical diversity in this area and the atheoretical development of some assessment devices appear to have hindered communication for both researchers and clinicians.

Because methodological development in the domain of stress and coping is so recent, a great deal of research is necessary to bring this area to maturity. In particular, the development of normative data will be essential so that clinicians and researchers will have baseline information on "normal" or "acceptable" levels of stress in comparison to levels that place individuals at risk. In addition, all nine measures reviewed in this chapter require extensive research to supplement the existing reliability and validity data.

Researchers who study family stress and coping must also acknowledge familial and cultural variations in the definition of stress and in the degree to which coping strategies are adaptive. As noted by Reiss and Oliveri (1980, p. 443): "In our fledgling science of family stress and coping we may be rushing to judgment, on very slender evidence, concerning which strategies are 'best'."

8

SELF-REPORT MEASURES OF PARENT–CHILD RELATIONSHIPS

with Paul A. Miller and Rhonda Hauser

The parent–child relationship is unique among family ties both in terms of the degree of obligation between parent and child throughout the life span and in terms of the initial asymmetry, and subsequent continuous demand for adjustment with maturation, of the reciprocal influence process between parents and their children (Maccoby & Martin, 1983). The responsibility and accommodation required of parenting, coupled with the importance of child outcomes—that is, the rearing of competent members of society—has given central importance to the measurement and study of the processes of socialization in child development and child clinical research and intervention.

The study of parent–child relationships has its origins in the study and treatment of children's clinical disorders, manifested most clearly in the child guidance movement in the early 1900s (Sears, 1975). Research and child clinical practice during this period was strongly influenced by the "social mold" traditions of psychoanalysis and, later, stimulus–response theory (Hartup, 1978). Studies carried out in this tradition assumed that parental attitudes and rearing practices "molded" children's later social and psychological adjustment. The socialization process was viewed as primarily unidirectional. Furthermore, little importance was given to the role of the child in his or her own socialization. Finally, because the mother was most frequently the primary caretaker, these early research efforts principally concerned the mother–child relationship.

Parent–child research during this period was also influenced by theories of personality that supported the notion that the emotional, cognitive, and motivational components of adult personality reflected stable characteristics over time and situations (Sears, 1975). Moreover, personality characteristics were believed to drive behavior. Regarding the parent–child relationship, parental patterns of attitudes and beliefs about the child-rearing process were thought to exert a consistent influence on parental behavior and were expected to delimit the range of social behaviors the child could acquire (Schaefer & Bell, 1958). Thus, one major focus of research on parent–child relations was the assessment of parental child-rearing attitudes and beliefs.

A final source of influence on the study of the parent–child relationship derived from the phenomenological tradition that emerged in response to psycho-analysis. In this tradition, the role of perception was viewed as central to per-sonality development, (e.g., Ausubel et al., 1954). In this view, *perceptions* of the parent or child regarding the other's behavior are seen as more influential in child adjustment than the *actual* behaviors of either the parent or child. Thus, parent–child researchers also focused on children's perceptions of paren-tal behavior and parent's perceptions of children's behavior toward them. Con-sonant with this view, as well as with the technology of the period, researchers relied on parent self-report interviews and questionnaires as primary sources of data (Maccoby & Martin, 1983).

The "social mold" view of parent–child relations reached its zenith in the 1950s, at which point it came under attack from a variety of disciplines, in-cluding psychiatry's focus on social interaction in the etiology of individual dysfunction, (e.g., Sullivan, 1953); ethology's emphasis on mutual regulation in the development of attachment between parent and child, (e.g., Bowlby, 1969); Mischel's (1968) critique of the situational stability of individual behav-ior; and ecological psychology's emphasis on the interaction of behavior with social context, (e.g., Barker, 1969; Hartup, 1978). Correspondingly, the meth-odology associated with the unidirectional "social mold" tradition received considerable criticism and resulted in a decline in socialization research during the 1960s. The use of parents as respondents was criticized because of the lack of awareness parents might possess regarding their own motives and behavior, the individual variability in response sets of parents, the unreliability of retro-spective reports, and the limited utility of self-report for clarifying parent–child behavioral contingencies (Maccoby & Martin, 1983).

Interest in socialization research reemerged in the 1970s and appears quite different from parent–child research of earlier decades (Hartup, 1978). Both the questions being posed and the answers being considered reflect increased sophistication in research design methodological complexity. For example, in determining child outcomes, socialization researchers are asked to consider the roles of (1) biology; (2) cognition and perception; (3) mutual regulation of parent–child interaction; (4) gender differences of boys, girls, fathers, and mothers; (5) social or situational context variability; (6) cross-cultural variabil-ity; and (7) developmental changes of the relationships within the family. The most recent conceptualizations of socialization view relationships as the context in which most of socialization takes place. Furthermore, parent–child relation-ships serve not only as contexts of social learning but also as critical templates for the child's construction of future relationships (Hartup, 1986; Sroufe & Fleeson, 1986).

The purpose of this chapter is to provide family and child development re-searchers and clinicians with an up-to-date, comparative analysis and critical evaluation of recently developed or currently used self-report measures for the assessment of parent–child relations. Although a variety of methods have been utilized in the study of parent–child relationships, the scope of this chapter is limited to the evaluation of self-report measures—that is, questionnaires that provide information about either the parent's or the child's subjective reality or experience, including attitudes and perceptions of self or other in the parent–child relational context. Standardized interview schedules, checklists, or daily/weekly reports of behavior were omitted. Measures developed prior to 1976 are included in the review only when considerable data have been amassed, as evident from a literature search subsequent to 1976, regarding the reliability and validity of the measure or when the measure has been revised since it was previously reviewed. Thus, the focus of this chapter is the critical review of recently developed parent–child self-report measures.

We will begin with descriptions and critical evaluations of 19 parent–child self-report measures. Because of the availability of multiple versions of some of these measures, 23 abstracts of parent–child measures appear in Part II. (The reader is referred to Chapter 5 for a discussion of the psychometric issues relevant to self-report measurement and for a review of the criteria used to evaluate the measures.) A comparative analysis of the parent–child self-report measures will follow. The chapter will conclude with an integrative discussion, guidelines for use, and issues to be addressed in the future development and refinement of parent–child self-report measures.

DESCRIPTIONS AND EVALUATIONS OF MEASURES

Adult–Adolescent Parenting Inventory (AAPI)

The AAPI (Bavolek, 1984) is a 32-item measure designed to assess high-risk parenting attitudes and child-rearing practices of adolescents and adults. Data from the AAPI provide an index of risk (high, medium, low) for the use of abusive and neglecting parenting and child-rearing behaviors. Based on socialization theory, the AAPI is appropriate for adolescents aged 12 to 19 and adults over age 20. The AAPI includes four parenting scales: Inappropriate Expectations, Empathy, Corporal Punishment, and Parent–Child Family Role Reversal. Extensive normative data are available, based on a sample of more than 8,800 adults and adolescents from multiple settings. The AAPI demonstrates test–retest reliability coefficients ranging from .39 to .89. Cronbach alpha coefficients within the four AAPI scales range from .70 to .86, with the alphas generally higher for the adults than for adolescents. Extensive evidence of criterion validity has been collected, with significant differences being found between male and female, abused and nonabused adolescents and adults, and younger and older mothers (Bavolek, 1984). Construct validity has been demonstrated by the findings of relations between AAPI scores and male children's exposure to violent, fantasy, superhero, and loner TV programs (Price, 1985). Further predictive and construct validity studies are currently in progress (Gordon & Gordon, undated). The AAPI is most useful as a clinical diagnostic tool in identifying individuals who are at higher risk for abusive behavior. The

AAPI's potential *proactive,* rather than reactive, approach to child abuse makes this measure a valuable addition to the pool of self-report family assessment measures.

Child Abuse Potential (CAP) Inventory

The CAP Inventory (Milner, 1986), which is grounded in psychiatric and interpersonal theories concerning family stress and mental health, is designed as a screening tool for the detection of physical child abuse. The 160-item inventory is responded to in a 2-point Likert agree/disagree format. The CAP Inventory included 77 items that tap seven abuse scales: Abuse, Distress, Rigidity, Unhappiness, Problems with Child and Self, Problems with Family, and Problems from Others. It also includes three validity scales: a lie scale, a random-response scale, and an inconsistency scale. Experimental items were added to bring the total to 160 items. Normative data are available from multiple samples. Internal consistency reliabilities for the abuse subscales range from .50 to .90, with split-half reliability for the measure in the .90's across various groups. Test–retest reliabilities across 1-day to 1-week intervals and 1- and 3-month intervals range from .53 to .90 (Milner, 1986). The CAP Inventory has been carefully validated, and extensive data are available from studies in which the CAP Inventory was used to discriminate abusing from nonabusing parents (Milner, 1986). The Child Abuse Potential Inventory has demonstrated considerable clinical and research utility and is a significant addition to the group of measures used to assess parenting behavior.

Child Behavior Toward Parent Inventory (CBTPI)

The CBTPI (Schaefer & Finkelstein, 1975) is a questionnaire designed to complement the Child's Report of Parental Behavior Inventory (CRPBI) (Schaefer, 1965) so that the *reciprocity* in parent–child interaction can be measured. The measure is based on theories of phenomenology and cognitive-developmental psychology. The CBTPI is a 155-item inventory in which parents describe their child's behavior on a 4-point Likert scale ranging from "very much like" to "not at all alike." A short version (25 items) of the CBTPI has also been developed (Schaefer & Edgerton, 1977). From the 155 items, 31 five-item subscales were derived. From the 31 subscales, three major dimensions were identified: Control, Acceptance versus Rejection, and Independence versus Dependence. The Acceptance versus Rejection dimension was further differentiated into three scales; Affection, Considerateness, and Helpfulness. The short form includes five 5-item scales: Positive Relationship, Control, Independence, Obedience, and Detachment. Norms are not available at this time for either form. The internal reliability and construct validity of the CBTPI have been demonstrated, though the authors indicate the need for further validity studies. Internal consistency coefficients range from .60 to.81 for the short version of the CPTPI, and split-half reliability coefficients range from .69 to .95 for the long version (Schaefer & Edgerton, 1977; Schaefer & Finkelstein, 1975). On the short form, significant correlations were found between CBTPI scales and parent and teacher ratings of children's behavior (Schaefer & Edgerton, 1977). Further psychometric evaluation would strengthen the utility of the CBTPI as both a research and a clinical assessment tool.

Child-Rearing Practices Report (CRPR)

The CRPR (J. H. Block, 1965), which is derived from social learning theory, is designed to measure maternal and paternal child-rearing attitudes, values, and goals through a method that minimizes the occurrence of possible response sets. The CRPR is a 91-item Q-sort that contains socialization-relevant, behaviorally anchored statements. Respondents arrange the 91 items on a 7-point scale ranging from "most descriptive" to "least descriptive," using a forced-choice Q-sort format with 13 items at each scale point. Both a first-person form (parent form) and a third-person form of the CRPR are available. The third-person form is completed by adolescents or young adults to describe their parents' child-rearing orientations. Twenty-eight scales depicting parental socialization practices have been developed out of the 91 CRPR item pool—for example, Encouraging Openness to Experience, Emphasis on Achievement, Authoritarian Control, and Affective Quality of Parent–Child Interaction (a complete listing of the scales can be found in Roberts, Block, & Block, 1984). The CRPR has been standardized and normed on a diverse sample of more than 6,000 persons from multiple settings. Test–retest reliability studies yielded high correlations, with a coefficient of .71 at a 1-year interval and .64 to .66 at a 3-year interval. Both criterion and predictive validity have been adequately established on the Child-Rearing Practices Report (e.g., J. H. Block, Block, & Morrison, 1981; J. H. Block & Gjerde, 1986). The CRPR is a widely used assessment tool and is appropriate for use in cross-cultural studies. The measure is a valuable clinical and research tool, and the Q-sort format is one of its primary strengths.

Home Environment Questionnaire (HEQ)

The Home Environment Questionnaire (HEQ-1R, HEQ-2R) (Sines, 1983) assess the psychosocial environments of fourth- to sixth-grade children in one- and two-parent families. The measure is designed to identify environmental factors relevant to the clinical and social behaviors of children. Although the HEQ-2R contains a greater number of items (134 items) than the HEQ-1R (76 items), both forms include 10 subscales: Achievement, Aggression—External, Aggression—Home, Aggression—Total, Supervision, Change, Affiliation, Separation, Sociability, and Socioeconomic Status. Six of the 10 HEQ-2R subscales have adequate internal consistency coefficients (.69 to .89); four subscales are low (.27 to .49). Five of the HEQ-1R subscales have internal consistency coefficients in the .60 to .79 range, with the remaining five subscales in the .26 to .56 range. Across forms, the three Aggression subscales and the Affiliation, and Socioeconomic Status subscales demonstrate higher internal consistency. A social desirability response bias has been reported (Sines, 1983; Sines, Clarke, & Lauer, 1984). Validity data for the HEQ are limited. Thus, although the HEQ is designed to evaluate an aspect of the parent–child environment that is not assessed with other measures, further psychometric development is needed to improve its usefulness to clinicians and researchers.

Index of Parental Attitudes (IPA)

The IPA (Hudson, 1982) is designed to measure the degree, severity, and magnitude of a problem in a parent–child relationship. The measure is one of nine short-form scales that make up the Clinical Measurement Package (see, also, descriptions of Index of Family Relations description in Chapter 6 and Child's Attitude toward Mother/Child's Attitude toward Father in this chapter.). The measure is a 25-item questionnaire that is responded to on a 5-point scale ranging from "rarely or none of the time" to "mostly or all of the time." One score of Problem Severity is derived by the summation of the 25 items, higher scores indicate more severe problems, and lower scores indicate the relative absence of problems. Reliability for the IPA across three studies yielded alpha coefficients ranging from .91 to .98; thus, the IPA is a highly reliable measure. Research supporting the discriminant and construct validity of the IPA has been conducted (Hudson, 1982). According to the author, the IPA is a unidimensional measure of a personal or social problem and should not be taken as an assessment of cause, type, or origin of a problem. In addition, the author notes that the IPA is most useful as an evaluation tool and a monitor of treatment.

Although further psychometric validation is appropriate, the existing data indicate that the Index of Parental Attitudes is both a reliable and a valid measure for use in monitoring and assessing the parental perspective on parent–child relationship problems in the clinic setting.

Maryland Parent Attitude Survey (MPAS)

The MPAS (Pumroy, 1966), which is based on socialization theory, measures parent attitudes toward child rearing while controlling for the effects of social desirability. The MPAS consists of 95 forced-choice item pairs, with the first five item pairs left unscored. The MPAS includes four parenting style scales: Disciplinarian, Indulgent, Protective, and Rejecting. The instrument was standardized on a sample of 197 male and 186 female college students. Although no reliability data are available for a population consisting of parents, a 3-month test–retest reliability study on college students yielded moderately high coefficients, ranging from .62 to .73 for the four parenting styles. In a separate sample of college students, split-half reliability coefficients were also high, ranging from .67 to .84. Intercorrelations (.07 to .74) among the four parenting styles indicate that several of the scales may represent different aspects of the *same* construct, calling for a reexamination of the scale definitions (Pumroy, 1966; Tolor, 1967). Validity studies indicate that mothers with high Disciplinarian ratings were more directing and restricting in their interactions with their children than mothers with low scores. Mothers' prohibitions were also positively related to their scores on the Rejecting scale (Pumroy, 1966). Generalization from the validity findings should be made with caution, as males' and females' scores on the MPAS corresponded somewhat to typical sex role socialization patterns and were based on college samples. As an assessment device, the MPAS was designed primarily for research purposes. Its chief advantage is the minimizing of socially desirable response patterns, and its chief disadvantage is inadequate psychometric research and development.

Parent as a Teacher Inventory (PAAT)

The PAAT (Strom, 1984) is designed to measure parents' attitudes about their role in their children's creativity, play, and learning and their levels of frustration and need for control over their children's behavior. The measure was initially developed for determining parents' needs in a parent education curriculum. Theoretically, the PAAT is consistent with views examining parental influence on child development, with an emphasis on Torrance's work on creativity and Strom's work on the role of play in development. The PAAT, intended for parents of children aged 3 to 9, includes 50 items, each of which is responded to on a 4-point Likert scale ranging from "strong yes" to "strong no." Five subscales are assessed: Creativity, Frustration, Control, Play, and Teaching-Learning. Internal reliability of the PAAT has been established in a series of studies, producing alpha coefficients ranging from .77 to .88. Tests of construct validity yield high consistency levels (66%–85%) between observed parental behavior and parents' reports of their behavior with their child on the PAAT (Johnson, 1975; Panetta, 1980). In a study of criterion-related validity, in which the PAAT was used as a pre–post assessment instrument, posttest results showed that parents made significant gains on all five subscales of the PAAT and on the total score (Strom, 1984). The Parent as a Teacher Inventory is a useful, concise instrument that can be used in prevention and intervention programs as well as in research.

Parent Attitude Research Instrument (PARI)

The Parent Attitude Research Instrument (PARI) was originally published by Schaefer & Bell (1958). The theoretical base of the instrument comes from social and developmental psychology. Because of problems with response bias, the PARI has been revised several times (Schludermann & Schludermann, 1971, 1977; Zuckerman, 1958). The most recent version of the PARI, the PARI Q4, is a 115-item self-report questionnaire designed to assess paternal and maternal attitudes toward child rearing and family life. There are 23 5-item scales, which load on two major factors, Authoritarian Control and Family Disharmony (mother form) and Democratic Attitudes and Paternal Detachment (father form). The response format is a 4-point Likert scale to which parents indicate the extent to which they agree or disagree with the item. Test–retest reliability coefficients of both forms range from .52 to .81, and the reliability of the factor scores ranges from .75 to .81 (specific scale reliabilities are available from the author). Few validity data are available on the PARI Q4. Although the influence of acquiescence and opposition response sets has been reduced, response bias problems remain. In summary, the PARI Q4 assesses several domains of parental attitudes relevant to children's social and personality development. Reduction of response bias and further validity studies would enhance the potential of the instrument for research.

Perceptions of Parental Role Scales (PPRS)

The purpose of the PPRS (Gilbert & Hanson, 1982) is to provide a comprehensive measure of perceived parental role responsibilities that reflects the views of both male and female working parents. Based on a role theory perspective, the PPRS is a 78-item inventory consisting of 13 scales in three major domains: Teaching the Child, Meeting the Child's Basic Needs, and Family as an Interface with Society. The items are responded to on a 5-point Likert scale ranging from "not at all important as a parental responsibility" to "very important as a parental responsibility." In the Teaching the Child domain, the subscales included are Cognitive Development, Social Skills, Handling of Emotions, Physical Health, Norms and Social Values, Personal Hygiene, and Survival Skills. In the Basic Needs domain, the subscales consist of Health Care; Food, Clothing, and Shelter; Child's Emotional Needs; and Child Care. The subscales included in the Family as an Interface with Society domain are Social Institutions and the Family Unit. Studies of reliability have demonstrated both high internal consistency, with alphas in the .81 to .91 range, and high 1-month test–retest reliability, with coefficients ranging from .73 to .90 across subscales. In one study of criterion validity, females scored significantly higher than males on a majority of the parenting responsibilities (Gilbert & Hanson, 1982). The 13 scales were found to be moderately intercorrelated, suggesting that the scales may be measuring aspects of the same construct. The PPRS was developed primarily as a research tool; however, the comprehensiveness of the measure also makes it useful in educational and counseling settings. A wide variety of parental role perceptions in *dual-working* families are addressed in the PPRS. The Perceptions of Parental Role Scales was developed from a white, middle-class, university-employed sample, so caution must be taken when generalizing from the measure.

Parenting Stress Index (PSI)

The PSI (Abidin, 1983) is a self-report questionnaire designed for screening and diagnosis of stress in parents of children under ago 10. Based on attachment, temperament, and stress theories, the PSI is useful for early identification screening, individual diagnostic assessment, pre–post measures of intervention effectiveness, and research on effects of stress. The PSI is composed of 101 items, which are responded to on a 5-point Likert scale ranging from "strongly agree" to "strongly disagree." Nineteen optional items are also included to assess the presence of specific stressful family events. The PSI includes both a Child domain and a Parent domain. In the Child domain, the six subscales are Adaptability, Acceptability of the Child to the Parent, Child Demandingness, Child Mood, Child Distractability/Hyperactivity, and Child Reinforces Parent. The Parent domain includes seven subscales: Parent Depression or Unhappiness, Parent Attachment, Restrictions Imposed by the Parental Role, Parent's Sense of Competence, Social Isolation, Relationship with Spouse, and Physical Health. Norms based on a sample of 534 parents of both normal and problem children visiting small group pediatric clinics are available, but the norm group is not entirely representative of the U.S. population, and generalizations must be made with caution. Susbstantial evidence has been collected regarding the test–retest and internal reliability of the PSI. Alpha coefficients range from .55 to .80 for the parent and child subscales and .89 to .93 for the total scales. Test–retest reliability coefficients range from .69 to .91 over time periods of 3 weeks to 3 months. Numerous studies have successfully demonstrated the PSI's validity. The PSI discriminated between physically abusive and nonabusive mothers (Mash & Johnston, 1983), and significant decreases were found in parental stress in two groups of parents who were receiving parent training courses (Lafferty, Cote, Chafe, Kellar, & Robertson, 1980). Although the factors are not completely independent, as shown by factor-analytic studies, most items load primarily on the appropriate subscales. The PSI is a straightforward measure with multiple potential clinical and research uses.

Pleasure-Arousal and Dominance-Inducing Scales of Parental Attitudes (PADSPA)

The PADSPA (Falender & Mehrabian, 1979) is a 46-item questionnaire that assesses parental child-rearing attitudes that create an emotional climate for children. Emotional climate is measured on three scales: Pleasure–Displeasure, Arousal–Nonarousal, and Dominance–Submisiveness. Parents respond to the questionnaire on a 9-point Likert format ranging from "very strong agreement" to "very strong disagreement." The scales were developed on a sample of 246 mothers with children between the ages of 3 months and 8 years. Internal consistency coefficients for the three scales range from .62 to .77. Although few validity studies have been conducted, interscale correlations were low, suggesting that the scales are assessing independent dimensions. Although the measure addresses the theoretically compelling concept of emotional climate created by child-rearing attitudes, the psychometric properties of the instrument need further development, not only to support its reliability and validity but also to ascertain its clinical and research utility.

Family–Peer Relationship Questionnaire (FPRQ)

The FPRQ (Ellison, 1983) is designed primarily to assess the quality of parental support as perceived by *both* the parent and the child. A secondary purpose of the measure is to assess children's peer relations. The FPRQ is based theoretically on an ecological model of social support and is developed for children aged 7 to 12 and their parents. The FPRQ is an 18-item self-report measure in which the majority of responses appear in a 5-point Likert format ranging from low frequency to high frequency of a behavior. Some questions ask for time estimates, while others require peer relationship information (e.g., names, length of friendship). The Parent domain includes three scales: Togetherness, Nurturance–Disclosure, and Peer Relationships. Similar scales are included in the Child domain, but the number of items within each scale differs from those in the Parent Domain. Cronbach alpha coefficients ranged from .65 to .92, suggesting that the FPRQ is internally consistent (Ellison, 1985a). Test–retest reliability on the parental support scales was .64 for the Togetherness scale and .85 for the Nurturance scale, with the time interval unspecified (Ellison, undated). Construct validity was reported in one study (Ellison, Kieckhefer, Houck, & Wallace, undated), and further criterion validity studies are in progress (Ellison, 1985b).

The FPRQ is a concise and easily administered measure, making it a valuable tool for use in a health care setting. The measure recognizes and addresses the importance of the inclusion of the child's perspective in the emotional health of the family environment. Continued work regarding the measure's validity would strengthen the FPRQ as both a clinical and a research assessment tool.

Parental Acceptance–Rejection Questionnaire (PARQ)— Child, Mother, and Adult

The PARQ (Rohner, 1980, 1984) is a 60-item questionnaire for the cross-cultural assessment of parental accepting–rejecting behaviors. The PARQ is available in Spanish, Czechoslovakian, Hindi, Korean, Swedish, and several African languages. The PARQ has three forms: a Child scale for children aged 9 to 11 years; a Mother scale; and an Adult scale to assess adults' reports of their own parents' behavior. (Separate abstracts of the three forms are included in Part Two.) Items are identical on all forms, although there are some minor wording changes to reflect respondent viewpoint. Respondents indicate the frequency of each parental behavior, using a 4-point Likert scale ranging from "almost always true" to "almost never true." Each form has four scales: Warmth/Affection; Aggression/Hostility; Neglect/Indifference; and (Undifferentiated) Rejection. Reliability and validity data are available for the Child and Adult forms of the PARQ. For the Adult form, internal consistency coefficients range from .86 to .95 across two samples of male and female undergraduate students and from .71 to .96 for the Spanish version of the scale. On the Child form, internal consistency of the scales ranges from .72 to .90 for a sample of American children in the fourth and fifth grades. Validity of the instrument is supported by a number of research studies (Rohner, 1984). Although developed on American samples and nonparent populations, the PARQ has demonstrable value (see Rohner, 1984) for use by clinicians and researchers interested in parental acceptance–rejection in different cultures.

Child's Attitude toward Mother (CAM)/Child's Attitude toward Father (CAF)

The CAM and CAF scales are designed to measure the degree, severity, or magnitude of a problem a child has with his or her mother or father. The CAM and CAF scales are two of nine scales included in the Clinical Measurement Package (Hudson, 1982) (see, also, earlier discussion in this chapter of the Index of Parental Attitudes) and are suitable for adolescents (aged 12 and above) and adult children. Like the other scales in the Clinical Measurement Package, the CAM and CAF are 25-item scales, with a 5-point Likert response format ranging from "rarely" to "most of the time." The scales are unidimensional; thus, a single "problem severity" score is derived by summing the responses. The CAM and CAF scales have been determined to be highly reliable, with alpha coefficients ranging from .93 to .97 (Hudson, 1982; Saunders & Schuchts, 1987). The differential construct validity of the CAM and CAF has been established in two studies using a known-groups approach (Hudson, 1982; Saunders & Schuchts, 1987). Thus, the CAM and CAF appear to be reliable and valid measures of parent–child relationship problems that are useful for both clinicians and researchers.

Cornell Parent Behavior Inventory (CPBI)

The CPBI (Devereux, Bronfenbrenner, & Rodgers, 1969) is a 30-item questionnaire designed to assess children's and adolescents' perceptions of their mothers' and fathers' child-rearing attitudes and behavior. It is a revision of the Bronfenbrenner Parent Behavior Questionnaire (Devereux, Bronfenbrenner, & Suci, 1962; see also Siegelman, 1965). In addition to the CPBI, a shorter 21-item version, the Perceived Parenting Questionnaire (PPQ) (MacDonald, 1971) has also been developed to assess parental behaviors retrospectively. (A separate abstract for the PPQ is included in Part Two.) The CPBI contains 14 subscales (the first 9 are contained in the PPQ): Nurturance, Instrumental Companionship, Principled Discipline, Predictability of Standards, Protectiveness, Physical Punishment, Achievement Pressure, Deprivation of Privileges, Affective Punishment, Encouragement of Autonomy, Indulgence, Prescription of Responsibilities, Control, and Scolding. Respondents indicate how frequently their parents do each of the behaviors described, using three different 5-point Likert response scales. Factor analyses yield similar factor structures for the CPBI (Loving, Demanding, Punishing, and Control) (Gfellner, 1986) and the PPQ

(Support, Discipline, and Covert Control) (Aguilino, 1986). Internal consistency coefficients range from .48 to .82 for the nine PPQ subscales (MacDonald, 1971; Halpin, Halpin, & Whiddon, 1980), and .70 to .82 for the factors derived from the CPBI (Aguilino, 1986). Validity data are available for both the CPBI and PPQ across multiple samples, including cross-cultural groups. Although there is a clear need for test–retest reliability data on both measures, the factorial consistency and validity evidence for the PPQ and CPBI across various samples and cultural groups suggests that the scales are assessing robust child-rearing behaviors.

Child's Report of Parental Behavior Inventory (CRPBI)

The CRPBI (Schaefer, 1965) was developed on the theoretical assumption that children's perceptions of parental behavior directed toward them influence their social and personality development. Although the original CRPBI appears to be no longer in use, several revisions are available, including a 56-item, 6-subscale version (Burger & Armentrout, 1971; Burger, Armentrout, & Rapfogel, 1973) and a 108-item, 18-subscale version (Schludermann & Schludermann, 1970, 1983). Separate abstracts of these two versions are included in Part II. For each version, children and adolescents indicate on a 3-point Likert scale the degree to which the behavior depicted is "like" their mother or father. The shorter version of the CRPBI (Burger & Armentrout, 1971; Burger et al., 1973) includes six subscales: Acceptance, Control through Guilt, Nonenforcement, Lax Discipline, Childcenteredness, and Instilling Persistent Anxiety. The longer version adds the subscales Possessivness, Rejection, Control, Enforcement, Positive Involvement, Intrusiveness, Hostile Control, Inconsistent Discipline, Acceptance of Individuation, Hostile Detachment, Withdrawal of Relations, and Extreme Autonomy. Factor analyses of both CRPBI versions consistently yield three factors, Acceptance versus Rejection, Psychological Autonomy versus Psychological Control, and Firm versus Lax Control (Burger et al., 1973; Margolies & Weintraub, 1977; Schludermann & Schludermann, 1983). Internal consistency data are unavailable for either form of the CRPBI; test–retest reliability ranges from .50 to .96 for the three-factor solution of the short version (Margolies & Weintraub, 1977). Criterion-related validity has been demonstrated for both versions of the CRPBI (Litovsky & Dusek, 1985; Schludermann & Schludermann, 1983). Nonwithstanding the need for further reliability data, these two adaptations of the CRPBI provide researchers with shorter and more psychometrically grounded versions of the original CRPBI for the study of child and adolescent views of parental child-rearing behaviors.

Inventory of Parent and Peer Attachment (IPPA)

The IPPA (Armsden & Greenberg, 1984) assesses adolescents' perceptions of the quality of their attachments with their parents and friends. Based on ethological-organizational attachment theory, the IPPA is a 75-item questionnaire.

Adolescents aged 16 to 20 rate their feelings of attachment to mother, father, and close friends on a 5-point Likert scale ranging from "never true" to "always true." The three scales for the Parent and Peer sections of the IPPA are Trust, Communication, and Alienation. Internal consistency for the three scales for the Parent and Peer sections of the IPPA ranges from .72 to .91. Test–retest realiability over a 3-week interval yielded a coefficient of .86 for the Peer form and .93 for the Parent form. Significant intercorrelations among the Parent and Peer IPPA scales indicate that the three scales may be assessing aspects of the same attachment construct. Combining the scale scores may be more appropriate than evaluating them individually. The validity data on the IPPA have been adequately reported in several studies (Armsden, 1986; Armsden & Greenberg, 1984). The IPPA has potential clinical and research utility; its usefulness would be enhanced by the collection of standardization and normative data.

Parent Perception Inventory (PPI)

The PPI (Hazzard, Christensen, & Margolin, 1983) assesses children's perceptions of positive and negative parental behaviors. The PPI is a measure for young children that taps perceptions of parental behavior rather than attitudinal dimensions. Based on social learning theory, the PPI includes 18 items, which are responded to on a 5-point Likert scale ranging from "never" to "a lot." The PPI contains two 9-item dimensions: Positive Parental Behaviors and Negative Parental Behaviors. Included in the positive parental behaviors are positive reinforcement, comfort, talk time, involvement in decision making, time together, positive evaluation, allowing independence, and assistance and non-verbal affection. The negative parental behaviors include privilege removal, criticism, command, physical punishment, yelling, threatening, time-out, nagging, and ignoring. The parental behaviors form four subscales: Mother Positive, Mother Negative, Father Positive, and Father Negative. Cronbach alpha reliability coefficients for the four subscales range from .78 to .88, and convergent validity indicates moderate correlations between PPI scale scores and child's self-esteem and parental perceptions of child conduct disorder (Hazzard et al., 1983). The PPI shows promise as an efficient measure of children's perceptions of parental behaviors, but it is still largely untested.

COMPARATIVE EVALUATIONS OF MEASURES

Measurement Focus and Perspective

The parent–child measures in this review varied considerably, both in measurement perspective (i.e., parent or child as respondent) and in the primary focus of questionnaire content. Regarding measurement perspective, as shown in Table 8–1, parents are the respondents in the majority (12) of the parent–child measures. Only two measures have parallel parent and child forms.

TABLE 8–1. Measurement Perspectives of Subscales of the Parent–Child Relationship Measures

Measure (Author, Date); Emphasis	Parent Evaluation	Parent Child-Rearing Attitudes	Report of Parent Behavior	Child Evaluation	Family/Other Relationships
Parent as Respondent					
Adult–Adolescent Parenting Inventory (Bavolek, 1984); child abuse		Role Reversal Corporal Punishment Inappropriate Expectations Empathy			
Child Abuse Potential Inventory (Milner, 1986); child abuse/family stress	Distress Unhappiness Problems with Child and Self	Rigidity			Problems with Family Problems from Others
Child Behavior Toward Parent Inventory (Schaefer, 1975, 1977); bidirectional influence				Independence/ Dependence Acceptance/Rejection Control	
Child-Rearing Practices Report (Block, 1965); social learning		Q-sort items			
Home Environment Questionnaire (Sines, 1983); environmental press	Affiliation		Supervision Aggression—Home	Aggression—External	Sociability Separation Affiliation Change Socioeconomic Status
Maryland Parent Attitude Survey (Pumroy, 1966); social-developmental		Disciplinarian Rejecting Indulgent Protective			

Instrument (reference); orientation					
Parent as a Teacher Inventory (Strom, 1984); creativity, play	Teaching-Learning	Teaching-Learning, Play, Control, Creativity		Frustration	Family Disharmony (factor scale)
Parent Attitude Research Instrument (Schaefer & Bell, 1958); social developmental		Authoritarian Control (factor scale)			
Perceptions of Parental Role Scales (Gilbert & Hanson, 1982) role theory		Teaching, Basic Needs, Family Interface			
Parenting Stress Index (Abidin, 1983); attachment, temperament, family stress	Depression, Unhappiness, Restriction of Role, Sense of Competence, Social Isolation, Parental Health	Attachment	Adaptability, Acceptability, Mood, Demandingness, Distractability/Hyperactivity, Reinforces Parent		
Pleasure-Arousal and Dominance-Inducing Scales of Parental Attitudes (Falender & Mehrabian, 1979); emotional climate	Pleasure-Displeasure	Dominance-Submisiveness, Arousal-Nonarousal			
Parent or Child as Respondent (equivalent forms)					
Clinical Measurement Package (Hudson, 1982); clinical					

(continued)

TABLE 8–1. CONTINUED

Measure (Author, Date); Emphasis	Parent Evaluation	Parent Child-Rearing Attitudes	Report of Parent Behavior	Child Evaluation	Family/Other Relationships
Index of Parental Attitudes Child's Attitude toward Mother/Father	Problem Severity			Problem Severity	
Family–Peer Relationship Questionnaire (Ellison, 1983); ecological			Togetherness Nurturance–Disclosure	Peer Relations (parent form)	Peer Relations (child form)
Parental Acceptance–Rejection Questionnaire—Adult, Mother, & Child Forms (Rohner, 1980); cross-cultural			Rejection Aggression/Hostility Neglect/Indifference Warmth/Affection (Mother and Child Forms)		Rejection Aggression/Hostility Neglect/Indifference Warmth/Affection (Adult Form)
Child as Respondent					
Cornell Parent Behavior Inventory (Devereux, Bronfenbrenner, & Rodgers, 1969); phenomenology, cognitive development			Nurturance Principled Discipline Instrumental Companionship Consistency of Expectations Encouragement of Autonomy Indulgence Prescription of Responsibility Achievement Demands Control Protectiveness Affective Punishment Deprivation of Privileges Scolding Physical Punishment		

Instrument	Dimensions
Perceived Parenting Questionnaire (McDonald, 1971) (CPBI adaptation)	Nurturance Predictability of Standards Protectiveness Deprivation of Priveleges Affective Punishment Instrumental Companionship Principled Discipline Achievement Pressure Physical Punishment
Child's Report of Parental Behavior Inventory—Revised[a] (192-item version: Burger & Armentrout, 1971) (108-item version: Schludermann & Schludermann, 1970, 1983) (56-item version: Margolies & Weintraub, 1977); phenomenology cognitive development	Acceptance vs. Rejection Firm vs. Lax Control Psychological Autonomy vs. Control (Factor Scales)
Inventory of Parent and Peer Attachment (Armsden, 1986); attachment theory	Trust Communication Alienation

Parent Perception Inventory (Hazzard & Christensen, 1983); social learning	Mother
	  Positive
	  Negative
	Father
	  Positive
	  Negative

[a]The original CRPBI (Schaefer, 1965) included 260 items.

The assessment focus of questionnaire items and subscales among the parent–child measures was also somewhat heterogeneous. To facilitate subsequent theoretical and conceptual comparisons, the parent–child measures were grouped by subscale into rationally derived item content categories. Five item categories were identified: parent self-evaluation of behavior, mood, or competence; child evaluation of behavior, mood, or competence, either by self or parent; attitudes toward child rearing; report of parent behaviors; and evaluation of other relationships. Although the subscales of any given measure might include items reflecting multiple categories, subscales were placed in the category that was represented by the majority of items. The results, which appear in Table 8–1, indicate that most of the parent–child measures reflect a mixture of measurement foci. Five questionnaires (Adult–Adolescent Parenting Inventory, Maryland Parent Attitude Survey, Parent Attitude Research Instrument, Perceptions of Parental Role Scales, and Pleasure-Arousal and Dominance-Inducing Scales of Parental Attitudes) are measures primarily, though not exclusively, of parental attitudes toward child rearing. Measures with the child as respondent assess primarily, but not exclusively, parent behavior. Although these represent exceptions, the mixed measurement foci of the majority of the parent–child measures indicates that most measures do not clearly differentiate attitudes, behavior, and feeling states.

Theoretical and Conceptual Comparisons

All of the parent–child measures can be viewed as theoretically driven by socialization theory, with *socialization* defined as the role of the parent–child relationship in the social, emotional, and cognitive development of children. Within the socialization framework, the parent–child measures differ considerably in their theoretical emphases (see Table 8–2), with consistencies the exception rather than the rule. Three measures emphasize risk for dysfunctional (abusive or stressed) parenting; however, the theoretical bases for these measures differ or are absent. Two measures derive from attachment theory; however, one is focused on preschool and young children, whereas the other focuses on adolescents.

Conceptual comparison of the constructs measured by the parent–child measures is hindered by the aforementioned heterogeneity in measurement perspective among instruments. Nevertheless, a conceptual grouping of the subscales of the parent–child measures appears in Table 8–2. The categories, rationally derived to facilitate comparison among the measures, reflect schemes previously utilized in this book and categories unique to this measurement area. The categories are roles, orientation, affect, communication, control, autonomy, and other. *Roles* refers to behavior patterns associated with normative expectations. *Orientation* refers to the general focus of the parent, as reflected in the continuums of parent-centeredness versus child-centeredness and acceptance versus rejection of the child. *Affect* refers to the expression and the experience of emotions. *Communication* refers to the quality of family interaction or discussion. *Control/autonomy* refers to parent behaviors that are intended to inhibit undesired child behavior (control) and that are intended to encourage child independence and mastery (autonomy). Subscales that could not reasonably be included in one of these six categories were placed in the ''other'' category.

The categorization of subscales (see Table 8–2), attests to both the conceptual similarity and the heterogeneity among the parent–child measures. Measures in which the parent is the respondent are most likely to have subscales that fall within the orientation and control/autonomy categories, closely followed by subscales reflecting affect. The predominance of these categories across various instruments suggests that these are somewhat consistently perceived key qualities of parenting. Deviations from this pattern are evident in parent-response measures that have unique theoretical emphases, such as the attachment and temperament theoretical focus of the Parenting Stress Index, the role theory focus of the Perceptions of Parental Role Scales, or the cognitive developmental focus of the Parent as a Teacher Inventory. Examination of the conceptual groupings of the constructs in the child-respondent measures reveals the influence of developmental stage. Whereas the categories assessed by measures developed for children as respondents appear similar to categories for the parent-respondent measures, adolescent measures are unique in the inclusion of communication subscales, suggesting the increased salience of this child-rearing strategy with maturation (Roberts, Block, & Block, 1984).

As was observed with the self-report measures of whole-family functioning (see Chapter 6), subscales of the parent–child measures are not always labeled consistently with their content. In Table 8–2, the subscales were categorized according to the domains that corresponded to the content reflected by the majority of items, rather than the association expected from the subscale title. For example, in the Parent as a Teacher Inventory, the item content of the subscale Frustration, which might be expected to refer to an affective state, reflects a child-centered orientation on the part of the parent that accepts the inconveniences associated with a view of the child as an active learner. Thus, examination of item content remains essential in the selection of instruments to ensure that the construct of importance is being measured as intended.

The parent–child measures also reveal considerable similarity of constructs across measures. This may reflect a greater consensus within the socialization literature regarding the salience of theoretical child-rearing variables than is evident in the family process literature (Beavers & Voeller, 1983; Carlson & Grotevant, 1987b). On the other hand, the parent–child measures reveal greater heterogeneity regarding operationalization of theoretical variables (i.e., variables reflecting mixtures of attitudes, behaviors, and feeling states) than whole-family self-report measures that assess qualities of the family as a whole.

Physical and Administrative Comparisons

The parent–child measures were evaluated according to the criteria discussed in Chapter 5. Physical and administrative criteria include the availability and

TABLE 8–2. Conceptual Groupings of Subscales of the Parent–Child Relationship Measures

Measure	Roles	Orientation	Affect	Communication	Control/Autonomy	Other
Parent as Respondent						
Adult–Adolescent Parenting Inventory	Empathy Role Reversal				Inappropriate Expectations Corporal Punishment	
Child Abuse Potential Inventory			Distress Unhappiness			Rigidity Problems with Self and Child Problems with Family Problems from Others
Child Behavior Toward Parent Inventory		Acceptance/Rejection			Control Independence/Dependence	
Child-Rearing Practices Report	Achievement Health	Investment in Child Parental Independence Inconsistency	Worries Negative Affect Expression of Affect	Rational Guidance	Independence Control Suppression of Aggression Suppression of Sex Control by Anxiety Induction Control by Guilt Induction Openness to Experience Protectiveness Supervision Nonphysical punishment	
Home Environment Questionnaire	Achievement Socioeconomic status	Aggression—Home Affiliation			Supervision	Aggression—External Change Separation Sociability

(continued)

Measure					
Maryland Parent Attitude Survey	Rejecting Indulgent Protective			Disciplinarian	
Parent as a Teacher Inventory	Frustration			Control	Creativity Play Teaching-Learning
Parent Attitude Research Instrument	Family Disharmony			Control	
Perceptions of Parental Role Scales	Teaching Basic Needs Interface Role			Authoritarian Control	
Parenting Stress Index	Acceptability Demandingness	Depression/Unhappiness Attachment Mood Reinforces Parent	Restriction Imposed by Role		Parental Health Sense of Competence Social Isolation Relationship with Spouse Distractibility/Hyperactivity Adaptability
Pleasure-Arousal and Dominance-Inducing Scales of Parental Attitudes		Pleasure–Displeasure Arousal–Nonarousal		Dominance–Submissiveness	
Parent or Child as Respondent (equivalent forms)					
Clinical Measurement Package (Index of Parental Attitudes, Child's Attitude toward Mother/Father)		Problem Severity			

TABLE 8–2. CONTINUED

Measure	Roles	Orientation	Affect	Communication	Control/Autonomy	Other
Family–Peer Relationship Questionnaire		Togetherness			Nurturance/ Disclosure	
Parental Acceptance– Rejection Questionnaire		Undifferentiated Rejection Neglect/ Indifference	Aggression/Hostility Warmth/Acceptance			
Child as Respondent						
Cornell Parent Behavior Inventory	Prescription of Responsibili- ties	Nurturance Instrumental Companionship Consistency of Expectations			Principled Discipline Encouragement of Autonomy Indulgence Achievement Demands Control Protectiveness Affective Punishment Deprivation of Privileges Scolding Physical Punishment	

Instrument			
Perceived Parenting Questionnaire (adaptation of CPBI for older children)	Nurturance Instrumental Companionship		Predictability of Standards Protectiveness Affective Punishment Deprivation of Priveleges Principled Discipline Achievement Pressure Physical Punishment Firm vs. Lax Control Psychological Autonomy vs. Control
Child's Report of Parental Behavior Inventory—Revised (two versions; same factors)		Acceptance vs. Rejection	
Inventory of Parent and Peer Attachment	Trust	Alienation	Commu-nication
Parent Perception Inventory	Mother/Father Positive		Mother/Father Negative

adequacy of norms, the availability and adequacy of a manual, and the adequacy of test construction, including item response bias, reading level, and response format. Table 8–3 summarizes the physical and administrative characteristics that differentiate the measures. Variability among measures was noted in the areas of response format, response set, and availability of standardized administration and scoring procedures, norms, and manuals. Unique strengths and weaknesses associated with each instrument are provided in the "Notes" column of the table.

Norms provide a basis for interpreting the test performance of a person or group in relation to a defined population (*Standards*, 1985). The collection of an adequate normative sample is recognized to be costly; therefore, the evaluation of the adequacy of test norms varies, depending on the purpose of the test. Measures designed for research purposes and measures in the test development phase are not expected to have representative norms (*Standards*, 1985); clearly defined descriptive statistics regarding the various populations of research interest can suffice. In contrast, measures designed for clinical use or for classification purposes demand an adequate normative sample, usually based on probability sampling techniques across geographic, socioeconomic, and cultural groups.

Most of the parent–child measures are designed primarily for research use (see Table 8–4). Although requirements for normative data are less stringent for these measures, provision of adequate descriptive information regarding samples (either published or available from the author) is problematic, and the administration of measures to multiple samples is limited. Measures that have been administered to multiple samples include the Child-Rearing Practices Report (J. H. Block, 1965), the Cornell Parent Behavior Inventory (Devereux et al., 1969), the Parent as a Teacher Inventory (Strom, 1984), the Parent Acceptance–Rejection Questionnaire (Rohner, 1980, 1984), the Parent Attitute Research Instrument (Schaefer & Bell, 1958; Schludermann & Schludermann, 1977), and the revised versions of the Child's Report of Parental Behavior (Margolies & Weintraub, 1977; Schaefer, 1965; Schludermann & Schludermann, 1970, 1983). It should be noted that criterion referencing is considered more appropriate than norm referencing for the Child-Rearing Practices Report, which utilizes a Q-sort methodology (Block, 1965). Regarding parent–child measures designed for clinical use (Index of Parental Attitudes and Child's Attitude toward Mother/Father (Hudson, 1982), Parenting Stress Index (Abidin, 1983), Child Abuse Potential Inventory (Milner, 1986), and the Adult–Adolescent Parenting Inventory (Bavolek, 1984), most have established norms. Only the Index of Parental Attitudes lacks normative data. Regarding the adequacy of normative samples, only the Parenting Stress Index would appear to benefit from a more representative normative sample.

The manual of a measure—which should include standardized administration and scoring instructions, interpretation guidelines, theoretical premises, and normative and psychometric data—assures appropriate use of the measure and reduces error that may lower test reliability. Manuals are available for 9 of the

TABLE 8–3. Physical and Administrative Properties of the Parent–Child Relationship Measures

Measure	Age Range	Norms	Manual	Response Format	Response Problems	Notes
Parent as Respondent						
Adult–Adolescent Parenting Inventory	Adolescents–adult (6th-grade reading)	Yes	Yes	5-choice	Susceptible to social desirability	All abuse-related measures susceptible to social desirability; needs investigation; sex bias favors females
Child Abuse Potential Inventory	Adult (3rd-grade reading)	Yes	Yes	2-choice	None noted	Uncorrelated with social desirability
Child Behavior Toward Parent Inventory	Adult	No	No	4-choice	None noted	
Child-Rearing Practices Report	16–adult	No	Yes	Q-sort	No	Two forms: parent and young adult/nonparent; criterion vs. norm referencing is advised; Q-sort minimizes response bias; available in many languages
Home Environment Questionnaire	Adult	Limited	Yes	2-choice	Susceptible to social desirability	Items behaviorally specific
Maryland Parent Attitude Survey	Adult	No	Limited	2-choice		Social desirability has been controlled
Parent as a Teacher Inventory	Parents of children aged 3–9 yrs	Unpublished, available	Yes	4-choice	None noted	Available in 15 languages
Parent Attitude Research Instrument	Adult	No	No	4-choice	Extreme response set	Acquiescence and oppositional response bias has been reduced

(continued)

135

TABLE 8–3. CONTINUED

Measure	Age Range	Norms	Manual	Response Format	Response Problems	Notes
Perceptions of Parental Role Scales	Adult	No	Yes	5-choice	None noted	Role responsibilities are expected to vary with child age; thus, role scores are difficult to interpret without norms
Parenting Stress Index	Parents of children under 10 (5th grade reading)	Yes	Yes	5-choice	None noted	Low correlation with social desirability; normative group is not representative
Pleasure-Arousal Dominance Inducing and Scales of Parental Attitudes	Adult	Very limited	No	9-choice	None noted	Item content reflects a mixture of self and child evaluation and parent attitudes
Parent or Child as Respondent (equivalent forms)						
Clinical Measurement Package						
Index of Parental Attitudes	Adult	No	Yes	5-choice	Susceptible to social desirability	Item content reflects a mixture of self and other evaluation; available in four languages
Child's Attitude toward Mother/Father	12 yrs min.	Yes	Yes	5-choice		
Family–Peer Relationship Questionnaire	Adults; Child form, 7 yrs min.	No	No	5-choice	None noted	Relies on recall for completion of items; Peer Relations Form

Parental Acceptance–Rejection Questionnaire						
Mother Form	Adult	No	Yes	4-choice	Expected social desirability	z-score conversions recommended but no tables provided; items limited to mother's behavior; multiple language versions
Child Form	9–10 yrs min.	No	Yes	4-choice	None noted	
Adult Form	Adult	No	Yes	4-choice	None noted	Retrospective report
Child as Respondent						
Cornell Parent Behavior Inventory	8 yrs–adult	No	No	5-choice	None noted	Reading level and response format may be too difficult for some 8-yr-olds
Perceived Parenting Questionnaire (CPBI adaptation)	Adolescents	No	No	5-choice	None noted	
Child's Report of Parental Behavior–Revised	7 yrs–college	No	No	3-choice	None noted	
Inventory of Parent and Peer Attachment	Adolescents	No	No	5-choice	None noted	Scales nonindependent; Peer Relations Form
Parent Perception Inventory	5–13 yrs	No	No	5-choice	None noted	Verbal report format may increase social desirability; no age differences obtained

19 parent–child measures reviewed, with all of the clinically oriented measures providing manuals. The available manuals were clearly written and comprehensive. Only the manual for the Maryland Parent Attitude Survey suffered in this regard. Information typically contained in a manual can be gleaned to some extent from the references for most of the measures that do not have manuals. However, this procedure is haphazard and time-consuming and may lead to the use of outdated information, which could seriously hinder comparison of results across studies that presumably use the same measure. In sum, manuals should be available for all published measures, including those that are designed primarily for research purposes.

As noted earlier (see Chapter 5), the response format of a measure influences its reliability, with the enhancement of reliability leveling off at about seven response choices (Nunnally, 1978). Response formats of the parent–child measures range from two (forced-choice format) to nine, with most of the instruments adopting a five-choice format. Only the Mehrabian scale appears problematic regarding the complexity of response choices, and this complexity is increased with the measure's physical design, which provides the response key only in the instructions. Including defined anchor points in the response format to each item is recommended to reduce response error (Anastasi, 1982). Also, the Cornell Parent Behavior Inventory uses three different 5-point response formats, which may be confusing to children.

Various response set problems have the potential for introducing systematic error into scores in self-report measures (see Chapter 5 for a discussion of response set problems). Although all response set errors are applicable to the parent–child measures reviewed, social desirability is a particular concern because parents, as a result of the social pressure exerted to be "good parents," are expected to "fake good" reports of their parenting practices. For the majority of these recently developed parent–child measures, response set problems generally were not found. However, very few measures have empirically investigated response bias in their test development. The potential for social desirability response bias was present in the minds of the reviewers for the Parental Acceptance–Rejection Questionnaire, the Adult–Adolescent Parenting Inventory, and the Index of Parental Attitudes, because the items tap undesirable behavior, and for the Parent Perception Inventory, which does not protect the anonymity of the respondent with its verbal report format. In contrast to the concerns noted, several measures are commendable in their efforts to reduce, eliminate, and investigate response set bias. Selection of response format minimizes response bias for the Child-Rearing Practices Report (a Q-sort) and for the Maryland Parent Attitude Survey (a forced-choice format); however, the response bias gains derived from measures using a forced-choice format must be balanced against the inherent loss of information (Anastasi, 1982; Nunnally, 1978). The Child Abuse Potential Inventory includes three validity scales to evaluate error due to lying, random responding, and inconsistency. This is particularly appropriate given the clinical use of this measure and the potential reactivity of item content. Social desirability response bias has been reduced

TABLE 8–4. Comparative Reliability and Validity of the Parent–Child Relationship Measures

Measure	Purpose[a]	Reliability		Validity	
		Test-Retest[b]	Internal Consistency	Criterion-Related	Construct-Related
Adult as Respondent					
Adult–Adolescent Parenting Inventory	1, 2	1 wk: .39–.89 for factors (Bavolek, 1984)	Alphas: .70–.86 for factors (Bavolek, 1984)	Empathy discriminated abused vs. nonabused adolescents; all factors discriminated abused vs. nonabused adults (Bavolek, 1984); parent scores predict males exposure but not preference for violent, fantasy, superhero, and loner TV programs (Price, 1985)	Items loading on each factor are distinct (Bavolek, 1984)
Child Abuse Potential Inventory	1, 2, 3	1 day–3 mo: .53–.90 across subscales (Milner, 1986)	Total KR-20: .90's for various groups; .50–.90 for subscales (Milner, 1986)	Differentiated normal and clinical families in multiple studies (Milner, 1986); abusers discriminated from nonabusers with 85%–93% accuracy (Milner et al., 1986)	Parent subscale scores correspond to Parent Stress Index, to relevant MMPI and Mental Health Index subscales; child scores relate to maternal ratings of conduct disorders and problems (Milner, 1986)
Child Behavior Toward Parent Inventory	2	Unknown	KR-20: .69–.95 (long form); Alphas: .60–.81 (short form)	Scales correlate significantly with parent and teacher ratings (Schaefer & Edgerton, 1977) (short form)	Scales load separately on three factors (Schaefer & Finkelstein, 1975) (long form)
Child-Rearing Practices Report	2	1 yr: .71, young adult; 3 yr: young adult = .66, mother = .64, father = .65 (Block, undated)	Unknown	Adults' agreement on CRPR items predicted marriage success/termination and quality of their children's psychological functioning (Block, Block, & Morrison, 1981); parent CRPR scores differentiate undercontrolled from antisocial adolescents (Block & Gjerde, 1986)	Unknown

(continued)

139

TABLE 8-4. CONTINUED

Measure	Purpose[a]	Reliability		Validity	
		Test–Retest[b]	Internal Consistency	Criterion-Related	Construct-Related
Maryland Parent Attitude Survey	2	3 mo: .67–.73 (Pumroy, 1966)	Split-half: .67–.84 across scales (Pumroy, 1966)	Disciplinarian scale differentiated high vs. low restrictive and directing mothers; rejecting scale significantly related to use of prohibitions by mothers (Pumroy, 1966)	Interscale correlations are high, suggesting nonindependent scales (Tolor, 1967)
Parent as a Teacher Inventory	2, 4	Unknown	Total alphas: .77–.88 in 17 samples; subscale alphas not reported (Strom, 1984)	Parent PAAT scores significantly increased after a parent education program (Strom, 1984); Maternal Control subscale significantly predicted McCarthy Scales of Children's Abilities, Cognitions and Motor scores (Strom et al., 1981)	75%–85% concordance between parents' PAAT and home teaching behaviors (Strom, 1984)
Parent Attitude Research Instrument	2	1 wk: .52–.81 for 23 scales; .75–.81 for factor scales (PARI Q[4]) (Schludermann & Schludermann, 1977)	KR-20: .34–.76 in two samples (Schaefer & Bell, 1958); PARI Q[4] unknown	Differentiated normal mothers from those with problem children; scores correlate significantly with children's Mooney Problem Cklst scores and ratings of adjustment (Becker & Krug, 1965); PARI Q[4] unknown	PARI Q[4] unknown
Perceptions of Parental Role Scales	1, 2	1 mo: .73–.90 for 13 subscales (Gilbert & Hansen, 1982)	Alphas: .81–.91 for 13 subscales (Gilbert & Hansen, 1982)	Females score higher than males in parenting responsibilities (Gilbert & Hansen, 1982)	Unknown

Instrument	Respondent	Reliability	Internal consistency	Validity	Construct validity
Parenting Stress Index	1, 3	3 wk, 1–3 mo., 3 mo intervals; Child: .82, .63, 77; Parent: .71, .91, .69 (Abidin, 1983)	Alphas: .62–.70; Child subscales = .63–.70; Parent subscales = .55–.80; total child = .89; total parent = .93 (Abidin, 1983)	Child and Parent domain scores discriminated mothers of mentally and physically handicapped vs. nonhandicapped children; abusive vs. nonabusive mothers; single vs. married mothers of infants (Abidin, 1983)	Total child is significantly related to Child Behavior Cklst and Achenbach Child Behavior Cklst scores; total adult significantly related to State-Trait Anxiety in two studies; factor analysis yields two distinct constructs (Abidin, 1983)
Pleasure-Arousal and Dominance Inducing Scales of Parental Attitudes	2	Unknown	KR-20's: Arousal = .62; Pleasure = .79; Dominance = .77 (Falendar & Mehrabian, 1980)	Unknown	Interscale correlations .03–.14, indicating scales assess separate aspects of emotional climate (Falendar & Mehrabian, 1980)

Parent and Child as Respondent (equivalent forms)

Clinical Measurement Package

Instrument	Respondent	Reliability	Internal consistency	Validity	Construct validity
Index of Parental Attitudes	1, 3	Unknown	Alpha: .93 (Hudson, 1982)	Discriminated parent–child discord groups (Hudson, 1982)	Relates to relevant items on the Psychosocial Screening Package (Hudson, 1982)
Child's Attitude Toward Mother/Father	1, 3	Unknown	Alphas: .93–.95 (Hudson, 1982); .95–.97 (Saunders & Schuchts, 1987)	Discriminated parent–child discord groups (Saunders & Schuchts, 1987)	Unknown
Family–Peer Relationship Questionnaire	1, 2	Togetherness = .64; Nurturance = .85 (Ellison et al., undated) (test-retest interval not specified)	Alphas: .65–.86, (mother/child); .72–.92 (father/child) (Ellison, 1985a)	Child Nurturance related to reported feeling informed and reassured about mother's illness; Child Togetherness negatively related to fears regarding mother's illness (Ellison et al., undated)	In progress (see Ellison, 1985b)
Parental Acceptance–Rejection Questionnaire	2	Unknown	Alphas: Child scale: .72–.90; adult scale: .86–.95; Mother scale not reported	Adult scale: adolescent's report of parental warmth related to self-esteem and self-adequacy (Saavedra, 1980)	Child and Adult scales correlate with the CRPBI (Schaefer, 1965) and PBQ scales (Siegelman, 1965); Mother scale unknown

(continued)

TABLE 8-4. CONTINUED

		Reliability		Validity	
Measure	Purpose[a]	Test–Retest[b]	Internal Consistency	Criterion-Related	Construct-Related
Child as Respondent					
Cornell Parent Behavior Inventory	2	Unknown	Alphas: .70–.82 for factors (Aguilino, 1986)	Perception of quality of marital interaction related to levels of parental support vs. punishment (Aguilino, 1986); maternal demandingness and support related to internal locus of control for Anglo- and Mexican-American children; internal control varies by ethnic group for paternal control and demandingness (Buriel, 1981)	Child perceptions of parent rearing behaviors consistent with observational data (Devereux et al., 1969)
Perceived Parenting Questionnaire (CPBI adaptation)	2	Unknown	Alphas: .38–.84 (26-item scale) (Halpin, Halpin, & Whiddon, 1980)	Girls' report of parental loving related to higher ego stage development; boys' report of parental demanding related to ego stage development (Gfellner, 1986); self-esteem of adolescents related to perceived parental nurturance; external punishment; protectiveness and achievement pressure negatively related to self-esteem of adolescents (26-item version) (Halpen et al., 1980)	Factor structure consistent with BPB consistent with BPB longform factors (Siegelman, 1965) and with other measures of children's perceptions of parenting (Gfellner, 1986); factors did not replicate among a sample of adopted/nonadopted children using a 13-item version (Marquis & Detweiler, 1985)

Measure	Type[a]	Test–retest[b]	Internal consistency	Validity	Factor structure / other
Child's Report of Parental Behavior—Revised (1970)	2	Unknown	Unknown	Traditionally reared adolescents report more firm psychological control than less traditional; more psychological control among lower- and middle-class adolescents (Schludermann & Schludermann, 1983)	Factor structures of CRPBI items replicate across samples and cultures (Schludermann, 1971) (192-item version)
Child's Report of Parental Behavior—Revised (1971)	2	1 wk: .50–.96; 5 wk: .77–.93 for factors (4, 5, 6th graders) (Margolies & Weintraub, 1977)	Unknown	High-self-esteem young adolescents report more parental acceptance, less psychological and less firm control than low-self-esteem adolescents (Litovsky & Dusek, 1985)	Revised version yields same factors as the original CRPBI (Margolies & Weintraub, 1977; Burger, 1973)
Inventory of Parent and Peer Attachment	1, 2	3 wk: Peer = .86; Parent = .93 (Armsden, 1986)	Alphas: .72–.91 for Parent and Peer scales (Armsden, 1986)	Securely attached adolescents had higher self-esteem and life satisfaction scores, reported fewer negative life events than insecurely attached; attachment related to various measures of family functioning (Armsden & Greenberg, 1984; Armsden, 1986)	High interscale correlations suggest that scales are interdependent (Armsden & Greenberg, 1984)
Parent Perception Inventory	2	Unknown	Alphas: .78–.88 for 4 subscales (Hazzard & Christensen, 1983)	Children from distressed families rate mothers higher on negative behaviors (Hazzard & Christensen, 1983)	Negative PPI scores positively related to Child Behavior Cklst of Conduct Disorder Scale; PPI unrelated to WRAT and Becker Intellectual Inadequacy Scale (Hazzard, Christensen, & Margolin, 1983)

[a] 1 = clinical; 2 = research; 3 = screening; 4 = educational
[b] Test–retest coefficients are Pearson product moment correlations unless otherwise specified.

from recent revisions of the Parent Attitude Research Instrument (Q4); however, an extreme response set bias continues to plague this measure and would appear to be a function of the absolutist wording of the items (e.g., "A good wife never has to argue with her husband"). All but three measures (Adult–Adolescent Parenting Inventory, Perceptions of Parental Role Scales, Family–Peer Relationship Questionnaire) include reverse-scored items to offset response set bias.

In summary, the adequacy of the physical and administrative features of the parent–child measures is variable. Overall, the clinical measures demonstrate superior evaluations on physical and administrative criteria. Among these measures, however, both the Parenting Stress Index (PSI) and the Adult–Adolescent Parenting Inventory deserve empirical investigation of potential response set bias, and the PSI could benefit from a more representative normative sample. Regarding parent–child measures designed primarily for research, many could be improved with the provision of manuals, more comprehensive descriptive information regarding population samples, and investigation of potential response set problems. In contrast to the other family measurement areas reviewed in this book, the parent–child area is unique in that many measures have foreign-language translations, permitting cross-cultural research.

Comparisons of Reliability and Validity

The psychometric quality of the self-report parent–child measures (Table 8–4) is most clearly differentiated by their overall purpose (i.e., clinical or research use), with clinically oriented measures demonstrating superior reliability and validity.

Reliability

Most of the parent–child measures (18/19) report data on internal consistency. Of these, 12 estimated reliability using coefficient alphas, five used a split-half technique (predominantly KR-20's), and, one measure used an unspecified technique. Half of the measures (10/19) also evidence stability, ranging from 1 day to 3 months. However, the quality of these data was noticeably different for clinical and research measures.

For measures designed for clinical purposes, both internal consistency and stability data were more extensive. Of the six clinically oriented measures, the Child Abuse Potential Inventory and the Parenting Stress Index provided multiple studies on internal consistency across different groups and at total and subscale levels. Total scale coefficients were in the .80's and .90's. Subscale coefficients ranged from the .50's to the .90's, in part because of subscales with small numbers of items. The internal consistency of the six remaining measures (Adult–Adolescent Parenting Attitudes, Child's Attitude toward Mother/Father, Family–Peer Relationship Questionnaire, Inventory of Parent and Peer Attachment) ranged from the .60's to the mid- .90's, again typically with greater consistency for the total scales than for the subscales. Similarly, extensive data are provided on the stability of the CAP and the PSI. Test–retest coefficients (Pearson product moment correlations unless otherwise indicated) ranged from the .50's to the .90's across various subgroups on assessments made over 1-day to 3-month intervals. Of the remaining measures, four report stability information, with coefficients ranging from .39 to the .90's and generally falling in the .80's. Stability data were not provided for the Index of Parental Attitudes or the Child's Attitude toward Mother/Father. These measures are designed to capture change in treatment; therefore, test–retest reliability is considered inappropriate by the author (Hudson, 1982).

Overall, these coefficients are lower than what is recommended by Nunnally (1978) for measures designed for use in classification of individuals. Considerable variation was present, however. The Child Abuse Potential Inventory provided multiple studies of internal consistency and stability data over different groups of individuals and over different time intervals, and these data are adequate for the total scale scores and the subscales with larger sets of items. Adequate total score internal consistency was demonstrated for the Parenting Stress Index, the Index of Parental Attitudes, and the Child's Attitude Toward Mother/Father scales and was at acceptable limits for the subscales of the Perceptions of Parental Role Scales. More variability is present among the subscales of tests. Lower internal consistency and stability coefficients were often found for a particular subscale with a small number of items or for a particular subgroup over a single test–retest interval. Nevertheless, coefficients were not consistently above recommended criteria for classification tests (.90's); the interested user should examine the data for each subscale separately. For research purposes, however, the psychometric quality of the clinically oriented measures' total scale scores and majority of subscales scores is adequate.

Self-report parent–child measures that are designed for research purposes demonstrate weaker internal consistency and stability than the clinical measures. Most of the measures (9/12) report internal consistency data. Of those that do not, one was not designed for use with subscales (Child Rearing Practices Report) and internal consistency data have not been reported for the other two (Cornell Parent Behavior Inventory, Perceived Parenting Questionnaire). Of the nine measures remaining, internal consistency data are reported on four measures using split-half methods, with coefficients ranging from the .30's to the .90's. Only the Maryland Parent Attitude Survey has the requisite number of test items necessary for using the split-half method. The remaining five measures (Parent as a Teacher Inventory, Pleasure-Arousal and Dominance-Inducing Scales of Parental Attitudes, Parental Acceptance–Rejection Questionnaire, Parent Perception Inventory, and Child's Report of Parental Behavior Inventory—both versions) report alpha coefficients ranging from the .60's to the .90's, which is adequate for research purposes.

What is strikingly different from the clinical measures, however, is the lack of data on the stability of the measures. Test–retest data are available only for the Child-Rearing Practices Report, the Parent Attitude Research Instrument, and the Child's Report of Parental Behavior Inventory. These coefficients range from .50's to the .90's over 1-week to 3-month intervals. The dearth of stability data on these measures is a serious limitation. To the extent that these measures assume that parental socialization practices and attitudes determine children's personality and social development, it would seem critical to have evidence that the measure of socialization assessed parents' practices consistently over time. Although it may be argued that parents' practices should be expected to change with shifts in the developmental status of their children (e.g., Roberts et al., 1984), this form of shift covers a much wider age span than expected for traditional assessments of the stability of a test.

In general, the strongest evidence for reliability has come from the parent–child measures designed for clinical purposes and those that have been developed more recently. Research-oriented measures demonstrate acceptable internal consistency, except for measures without subscales (making such data inappropriate). Data on the stability of these measures is insufficient, however, which presents a serious measurement issue for those interested in conducting research on the influence of parental socialization practices and the role of parent–child interaction in children's social and personality development. Finally, the quality of the reliability data for a given measure does not appear to be affected by the respondent (parent or child) or the particular relationship assessed (i.e., the parent, child, or peer forms of the measures).

Validity

All of the parent–child measures provided some form of construct or criterion-related validity (see Table 8–4). The measures are most consistent in providing discriminant forms of criterion validity, and convergent and factorial forms of construct validity are available for some measures.

Five of the eight clinically relevant parent–child assessment measures demonstrate evidence of construct validity. The Child Abuse Potential Inventory, the Parenting Stress Index, and the Index of Parental Attitudes demonstrate theoretically consistent relationships with instruments that assess similar constructs. Factorial validity was demonstrated for the Adult–Adolescent Parenting Inventory. Construct validity data were not found for the Child's Attitude toward Mother/Father scales, the Perceptions of Parental Role Scales, or the Family–Peer Relationship Questionnaire, although Ellison (1985b) reports that such work is in progress for the latter measure. All eight of the clinical parent–child instruments report either discriminant or concurrent forms of criterion-related validity. Although evidence of validity for the clinically relevant parent–child measures is consistent across instruments, the number of studies remains limited. The recent development of some of these measures may be one contributing factor; however, continued validation of instruments appears warranted.

Validity evaluation of research-oriented parent–child measures shows data for 10 of 12 measures on construct validity, either factorial or convergent/divergent forms. The factor structure of the two adaptations of the Child's

Report of Parental Behavior Inventory (Schaefer, 1965) has been replicated over multiple samples and cultural groups (Burger & Armentrout, 1971; Margolies & Weintraub, 1977; Schludermann & Schludermann, 1970). The factor structure of the Cornell Parent Behavior Inventory (Devereux et al., 1969) and a shorter version of it (Perceived Parenting Questionnaire) has also been replicated, providing strong evidence of the construct validity of the original measures. Convergent validity evidence was found for 5 of the 12 research-oriented measures (Parental Acceptance–Rejection Questionnaire, Parent Perception Inventory, Perceived Parenting Questionnaire, Parent as a Teacher Inventory, Cornell Parent Behavior Inventory).

Almost all of the research-oriented parent–child measures provide evidence of criterion-related validity (the Pleasure-Arousal and Dominance-Inducing Scales of Parental Attitudes measure is the exception). The most extensive data are presented for the Child-Rearing Practices Report, the Parental Acceptance–Rejection Questionnaire, the Parent Attitude Research Instrument, and versions of the Child's Report of Parental Behavior Inventory. Criterion validity work is less extensive on the remaining measures.

Overall, the research-oriented measures all provide some evidence of validity, and several provide evidence of both criterion and construct validity. However, the fact that few of these measures provide evidence of measurement stability raises questions about the adequacy of the validity data. Judgments on the validity of several instruments must be viewed with caution, as they are based on a limited number of studies. Furthermore, evidence of reliability and/ or validity is sometimes reported for the original measure, but not for later revisions. It cannot be assumed that data on the original version of a measure support the psychometric quality of the revised forms. In summary, the stronger reliability data demonstrated by the clinically relevant measures provides a foundation for validity studies and is a model for the research-oriented parent–child measures.

DISCUSSION

A number of issues emerged from this review of current parent–child relationship measures: psychometric quality, including construct clarity and validity; comprehensiveness of assessment; theoretical diversity; and attention to developmental stage.

The psychometric quality of the parent–child measures reviewed in this chapter was variable. The clinically relevant measures generally demonstrated more comprehensive reliability and validity data, more adequate normative data, and standardized procedures for scoring and interpretation. Coefficients for reliability were at or somewhat below recommended guidelines for use in classification but were well above those required for research. Although measures designed for research typically provided evidence of internal reliability, evidence of stability was notably lacking. Lack of test–retest data is a serious limitation for measures of constructs that are assumed to be stable over time, such as parental attitudes toward child rearing. Regarding validity, almost all measures provide some evidence of criterion and/or construct-related validity; however, studies are limited in number. The lack of construct validation studies leaves open the question of the correspondence of constructs across measures within the field of parent–child relationship studies. In particular, the degree to which respondents' perceptions correspond with actual measures of behavior (the insider–outsider question) deserves investigation. An additional construct validity concern is the frequent merging of items that reflect both attitudes and behaviors in a single construct. Given the low correspondence between subjective attitudes and behavior found in previous research (e.g., Fishbein, 1967; Olson, 1977), it would appear that this practice would contribute to poor construct validity.

A second issue concerns the comprehensiveness of assessment of the parent–child relationship using these measures. By design, these measures focus on the dyadic relationship between a particular parent and child. A comprehensive assessment of parenting, therefore, might be expected to include the completion of a given measure for all possible parent–child dyadic combinations in a family. Reviews of the socialization literature, however, have found little evidence of assessment across multiple parent–child dyads; researchers appear to assume that parent practices are stable within the family across different children (Maccoby & Martin, 1983). Recent research suggests, however, that parental practices vary according to socialization context (Grusec & Kuczynski, 1980), parental values regarding different child behaviors (Costanzo & Fraenkel, 1986), and the child's own actions or reactions (R. Q. Bell & Chapman, 1986). Furthermore, it may be that combinations of different practices are more effective with particular children than any single style (Trickett & Kuczynski, 1986; Radke-Yarrow, Zahn-Waxler, & Chapman, 1983). Assessment of parent–child relationships can be criticized not only for too narrow a focus (e.g., a single parent–child dyad) but also for failure to focus broadly on the assessment of the context of parenting. Belsky (1984), for example, provides ample evidence of the multiple determinants of parenting, yet few of the measures reviewed measured the extrafamilial relationships of either parents or children.

The evaluation of comprehensiveness is linked with the issue of measurement focus. This review found that when the parent is the respondent, in parent–child measures, the most frequently assessed constructs are child-rearing attitudes regarding control–autonomy and acceptance–rejection. Fewer measures assess parents' reports of their actual behavior, personal characteristics, or relationships with others. The focus of parent measures attests to the importance ascribed to these parent attitudes by socialization researchers, starting over three decades ago. For children and adolescents, the measurement focus is almost exclusively behavioral. Thus, for both types of respondents, few measures explore the experience and expression of affect in the family. This is in direct contrast to measures of whole-family functioning, which derive primarily from the clinical literature. Given the importance of affective exchanges in children's development of moral and prosocial behavior (Eisenberg & Miller, 1987; Miller & Eisenberg, in press), this would appear to be a shortcoming of many existing parent–child relationship measures.

The issue of attitudinal versus behavioral item content evident in the parent–child measures raises another issue—the meanings of current measures of the parent–child relationship and their theoretical premises. The item content of several measures (e.g., Parenting Stress Index, Child Behavior Toward Parent Inventory), as well as the appearance of child-as-respondent measures, acknowledges the emergent theoretical trend in developmental psychology toward viewing the socialization process as bidirectional (e.g., R. Q. Bell & Chapman, 1986) or transactional (e.g., Sameroff, 1987). A limitation of current measures, within either a bidirectional or a transactional framework, is the failure to assess the parent and child(ren) simultaneously on the same set of dimensions—that is, to develop parallel forms of the same test. Thus, it would appear that the theoretically powerful transactional view of socialization processes has not yet been matched in terms of measurement technology.

Finally, despite the embeddedness of measurement of the parent–child relationship in the field of developmental psychology, existing measures are noteworthy for their lack of attention to developmental processes. Parent-as-respondent measures are not, for the most part, designed to assess parenting associated with a particular child developmental stage, despite the fact that parenting behavior and attitudes shift across the developmental cycle (Roberts, et al., 1984). In addition, child-as-respondent measures include no psychometric evaluation of children's cognitive developmental stage as it affects their capacity to respond to test items or their views of parental child-rearing practices. Clearly, more conscientious assessment of the role of developmental processes in existing measures is warranted and should be considered central to the development of future measures.

REFERENCES

Abidin, R. R. (1983). *Parenting Stress Index Manual.* Charlottesville, VA: Pediatric Psychology Press.

Aguilino, W. S. (1986). Children's perceptions of marital interaction. *Child Study Journal, 16,* 159–172.

Alexander, J. F. (1973a). Defensive and supportive communication in family systems. *Journal of Marriage and the Family, 35,* 613–617.

Alexander, J. F. (1973b). Defensive and supportive communication in normal and deviant families. *Journal of Consulting and Clinical Psychology, 40,* 223–231.

Alexander, J. F., Barton, C., Schiavo, R. S., & Parson, B. V. (1976). Behavioral intervention with families of delinquents: Therapist characteristics and outcome. *Journal of Consulting and Clinical Psychology, 44,* 656–664.

Anastasi, A. (1982). *Psychological testing* (rev. ed.). New York: Macmillan.

Armsden, G. G. (1986, March). *Coping strategies and quality of parent and peer attachment in late adolescence.* Paper presented at the First Biennial Meeting of the Society for Research in Adolescence, Madison, WI.

Armsden, G. G., & Greenberg, M. T. (1984). *The Inventory of Parent and Peer Attachment: Individual differences and their relationship to psychological well-being in adolescence.* Unpublished manuscript, Department of Psychology, University of Washington, Seattle.

Ausubel, D. P., Balthazar, E. E., Rosenthal, I., Blackman, L. S., Schpoont, S. H., & Welkowitz, J. (1954). Perceived parent attitudes as determinants of children's ego structures. *Child Development, 25,* 173–183.

Bagarozzi, D. A. (1985). Dimensions of family evaluation. In L. L'Abate (Ed.), *Handbook of family psychology and therapy* (Vol. II). Homewood, IL: Dorsey Press.

Bakeman, R., & Brown, J. V. (1980). Early interactions: Consequences for social and mental development at three years. *Child Development, 51,* 437–447.

Bakeman, R., & Gottman, J. M. (1986). *Observing interaction: An introduction to sequential analysis.* New York: Cambridge University Press.

Baldwin, A. L., Cole, R. E., & Baldwin, C. (1982). Parental pathology, family interaction, and the competence of the child in school. *Monographs of the Society for Research in Child Development, 47*(5).

Bales, R. F. (1951). *Interaction process analysis.* Cambridge: Addison-Wesley.

Barbarin, O. A. (undated). *Measuring basic family processes: Development and use of the FPS.* Manuscript submitted for publication.

Barbarin, O. A., & Gilbert, R. (1979). *Family Process Scales.* Ann Arbor, MI: Family Development Project.

Barbarin, O. A. & Tirado, M. (1985). Enmeshment, family processes, and successful treatment of obesity. *Family Relations, 34,* 115–121.

Barker, R. G. (1969). Wanted: An eco-behavioral science. In E. P. Willems & H. L. Raush (Eds.), *Naturalistic viewpoints in psychological research.* New York: Holt, Rinehart & Winston.

Bavolek, S. J. (1984). *Adult–Adolescent Parenting Inventory.* Eau Claire, WI: Family Development Resources.

Beavers, W. R. (1982). Healthy, midrange, and severely dysfunctional families. In F. Walsh (Ed.), *Normal family processes.* New York: Guilford Press.

Beavers, W. R. (undated). *Beavers-Timberlawn Family Evaluation Scale and Family Style Evaluation Manual.* (Available from the Southwest Family Institute, 12532 Nuestra, Dallas, TX 75230)

Beavers, W. R., Hampson, R. D., & Hulgus, Y. F. (1985). Commentary: The Beavers Systems approach to family assessment. *Family Process, 24,* 398–405.

Beavers, W. R., & Voeller, M. N. (1983). Family models: Comparing and contrasting the Olson Circumplex Model with the Beavers Systems Model. *Family Process, 22,* 85–98.

Becker, W. C., & Krug, R. S. (1965). The Parent Attitude Research Instrument: A research review. *Child Development, 36,* 329–365.

Bell, D. C., & Bell, L. G. (1982, April). *Power and support processes in dual-career marriages.* Paper presented at the meeting of the Texas Council on Family Relations, San Antonio.

Bell, D. C., & Bell, L. G. (1983). Parental validation and support in the development of adolescent daughters. In H. D. Grotevant & C. R. Cooper (Eds.), *Adolescent development in the family; New directions for child development.* San Francisco: Jossey-Bass.

Bell, D. C., Bell, L. G., & Cornwell, C. (1982). *Interaction Process Coding Scheme.* Houston, TX: University of Clear Lake City.

Bell, L. G., Cornwell, C. S., & Bell, D. C. (1985). *Peer relationships of adolescent daughters as a reflection of family relationship patterns: A family systems approach.* Manuscript submitted for publication.

Bell, L. G., Ericksen, L., Cornwell, C., & Bell, D. C. (1984, June). *Experienced closeness and distance among family members.* Paper presented at the meeting of the American Family Therapy Association, New York.

Bell, R. Q., & Chapman, M. (1986). Child effects in studies using experimental or brief longitudinal approaches to socialization. *Developmental Psychology, 22,* 595–603.

Belsky, J. (1984). The determinants of parenting: A process model. *Child Development, 55,* 83–96.

Benjamin, L. S. (1987). *Use of Structural Analysis of Social Behavior (SASB) for operational definition and measurement of some dynamic concepts.* Manuscript submitted for publication.

Benjamin, L. S. (1984). Principles of prediction using Structural Analysis of Social Behavior. In R. A. Zucker, J. Aaronoff, & A. J. Rabin (Eds.), *Personality and the prediction of behavior.* New York: Academic Press.

Benjamin, L. S., Giat, L., & Estroff, S. E. (1981). *Manual for coding social interactions in terms of Structural Analysis of Social Behavior (SASB).* Unpublished manuscript, University of Wisconsin.

Berkowitz, M. W., & Gibbs, J. C. (1979). *A preliminary manual for coding transactive features of dyadic discussion.* Unpublished manuscript, Marquette University.

Block, J., Block, J. H., & Gjerde, P. F. (in press). Parental functioning and the home environment in families of divorce: Prospective and concurrent analyses. *Journal of the American Academy of Child Psychiatry.*

Block, J. H. (1965). *The Child-Rearing Practices Report (CRPR): A set of Q items for the description of parental socialization attitudes and values.* Unpublished manuscript, University of California, Berkeley, Institute of Human Development.

Block, J. H., Block, J., & Morrison, A. (1981). Parental agreement–disagreement on childrearing orientations and gender-related personality correlates in children. *Child Development, 52,* 965–974.

Block, J. H., & Gjerde, P. F. (1986). Distinguishing between antisocial behavior and undercontrol. In D. Olweus, J. Block, & M. Radke-Yarrow (Eds.), *Development of antisocial and prosocial behavior: Research theories and issues* (pp. 177–206). New York: Academic Press.

Bloom, B. L. (1985). A factor analysis of self-report measures of family functioning. *Family Process, 24,* 225–239.

Bowen, M. (1966). The use of family theory in clinical practice. *Comprehensive Psychiatry, 7,* 345–374.

Bowen, M. (1976). Family therapy and family group therapy. In D. H. L. Olson (Ed.), *Treating relationships.* Lake Mills, IA: Graphic.

Bowen, M. (1978). *Family therapy in clinical practice.* New York: Aronson.

Bowlby, J. (1969). *Attachment: Vol. I. Attachment and loss.* New York: Basic Books.

Boyce, W. T., Jensen, E. W., James, S. A., & Peacock, J. L. (1983). The Family Routines Inventory: Theoretical origins. *Social Science and Medicine, 17,* 193–200.

Bray, J. H., & Harvey, D. M. (undated). *A measure of family and peer relationships for college students.* Unpublished manuscript.

Bray, J. H., Harvey, D. M., & Williamson, D. S. (undated). *Intergenerational family relationships: An evaluation of theory and measurement.* Unpublished manuscript.

Broderick, C. B. (1971). Beyond the five conceptual frameworks: A decade of development in family theory. *Journal of Marriage and the Family, 33,* 139–159.

Brown, L. H., & Kidwell, J. S. (1982). Methodology in family studies: The other side of caring. In L. H. Brown & J. S. Kidwell (Eds.), Methodology: The other side of caring [Special issue]. *Journal of Marriage and the Family, 44,* (4), 833–839.

Burger, G. K., & Armentrout, J. A. (1971). A factor analysis of fifth and sixth graders' reports of parental child-rearing behavior. *Developmental Psychology, 4,* 483.

Burger, G. K., Armentrout, J. A., & Rapfogel, R. (1973). Estimating factor scores for children's reports of parental child rearing behaviors. *Journal of Genetic Psychology, 123,* 107–113.

Burger, G. K., Lamp, R. E., & Rogers, D. (1975). Developmental trends in child rearing behavior. *Developmental Psychology, 11*(3), 391.

Buriel, R. The relation of Anglo- and Mexican-American children's locus of control beliefs to parents' and teachers' socialization practices. *Child Development, 52,* 104–113.

Burns, R. C., & Kaufman, S. H. (1970). *Kinetic family drawings (K-F-D): An introduction to understanding children through kinetic drawing.* New York: Brunner/Mazel.

Burr, W. R., Hill, R., Nye, F. I., & Reiss, I. L. (Eds.). (1979). *Contemporary theories about the family* (Vols. 1 & 2). New York: Free Press.

Burr, W. R. & Leigh, G. K. (1983). Famology: A new discipline. *Journal of Marriage and the Family, 45,* 467–480.

Cairns, R. B. (Ed.). (1979). *The analysis of social interactions: Methods, issues and illustrations.* Hillsdale, NJ: Lawrence Erlbaum.

Cairns, R. B., & Green, J. A. (1979). Appendix A: How to assess personality and social patterns. In R. B. Cairns (Ed.), *The analysis of social interactions: Methods, issues, and illustrations* (pp. 209–255). Hillsdale, NJ: Erlbaum.

Carlson, C. I. (1987). Family assessment and intervention in the school setting. In T. R. Kratochwill (Ed.), *Advances in school psychology* (Vol. VI). New York: Erlbaum.

Carlson, C. I. & Grotevant, H. D. (1987a). A comparative review of family rating scales: Guidelines for clinicians and researchers. *Journal of Family Psychology, 1* (1), 23–47.

Carlson, C. I. & Grotevant, H. D. (1987b). Rejoinder: The challenges of reconciling family theory with method. *Journal of Family Psychology, 1* (1), 62–65.

Carter, E. A., & McGoldrick, M. (Eds.). (1980). *The family life-cycle: A framework for family therapy.* New York: Gardner Press.

Coleman, J. C. (1974). *Relationships in adolescence.* London: Routledge & Kegan Paul.

Condon, S. L., Cooper, C. R., & Grotevant, H. D. (1984). Manual for the analysis of family discourse. *Psychological Documents, 14,* 8. (M No. 2616)

Cone, J. D. (1982). Validity of direct observation assessment procedures. In D. P. Hartmann (Ed.), *Using observers to study behavior: New directions for methodology of social and behavioral science.* San Francisco: Jossey-Bass.

Constantine, L. L. (1978). Family sculpture and relationship mapping techniques. *Journal of Marriage and Family Counseling, 4,* 13–23.

Cooper, C. R., & Grotevant, H. D. (1987). Gender issues in the interface of family experience and adolescents' friendship and dating identity. *Journal of Youth and Adolescence, 16,* 247–264.

Cooper, C. R., Grotevant, H. D., & Ayers-Lopez, S. (1987). *Links between patterns of negotiation in adolescents' family and peer interaction.* Manuscript submitted for publication.

Cooper, C. R., Grotevant, H. D., & Condon, S. L. (1982). Methodological challenges of selectivity in family interaction: Assessing temporal patterns of individuation. *Journal of Marriage and the Family, 44,* 749–754.

Cooper, C. R., Grotevant, H. D., & Condon, S. L. (1983). Individuality and connectedness in the family as a context for adolescent identity formation and role taking skill. In H. D. Grotevant & C. R. Cooper (Eds.), *Adolescent development in the family: New directions for child development.* San Francisco: Jossey-Bass.

Costanzo, P. R., & Fraenkel, P. (1987). Social influence, socialization, and the development of social cognition: The heart of the matter. In N. Eisenberg (Ed.), *Developmental psychology* (pp. 273–291). New York: Wiley.

Coulthard, M. (1977). *An introduction to discourse analysis.* Essex, England: Longman House.

Cousins, P. C., & Power, T. G. (1986). Quantifying family process: Issues in the analysis of interaction sequences. *Family Process, 25*(1), 89–105.

Cowan, P. A. (1987). The need for theoretical and methodological integrations in family research. *Journal of Family Psychology, 1*(1), 48–50.

Coyne, J. C. (1987). Some issues in the assessment of family patterns. *Journal of Family Psychology, 1*(1), 51–57.

Cromwell, R. E., Olson, D. H., & Fournier, D. G. (1976). Diagnosis and evaluation in marital and family counseling. In D. H. Olson (Ed.), *Treating relationships.* Lake Mills, IA: Graphic.

Cromwell, R. E., & Peterson, G. W. (1983). Multisystem-multimethod family assessment in clinical contexts. *Family Process, 22,* 147–164.

Cronbach, L. S., Gleser, G. C., Nanda, H., & Rajaratnam, J. (1972). *The dependability of behavioral measures.* New York: Wiley.

Devereux, E. C., Bronfenbrenner, W., & Rodgers, R. R. (1969). Child-rearing in England and the United States: A cross-cultural comparison. *Journal of Marriage and the Family, 31,* 257–270.

Devereux, E. C., Bronfenbrenner, U., & Suci, G. (1962). Patterns of parent behavior in the United States and the Federal Republic of Germany: A cross-national comparison. *International Social Science Journal, 14,* 488–506.

Doane, J. A., Falloon, I. R. H., Goldstein, M. J., & Mintz, J. (1985). Parental affective style and the treatment of schizophrenia: Predicting course of illness and social functioning. *Archives of General Psychiatry, 42,* 34–42.

Doane, J. A., Goldstein, M. J., & Rodnick, E. H. (1981). Parental patterns of affective style and the development of schizophrenia spectrum disorders. *Family Process, 20,* 337–349.

Doane, J. A., West, K. L., Goldstein, M. J., Rodnick, E. H., & Jones, J. E. (1981). Parental communication deviance and affective style: Predictors of subsequent schizophrenic spectrum disorders in vulnerable adolescents. *Archives of General Psychiatry, 38,* 679–685.

Dore, J. (1979). Conversational acts and the acquisition of language. In E. Ochs & B. B. Schieffelin (Eds.), *Developmental pragmatics.* New York: Academic Press.

Eisenberg, N., & Miller, P. A. (1987). The relation of empathy to prosocial behavior. *Psychological Bulletin, 100,* 89–113.

Ellison, E. S. (1983). Parental support and school-aged children. *Western Journal of Nursing Research, 5*(2), 145–153.

Ellison, E. S. (1985a). A multidimensional, dual-perspective index of parental support. *Western Journal of Nursing Research, 7*(4). 401–424.

Ellison, E. S. (1985b). *Nursing research emphasis grant final report.* University of Washington, School of Nursing.

Ellison, E. S. (undated). *Family Peer Relationship Questionnaire: Scoring procedure and components.* Unpublished manuscript, University of Washington, School of Nursing.

Ellison, E. S., Kieckhefer, G., Houck, G., & Wallace, K. (undated). *Child's perception of mother's illness.* Unpublished manuscript, University of Washington, School of Nursing.

Emery, R. E., Weintraub, S., & Neale, J. M. (1980 August). *The Family Evaluation Form: Construction and normative data.* Paper presented at the annual meeting of the American Psychological Association, Montreal.

Epstein, N. B., Baldwin, L. M., & Bishop, D. S. (1982). *McMaster Clinical Rating Scale.* Unpublished manuscript, Brown/Butler Family Research Program, Providence, RI.

Epstein, N. B., Baldwin, L. M., & Bishop, D. (1983). The McMaster Family Assessment Device. *Journal of Marital and Family Therapy, 9* (2), 171–180.

Epstein, N. B., & Bishop, D. S. (1981). Problem-centered systems therapy of the family. In A. Gurman & D. Kniskern (Eds.), *Handbook of family therapy* (pp. 444–482). New York: Brunner-Mazel.

Epstein, N. B., Bishop, D. S., & Levin, S. (1978). The McMaster Model of Family Functioning. *Journal of Marital and Family Counseling, 4,* 19–31.

Falender, C. A., & Mehrabian, A. (1980). The emotional climate for children as inferred from parental attitudes: A preliminary validation of three scales. *Educational and Psychological Measurement, 40,* 1033–1042.

Farina, A., & Dunham, R. M. (1963). Measurement in family relationships and their effects. *Archives of General Psychiatry, 9,* 64–73.

Faunce, E. E., & Riskin, J. (1970). Family interaction scales: II. Data analysis and findings. *Archives of General Psychiatry, 22,* 513–526.

Filsinger, E. E. (1983a). Choices among marital observation coding systems. *Family Process, 22,* 317–335.

Filsinger, E. E. (Ed.)(1983b). *Marriage and family assessment.* Beverly Hills, CA: Sage.

Filsinger, E. E., & Lewis, R. A. (1981). *Asessing marriage: New behavioral approaches.* Beverly Hills CA: Sage.

Fineberg, B. L., & Lowman, J. (1975). Affect and status dimensions of marital adjustment. *Journal of Marriage and the Family, 37,* 155–160.

Fishbein, M. (1967). Attitude and the prediction of behavior. In M. Fishbein (Ed.), *Readings in attitude theory and measurement.* New York: Wiley.

Fishbein, M., & Ajzen, I. (1974). Attitudes toward objects as predictors of single and multiple behavior criteria. *Psychological Review, 81,* 59–74.

Fisher, L. (1976). Dimensions of family assessment: A critical review. *Journal of Marriage and Family Counseling, 2,* 367–382.

Fisher, L. (1982). Transactional theories but individual assessment: A frequent discrepancy in family research. *Family Process, 21,* 313–320.

Forman, B. D., & Hagan, B. J. (1983). A comparative review of total family functioning measures. *American Journal of Family Therapy, 11,* 25–40.

Fowler, P. C. (1981). Maximum likelihood factor structure of the Family Environment Scale. *Journal of Clinical Psychology, 37*(1), 160–164.

Fowler, P. C. (1982). Factor structure of the Family Environment Scale: Effects of social desirability. *Journal of Clinical Psychology, 38*(2), 285–292.

Galligan, R. J. (1982). Innovative techniques: Siren or rose. *Journal of Marriage and the Family, 44*(4), 875–888.

Garfinkel, P. E., Garner, D. M., Rose, J., Darby, P. L., Brandes, J. S., O'Hanlon, J., & Walsh, N. (1983). A comparison of characteristics in the families of patients with anorexia nervosa and normal controls. *Psychological Medicine, 13,* 821–828.

Gfellner, B. M. (1986). Changes in ego and moral development in adolescents: A longitudinal study. *Journal of Adolescence, 9,* 281–302.

Gibb, J. R. (1961). Defensive communications. *Journal of Communications, 3,* 141–148.

Gilbert, L. A., & Hanson, G. R. (1982). *Manual for Perceptions of Parental Role Scales.* Columbus, OH: Marathon Consulting and Press.

Gilbert, R., & Christensen, A. (1985). Observational assessment of marital and family interaction: Methodological considerations. In L. L'Abate (Ed.), *Handbook of family psychology and therapy* (Vol. II). Homewood, IL: Dorsey Press.

Gjerde, P. F. (1983, August). *Parent–adolescent interaction in family context: Importance of second-order effects.* Paper presented at the meeting of the American Psychological Association, Anaheim, CA.

Gjerde, P. F. (1985, April). *Adolescent depression and parental socialization patterns: A prospective study.* Paper presented at the meeting of the Society for Research in Child Development, Toronto.

Gjerde, P. F. (1986). *A family systems perspective on parent–adolescent interaction: Second-order effects and sex differences in family interaction.* Unpublished manuscript.

Gjerde, P. F., Block, J., & Block, J. H. (1983). *Parental interactive patterns in dyads and triads: Prospective relationships in adolescent personality characteristics.* Unpublished manuscript.

Good, M. D., Smilkstein, G., Good, B. J., Shaffer, T., & Arona, T. (1979). The Family APGAR INDEX: A study of construct validity. *Journal of Family Practice, 8,* 577–582.

Gordon, R. H., & Gordon, P. E. (undated). *The Adult–Adolescent Parenting Inventory and the MMPI "AT RISK" Scale: A clinical validity study.* Unpublished manuscript (Available from Applied Mental Health Consultants, 1341 N. Wright Road, Janesville, WI 53545)

Gottman, J. M. (1979). *Marital interaction: Experimental investigations.* New York: Academic Press.

Green, R. G., Kolevzon, M. S., & Vosler, N. R. (1985). The Beavers-Timberlawn Model of Family Competence and the Circumplex Model of Family Adaptability and Cohesion: Separate but equal? *Family Process, 24,* 385–398.

Grotevant, H. D. & Carlson C. I. (1987). Family interaction coding systems: A descriptive review. *Family Process, 26*(1), 49–74.

Grotevant, H. D., & Cooper, C. R. (1985). Patterns of interaction in family relationships and the development of identity exploration. *Child Development, 56,* 415–428.

Grotevant, H. D., & Cooper, C. R. (1986). Individuation in family relationships: A perspective on individual differences in the development of identity and role taking skill in adolescence. *Human Development, 29,* 82–100.

Grusec, J., & Kuczynski, L. (1980). Direction of effect in socialization: A comparison of the parent vs. child's behavior as determinants of disciplinary techniques. *Developmental Psychology, 16,* 1–9.

Gurman, A. S., & Kniskern, D. P. (1981a). Family therapy outcome research:

Knowns and unknowns. In A. S. Gurman & D. P. Kniskern (Eds.), *Handbook of family therapy* (pp. 742–775). New York: Brunner/Mazel.

Gurman, A. S., & Kriskern, D. P. (Eds.). (1981b). *Handbook of family therapy.* New York: Brunner/Mazel.

Haley, J. (Ed.). (1971). *Changing families: A family therapy reader.* New York: Grune & Stratton.

Halpin, G., Halpin G., & Whiddon, T. (1980). The relationship of perceived parental behaviors to locus of control and self-esteem among American Indian and white children. *Journal of Social Psychology, 11,* 189–195.

Hartmann, D. P. (Ed.). (1982a). *Using observers to study behavior: New directions for methodology of social and behavior science.* San Francisco: Jossey-Bass.

Hartmann, D. P. (1982b). Validity of direct observation assessment procedures. In D. P. Hartmann (Ed.), *Using observers to study behavior: New directions for methodology of social and behavior science.* San Francisco: Jossey-Bass.

Hartup, W. W. (1978). Perspectives on child and family interaction: Past, present, and future. In R. M. Lerner & G. B. Spanier (Eds.), *Child influences on marital and family interaction: A life-span perspective* (pp. 23–46). New York: Academic Press.

Hartup, W. W. (1986). On relationships and development. In W. W. Hartup & Z. Rubin (Eds.), *Relationships and development* (pp. 1–26). Hillsdale, NJ: Erlbaum.

Harvey, D. M., & Bray, J. H. (1986). *Evaluation of an intergenerational theory of personal development: Family process determinants of psychological health and distress.* Unpublished manuscript.

Harvey, D. M., Curry, C. J., & Bray J. H. (1986, August). *Individuation/intimacy in intergenerational relationships and health: Patterns across two generations.* Paper presented at the annual convention of the American Psychological Association, Washington, DC.

Hauser, S. T., Book, B. K., Houlihan, J., Powers, S., Weiss-Perry, B., Follansbee, D., Jacobson, A. M., & Noam, G. G. (1987). Sex differences within the family: Studies of adolescent and parent family interactions. *Journal of Youth and Adolescence, 16,* 199–219.

Hauser, S. T., Houlihan, J., Powers, S., Jacobson, A. M., Noam, G., Weiss-Perry, B., & Follansbee, D. (in press). Interaction sequences in families of psychiatrically hospitalized and non-patient adolescents. *Psychiatry.*

Hauser, S. T., Powers, S. I., Jacobson, A. M., Schwartz J., & Noam, G. (1982). Family interactions and ego development in diabetic adolescents. *Pediatric and Adolescent Endocrinology, 10,* 69–76.

Hauser, S. T., Powers, S. I., Noam, G. G., Jacobson, A. M., Weiss, B., & Follansbee, D. J. (1984). Familial contexts of adolescent ago development. *Child Development, 55,* 195–213.

Hauser, S. T., Powers, S. I., Schwartz, J., Jacobson, A. M., & Noam, G. G. (1980, October). *Familial contexts of adolescent development.* Paper presented at the Theory Construction and Methodology Workshop of the meeting of the National Council on Family Relations, Portland, OR.

Hauser, S. T., Powers, S. I., Weiss-Perry, B., Follansbee, D., Rajapark, D. C., & Greene, W. M. (1987). *Family constraining and enabling coding system (CECS) manual.* Unpublished manuscript, Harvard Medical School, Adolescent and Family Development Project.

Hazzard, A., Christensen, A., & Margolin, G. (1983). Children's perceptions of parental behavior. *Journal of Abnormal Child Psychology, 2*(1), 49–60.

Heller, A., Rafman, S., Zvagulis, I., & Pless, I. B. (1985). Birth defects and psychosocial adjustment. *American Journal of Diseases in Children, 139,* 257–263.

Henggeler, S. W., Borduin, C. M., & Mann, B. J. (1987). Intrafamily agreement: Association with clinical status, social desirability, and observational ratings. *Journal of Applied Developmental Psychology, 8,* 97–111.

Henggeler, S. W., Borduin, C. M., Rodnick, J. D., & Tavormina, J. B. (1979). Importance of task content for family interaction research. *Developmental Psychology, 15,* 660–661.

Henggeler, S. W., & Tavormina, J. B. (1980). Social class and race differences in family interaction: Pathological, normative, or confounding methodological factors? *Journal of Genetic Psychology, 137,* 211–222.

Hetherington, E. M., Stouwie, R. J., & Ridberg, E. H. (1971). Patterns of family interaction and child-rearing attitudes related to three dimensions of juvenile delinquency. *Journal of Abnormal Psychology, 78,* 160–176.

Hill, R. (1949). *Families under stress.* New York: Harper & Row.

Hill, R. (1958). Generic features of families under stress. *Social Casework, 39,* 139–150.

Hill, R., & Hansen, D. A. (1960). The identification of conceptual frameworks utilized in family study. *Marriage and Family Living, 22,* 299–311.

Holahan, C. J., & Moos, R. H. (1981). Social support and psychological distress: A longitudinal analysis. *Journal of Abnormal Psychology, 90,* 365–370.

Holahan, C. J., & Moos, R. H. (1982). Social support and adjustment: Predictive benefits of social climate indices. *American Journal of Community Psychology, 10,* 403–415.

Holahan, C. J., & Moos, R. H. (1986). Personality, coping, and family resources in stress resistance: A longitudinal analysis. *Journal of Personality and Social Psychology, 51,* 389–395.

Holman, A. M. (1983). *Family assessment: Tools for understanding and intervention.* Beverly Hills, CA: Sage.

Holman, T. B., & Burr, W. R. (1980). Beyond the beyond: The growth of family theories in the 1970's. *Journal of Marriage and the Family, 42,* 729–742.

Hudson, W. W. (1982). *The Clinical Measurement Package*. Homewood, IL: Dorsey Press.

Hudson, W. W., Acklin, J. D., & Bartosh, J. C. (1980). Assessing discord in family relationships. *Social Work Research and Abstracts,* 16(3), 21–29.

Hulgus, Y. F. (1985). *Scoring guide for the Beavers-Timberlawn Family Evaluation Scale and the Centripetal/Centrifugal Family Style Scale.* (Available from Southwest Family Institute, 12532 Nuestra, Dallas, TX 75230)

Hulgus, Y. (1986). *Results of the psychometric evaluation of the SFI.* Unpublished manuscript. (Available from Southwest Family Institute, 12532 Nuestra, Dallas, TX 75230)

Huston, T., & Robins, E. (1982). Conceptual and methodological issues in studying close relationships. In L. H. Brown & J. S. Kidwell (Eds.), Methodology: The other side of caring [Special issue]. *Journal of Marriage and the Family,* 44(4), 901–925.

Huston, T. L., Robins, E., Atkinson, J., & McHale, S. M. (1987). Surveying the landscape of marital behavior: A behavioral self-report approach to studying marriage. In S. Oskamp (Ed.), *Family processes and problems: Social psychological aspects* (Vol. 7). Beverly Hills, CA: Sage.

Jackson, D. D., Riskin, J., & Satir, V. (1961). A method of analysis of a family interview. *Archives of General Psychiatry, 5,* 29–45.

Jacob, T. (1974). Patterns of family conflict and dominance as a function of child age and social class. *Developmental Psychology, 10,* 1–12.

Jacob, T. (1975). Family interaction in disturbed and normal families: A methodological and substantive review. *Psychological Bulletin, 82,* 33–65.

Jacob, T. (Ed.). (1987). *Family interaction and psychopathology.* New York: Plenum.

Jacob, T., & Davis, J. (1973). Family interaction as a function of experimental task. *Family Process, 12,* 415–427.

Jay, S., & Farran, D. C. (1981). The relative efficacy of predicting IQ from mother–child interactions using ratings versus behavioral count measures. *Journal of Applied Developmental Psychology, 2,* 165–177.

Jensen, E. W., James, S. A., Boyce, W. T., & Hartnett, S. A. (1983). The Family Routines Inventory: Development and validation. *Social Science and Medicine, 17,* 201–211.

Johnson, A. (1975). *An assessment of Mexican-American parent child-rearing feelings and behaviors.* Unpublished doctoral dissertation, Arizona State University.

Johnson, O. G. (1976). *Tests and measurements in child development.* San Francisco: Jossey-Bass.

Kelsey-Smith, M., & Beavers, W. R. (1981). Family assessment: Centripetal and centrifugal family systems. *American Journal of Family Therapy, 9,* 3–12.

Kerlinger, F. N. (1973). *Foundations of behavior research* (2nd ed.). New York: Holt, Rinehart & Winston.

L'Abate, L. (1983). *Family psychology: Theory, therapy, and training.* Washington, DC: University Press of America.

L'Abate, L. (1985). Preface. In L. L'Abate (Ed.), *Handbook of family psychology and therapy* (Vols. I & II). Homewood, IL: Dorsey Press.

Lafferty, W., Cote, J., Chafe, P., Kellar, L., & Robertson, H. (1980). *The use of the Parenting Stress Index (PSI) for the evaluation of a systematic training for effective parenting (STEP) programme.* Unpublished manuscript, Beachgrove Regional Children's Center, Toronto.

Larzelere, R. E., & Klein, D. M. (1986). Methodology. In M. B. Sussman & S. K. Steinmatz (Eds.), *Handbook of marriage and family* (pp. 125–155). New York: Plenum.

Lazarus, R. (1966). *Psychological stress and the coping process.* New York: McGraw-Hill.

Leary, T. (1957). *Interpersonal diagnosis of personality: A functional theory and methodology for personality evaluation.* New York: Ronald Press.

Lee, C. (1988). Theories of family adaptability: Toward a synthesis of Olson's circumplex and the Beavers Systems models. *Family Process, 27,* 73–84.

Levy, J., & Epstein, N. B. (1964). An application of the Rorschach test in family investigation. *Family Process, 3,* 344–376.

Lewis, J. M., Beavers, W. R., Gossett, J. T., & Phillips, V. A. (1976). *No single thread: Psychological health in family systems.* New York: Brunner/Mazel.

Litovsky, V. G., & Dusek, J. B. (1985). Perceptions of child rearing and self-concept development during the early adolescent years. *Journal of Youth and Adolescence, 14,* 373–387.

Loevinger, J. (1976). *Ego development: Conceptions and theories.* San Francisco: Jossey-Bass.

Lowman, J. (1980). Measurement of family affective structure. *Journal of Personality Assessment, 44* (2), 130–141.

Lowman, J. (1981). Love, hate, and the family: Measures of emotion. In E. E. Filsinger & R. A. Lewis (Eds.), *Assessing marriage: New behavioral approaches* (pp. 55–73). Beverly Hills, CA: Sage.

Maccoby, E. E., & Martin, J. A. (1983). Socialization in the context of the family: Parent–child interaction. In F. M. Hetherington (Ed.), *Handbook of child psychology: Vol. 4. Socialization, personality, and social development* (pp. 1–102). New York: Wiley.

MacDonald, A. P., Jr. (1971). Internal–external locus of control: Parental antecedents. *Journal of Consulting and Clinical Psychology, 37,* 141–147.

Margolies, P. J., & Weintraub, S. (1977). The revised 56-item CRBPI as a research instrument: Reliability and factor structure. *Journal of Clinical Psychology, 33,* 472–476.

Margolin, G., & Fernandez, V. (1983). Other marriage and family questionnaires. In F. F. Filsinger (Ed.), *Marriage and family assessment: A sourcebook for family therapy* (pp. 317–338). Newbury Park, CA: Sage.

Markman, H. J., & Notarius, C. I. (1987). Coding marital and family interaction: Current status. In T. J. Jacob (Ed.), *Family interaction and psychopathology*. New York: Plenum.

Mash, E. J., & Johnston, C. (1983). The prediction of mothers' behavior with their hyperactive children during play and task situations. *Child and Family Behavior Therapy, 5*, 1–14.

McCubbin, H. I., & Boss, P. G. (Eds.). (1980). Family stress, coping, and adaptation [Special issue]. *Family Relations, 29*(4).

McCubbin, H. I., & Figley, C. R. (1983). *Stress and the family* (Vols. I & II). New York: Brunner/Mazel.

McCubbin, H. I., & Patterson, J. M. (1983). Family transitions: Adaptation to stress. In H. I. McCubbin & C. R. Figley (Eds.), *Stress and the family: Vol. I: Coping with normative transitions* (pp. 5–25). New York: Brunner/Mazel.

McGoldrick, M., & Gerson, R. (1986). *Genograms in family assessment*. New York: Guilford Press.

Merton, R. K. (1945). Sociological theory. *American Journal of Sociology, 50*, 462–473.

Mikhail, A. (1981). Stress: A psychophysiological conception. *Journal of Human Stress, 7*, 9–15.

Milkowitz, D. J., Goldstein, M. J., Neuchterlein, K. H., Snyder, K. S., & Doane, J. A. (1986). Expressed emotion, affective style, lithium compliance, and relapse in recent onset mania. *Psychopharmacology Bulletin, 22*, 628–632.

Miller, B. C., Rollins, B. C., & Thomas, D. L. (1982). On methods of studying marriages and families. In L. H. Brown & J. S. Kidwell (Eds.), Methodology: The other side of caring [Special issue]. *Journal of Marriage and the Family, 44*(4), 851–873.

Miller, I. V., Epstein, N. B., Bishop, D. S., & Keitner, G. I. (1985). The McMaster Family Assessment Device: Reliability and validity. *Journal of Marital and Family Therapy, 11*(4), 345–356.

Miller, P. A., & Eisenberg, N. (in press). The relation of empathy to aggressive and externalizing/antisocial behavior. *Psychological Bulletin*.

Milner, J. S. (1986). *The Child Abuse Potential Inventory manual* (2nd ed.) Webster, NC: Psytech.

Minuchin, S. (1974). *Families and family therapy*. Cambridge: Harvard University Press.

Minuchin, S., Rosman, B. L., & Baker, L. (1978). *Psychosomatic families: Anorexia nervosa in context*. Cambridge: Harvard University Press.

Mischel, W. (1968). *Personality and assessment*. New York: Wiley.

Mishler, E. G., & Waxler, N. E. (1968). *Interaction in families: An experimental study of family processes and schizophrenia*. New York: Wiley.

Montemayor, R. (1982). The relationship between parent–adolescent conflict and the amount of time adolescents spend alone with parents and peers. *Child Development, 53*, 1512–1519.

Moos, R. H. (1974). *Combined preliminary manual for the Family, Work, and*

Group Environment Scales. Palo Alto, CA: Consulting Psychologists Press.

Moos, R. H., Clayton, J., & Max, W. (1979). *The Social Climate Scales: An annotated bibliography.* Palo Alto, CA: Consulting Psychologists Press.

Moos, R. H., & Moos, B. S. (1984). *Family Environment Scale manual* (rev. ed.). Palo Alto, CA: Consulting Psychologists Press.

Moos, R. H., & Spinrad, S. (1984). *The Social Climate Scales: An annotated bibliography.* Palo Alto, CA: Consulting Psychologists Press.

Morrison, A. L., Gjerde, P. F., & Block, J. H. (1983a, April). *A prospective study of divorce and its relationship to family functioning.* Paper presented at the meeting of the Society for Research in Child Development, Detroit.

Morrison, A. L., Gjerde, P. F., & Block, J. H. (1983b, August). *Interaction in families characterized by parental disagreement: Mother–father differences.* Paper presented at the meeting of the American Psychological Association, Anaheim, CA.

Murray, H. A. (1938). *Explorations in personality.* New York: Oxford University Press.

Nelson, G. (1984). The relationship between dimensions of classroom and family environments and the self-concept, satisfaction, and achievement of grade 7 and 8 students. *Journal of Community Psychology, 12,* 276–287.

Newcomb, T. (1931). An experiment designed to test the validity of a rating technique. *Journal of Educational Psychology, 22,* 279–288.

Nunnally, J. C. (1978). *Psychometric theory* (2nd ed.). New York: McGraw-Hill.

Oliveri, M. E., & Reiss, D. (1982). Family styles of construing the social environment: A perspective on variation among nonclinical families. In F. Walsh (Ed.), *Normal family processes* (pp. 94–114). New York: Guilford Press.

Olson, D. H. (1977). Insiders' and outsiders' views of relationships: Research studies. In G. Levinger & H. Rausch (Eds.), *Close relations.* Amherst: University of Massachusetts Press.

Olson, D. H. (1986). Circumplex Model VII: Validation studies and FACES III. *Family Process, 25,* 337–351.

Olson, D. H., & Killorin, E. (1985). *Clinical Rating Scale for the Circumplex Model of Marital and Family Systems.* St. Paul: University of Minnesota, Department of Family Social Science.

Olson, D. H., McCubbin, H. I., Barnes, H., Larsen, A., Muxen, M., & Wilson, M. (1982). *Family inventories: Inventories used in a national survey of families across the family life cycle.* (Available from Family Social Science, 290 McNeal Hall, University of Minnesota, St. Paul, MN 55108)

Olson, D. H., Portner, J., & Lavee, Y. (1985). *FACES III manual.* Unpublished manual. (Available from D. H. Olson, Family Social Science, 290 McNeal Hall, University of Minnesota, St. Paul, MN 55108).

Olson, D. H., Russell, G. S., & Sprenkle, D. H. (1983). Circumplex Model VI: Theoretical update, *Family Process, 22,* 69–83.

Olson, D. H., Sprenkle, D. H., & Russell, C. S. (1979). Circumplex Model of Marital and Family Systems I: Cohesion and adaptability dimensions, family types, and clinical applications. *Family Process, 18,* 3–28.

O'Rourke, J. F. (1963). Field and laboratory: The decision-making behavior of family and group in two experimental conditions. *Sociometry, 26,* 422–435.

Panetta, S. J. (1980). *An exploration and analysis of parental behaviors which may be related to a child's problem-solving abilities.* Unpublished doctoral dissertation, University of Northern California.

Patterson, G. R. (1976). The aggressive child: Victim and architect of a coercive system. In L. A. Hamerlynck, L. C. Handy, & E. J. Mash (Eds.), *Behavior modification and families: Theory and research* (Vol. 1). New York: Brunner/Mazel.

Patterson, G. R. (1982). *A social learning approach to family intervention: Vol. 3. Coercive family process.* Eugene, OR: Castalia.

Patterson, G. R. (1984). Microsocial process: A view from the boundary. In J. C. Masters & K. Yarkin-Levin (Eds.), *Boundary areas in social and developmental psychology.* New York: Academic Press.

Patterson, G. R., & Fleischman, M. J. (1979). Maintenance of treatment effects: Some considerations concerning family systems and follow-up data. *Behavior Therapy, 10,* 168–185.

Patterson, G. R., Ray, R. S., Shaw, D. A., & Cobb, J. A. (1969). *Manual for coding family interactions.* New York: Microfiche.

Patterson, G. R., & Reid, J. B. (1984). Social interaction processes within the family: The study of the moment-by-moment family transactions in which human social development is imbedded. *Journal of Applied Developmental Psychology, 5,* 237–262.

Perosa, L. M. (1986). *The revision of the Structural Family Interaction Scale.* Unpublished manuscript.

Perosa, L. M., Hansen, J., & Perosa, S. (1981). Development of the Structural Family Interaction Scale. *Family Therapy, 8(2),* 77–90.

Perosa, L. M., & Perosa, S. L. (1982). Structural interaction patterns in families with a learning disabled child. *Family Therapy, 9(2),* 175–187.

Peterson, G. W., & Cromwell, R. E. (1983). A clarification of multisystem-multimethod assessment: Reductionism versus wholism. *Family Process, 22,* 173–178.

Pino, C. J., Simons, N., & Slawinowski, M. J. (1984). The Children's Family Environment Scale. *Family Therapy, 9(1),* 85–86.

Pinsoff, W. M. (1981). Family therapy process research. In A. S. Gurman & D. P. Kniskern (Eds.), *Handbook of family therapy.* New York: Brunner/Mazel.

Pless, I. B., & Satterwhite, B. B. (1973). A measure of family functioning and its application. *Social Science and Medicine, 7,* 613–621.

Pless, I. B., & Satterwhite, B. B. (1975). Family functioning and family problems. In R. J. Haggerty, K. J. Roghmenn, & I. B. Pless (Eds.), *Child
health and the community* (pp. 41–54). New York: Wiley.

Powers, S. I. (1982). *Family interaction and parental moral development as a
context for adolescent moral development.* Unpublished doctoral dissertation, Harvard University.

Powers, S. I., Beardslee, W., Jacobson, A. M., Hauser, S. T., Noam, G. G.,
Hopfenbeck, J., & Macias, E. (1986, December). *Family influences on
the development of adolescent coping processes.* Paper presented at the
Family Systems and Life-span Development Conference, Max Planck
Institute for Human Development and Education, Berlin.

Powers, S. I., Hauser, S. T., Schwartz, J. M., Noam, G. G., & Jacobson,
A. M. (1983). Adolescent ego development and family interaction: A
structural-developmental perspective. In H. D. Grotevant & C. R. Cooper
(Eds.), *Adolescent development in the family: New directions for child
development.* San Francisco: Jossey-Bass.

Powers, S. I., Jacobson, A. M., & Noam, G. G. (1987, April). Parental influences on the development of adolescent coping processes. In W. A.
Collins (Chair), *Parental factors in family relations in adolescence.*
Symposium presented at the biennial meeting of the Society for Research in Child Development, Baltimore.

Price, J. (1985, August). *Aspects of the family and children's television viewing content preferences.* Paper presented at the annual meeting of the
American Psychological Foundation, Toronto.

Procidano, M. E., & Heller, K. (1983). Measures of perceived social support
from friends and family: Three validation studies. *American Journal of
Community Psychology, 11*(3), 1–24.

Pumroy, D. K. (1966). Maryland Parent Attitude Survey: A research instrument with social desirability controlled. *Journal of Psychology, 64,* 73–
78.

Radke-Yarrow, M., Zahn-Waxler, C., & Chapman, M. (1983). Children's prosocial dispositions and behavior. In P. H. Mussen (Ed.), *Handbook of
child psychology: Vol IV. Socialization, personality, and social development* (pp. 469–545). New York: Wiley.

Reid, J. B. (Ed.). (1978). *A social learning approach to family intervention:
Vol. 2. Observation in home settings.* Eugene, OR: Castalia.

Reid, J. B., Taplin, P. S., & Lober R. (1981). A social-interactional approach
to the treatment of abusive families. In R. Stuart (Ed.), *Violent behavior: Social learning approaches to prediction, management, and treatment.* New York: Brunner/Mazel.

Reiss, D. (1980). Pathways to assessing the family: Some choice points and a
sample routine. In C. K. Hofling & J. M. Lewis (Eds.), *The family:
Evaluation and treatment* (pp. 86–121). New York: Brunner/Mazel.

Reiss, D. (1981). *The family's construction of reality.* Cambridge: Harvard
University Press.

Reiss, D. (1983). Sensory extenders versus meters and predictors: Clarifying strategies for the use of objective tests in family therapy. *Family Process, 22*, 165–172.

Reiss, D., & Oliveri, M. E. (1980). Family paradigm and family coping: A proposal for linking the family's intrinsic adaptive capacities to its responses to stress. *Family Relations, 29*, 431–444.

Riskin, J. (1982). Research on "nonlabeled" families: A longitudinal study. In F. Walsh (Ed.), *Normal family processes*. New York: Guilford Press.

Riskin, J., & Faunce, E. E. (1969). *Family Interaction Scales scoring manual*. Palo Alto, CA: Mental Research Institute.

Riskin, J., & Faunce, E. E. (1972). An evaluative review of family interaction research. *Family Process, 11*, 365–456.

Roberts, C. S., & Feetham, S. L. (1982). Assessing family functioning across three areas of relationships. *Nursing Research, 31*, 231–235.

Roberts, G. C., Block, J. H., & Block, J. (1984). Continuity and change in parents' child-rearing practices. *Child Development, 55*, 586–597.

Robin, A. (1981). A controlled evaluation of problem-solving communication training with parent–adolescent conflict. *Behavior Therapy, 12*, 593–609.

Robin, A., & Canter, W. (1984). A comparison of the Marital Interaction Coding System and community ratings for assessing mother–adolescent problem-solving. *Behavioral Assessment, 6*, 303–313.

Robin, A., & Fox, M. (1979). *Parent–Adolescent Interaction Coding System: Training and reference manual for coders*. Unpublished manual. (Available from Dr. Arthur Robin, Dept. of Psychology, Children's Hospital of Michigan, Detroit Medical Center, 3901 Beaubien Blvd, Detroit, MI 48201.)

Robin, A., & Weiss, J. G. (1980). Criterion-related validity of behavioral and self-report measures of problem-solving communication skills in distressed and non-distressed parent–adolescent dyads. *Behavioral Assessment, 2*, 339–352.

Roelofse, R., & Middleton, M. R. (1985). The Family Functioning in Adolescence Questionnaire: A measure of psychosocial family health during adolescence. *Journal of Adolescence, 8*, 33–45.

Rogers, L. E., Millar, F. E., & Bavelas, J. M. (1985). Methods for analyzing marital conflict discourse. *Family Process, 24*(2), 175–187.

Rohner, R. P. (1980). Worldwide tests of parental acceptance–rejection theory. *Behavior Science Research, 15*, 1–21.

Rohner, R. P. (1984). *Handbook for the study of parental acceptance and rejection* (rev. ed.). Storrs: University of Connecticut, Center for the Study of Parental Acceptance and Rejection.

Rohner, R. P., & Pettengill, S. M. (1985). Perceived parental acceptance–rejection and parental control among Korean adolescents. *Child Development, 56*, 524–528.

Rosman, B. L. (1978). *Philadelphia Child Guidance Clinic Family Task and scoring*. (Available from Bernice L. Rosman, PhD, Director of Research & Evaluation, Two Children's Center, 34th St. & Civic Blvd., Philadelphia, PA 19104)

Rutter, M. (1983). Stress, coping, and development: Some issues and some questions. In N. Garmezy and M. Rutter (Eds.), *Stress, coping, and development in children* (pp. 1–42). New York: McGraw-Hill.

Saal, F. E., Downey, R. G., & Lahey, M. A. (1980). Rating the ratings: Assessing the psychometric quality of rating data. *Psychological Bulletin, 88*, 413–428.

Sameroff, A. (1987). The social context of development. In N. Eisenberg (Ed.), *Contemporary topics in developmental psychology* (pp. 90–215). New York: Wiley.

Satterwhite, B. B., Zweig, S. R., Iker, H. P., & Pless, B. (1976). The Family Functioning Index: Five-year test–retest reliability and implications for use. *Journal of Comparative Family Studies, 7*, 111–116.

Saunders, B. E., & Schuchts, R. A. (1987). Assessing parent–child relationships: A report of normative scores and revalidation of two clinical scales. *Family Process, 26*, 373–381.

Sawa, R. J., Falk, W. A., & Pablo, R. Y. (1986a). *Assessing the family in primary care*. Unpublished manuscript.

Sawa, R. J., Falk, W. A., & Pablo, R. Y. (1986b). *Family function questionnaire*. Unpublished manuscript.

Schaefer, E. S. (1964). *Child's Report of Parent Behavior Inventory*. Washington, DC: National Institutes of Health.

Schaefer, E. S. (1965). Children's reports of parental behavior: An inventory. *Child Development, 36*, 413–424.

Schaefer, E. S., & Bell, R. Q. (1958). Development of a parental attitude research instrument. *Child Development, 29*, 339–361.

Schaefer, E. S., & Edgerton, M. (1977). *Parent Report of Child Behavior to the Parent: Short form*. (Available from Department of Maternal and Child Health, School of Public Health, University of North Carolina, Chapel Hill, NC 27514).

Schaefer, E. S., & Finkelstein, N. W. (1975, August). *Child Behavior Toward Parent: An inventory and factor analysis*. Paper presented at the annual meeting of the American Psychological Association, Chicago.

Schludermann, S., & Schludermann, E. (1970). Replicability of factors in Children's Report of Parent Behavior (CRBPI). *Journal of Psychology, 39*, 39–52.

Schludermann, S., & Schludermann, E. (1971). Response set analysis of a Parental Attitude Research Instrument (PARI). *Journal of Psychology, 86*, 327–334.

Schludermann, S., & Schludermann, E. (1977). A methodological study of a revised maternal attitude research instrument: PARI Q4. *Journal of Psychology, 95*, 77–86.

Schludermann, S., & Schludermann, E. (1983). Sociocultural change and adolescents' perceptions of parent behavior. *Developmental Psychology, 19*, 674–685.

Schumm, W. R. (1982). Integrating theory, measurement and data analysis in family studies survey research. *Journal of Marriage and the Family, 44*, 983–998.

Schumm, W. R., Martin, M. J., Bollman, S. R., & Jurich, A. P. (1982). Classifying family violence, whither the woozle? *Journal of Family Issues, 3*, 319–341.

Sears, R. R. (1975). Your ancients revisited: A history of child development. In E. Mavis Hetherington (Ed.), *Child development and research* (Vol. V, pp. 1–74). Chicago: University of Chicago Press.

Seeman, L., Tittler, B. I., & Friedman, S. (1985). Early interactional change and its relationship to family therapy outcome. *Family Process, 24*, 59–68.

Selye, H. (1974). *Stress without distress*. Philadelphia: Lippincott & Corwell.

Siegelman, M. (1965). Evaluation of Bronfenbrenner's questionnaire for children concerning parental behavior. *Child Development, 36*, 163–174.

Simon, R. M. (1972). Sculpting the family. *Family Process, 11*, 49–57.

Sines, J. O. (1983). *Home Environment Questionnaire: Manual for administration and scoring*. (Available from Psychological Assessment and Services, P. O. Box 1031, Iowa City, IA 52244)

Sines, J. O. (1987). Influence of the home and family environment on childhood dysfunction. In B. B. Lahey & A. E. Kazdin (Eds.), *Advances in clinical child psychology* (Vol. 10). New York: Plenum.

Sines, J. O., Clarke, W. M., & Lauer, R. M. (1984). Home Environment Questionnaire. *Journal of Abnormal Child Psychology, 23*, 521–529.

Skinner, H. A. (1987). Self-report instruments for family assessment. In T. Jacob (Ed.), *Family Interaction and psychopathology* (pp. 427–452). New York: Plenum.

Skinner, H., & Steinhauer, P. D. (1986). *Family Assessment Measure Clinical Rating Scale*. Toronto: Addiction Research Foundation.

Skinner, H. A., Steinhauer, P. D., & Santa-Barbara, J. (1983). The Family Assessment Measure. *Canadian Journal of Community Mental Health, 2*(2), 91–103.

Skinner H. A., Steinhauer, P. D., & Santa-Barbara, J. (1984). *The Family Assessment Measure: Administration and interpretation guide*. Toronto: Addiction Research Foundation.

Smilkstein, G. (1978). The Family APGAR: A proposal for a family function test and its use by physicians. *Journal of Family Practice, 6*, 1231–1239.

Smilkstein, G., Ashworth, C., & Montano, D. (1982). Validity and reliability of the Family APGAR as a test of family function. *Journal of Family Practice, 15*, 303–311.

Smilkstein, G., Helsper-Lucas, A., Ashworth, C., Montano, D., & Pagel, M. (1984). Prediction of pregnancy complications: An application of the biopsychosocial model. *Social Science and Medicine, 18*, 315–321.

Snyder, J. J. (1977). A reinforcement analysis of interaction in problem and nonproblem families. *Journal of Abnormal Psychology, 86*(5), 528–535.

Speer, J. J., & Sachs, B. (1985). Selecting the appropriate family assessment tool. *Pediatric Nursing, 11,* 349–355.

Sprenkle, D. H., & Olson, D. H. (1978). Circumplex Model of Martial Systems IV: An empirical study of clinic and non-clinic couples. *Journal of Marriage and Family Counseling, 4,* 59–74.

Sprunger, L. W., Boyce, W. T., & Gaines, J. A. (1985). Family–infant congruence: Routines and rhythmicity in family adaptations to a young infant. *Child Development, 56,* 564–572.

Sroufe, L. A., & Fleeson, J. (1986). Attachment and the construction of relationships. In W. W. Hartup & Z. Rubin (Eds.), *Relationships and development* (pp. 51–72). Hillsdale, NJ: Erlbaum.

Sroufe, L. A., & Rutter, M. (1984). The domain of developmental psychopathology. *Child Development, 55*(1), 17–29.

Standards for educational and psychological testing. (1985). Washington, DC: American Psychological Association.

Steinberg, L. D. (1981). Transformations in family relations at puberty. *Developmental Psychology, 17,* 833–840.

Steinglass, P. (1987). A systems view of family interaction and psychopathology. In T. Jacob (Ed.), *Family interaction and psychopathology* (pp. 25–65). New York: Plenum.

Steinhauer, P. D., Santa-Barbara, J., & Skinner, H. (1984). The Process Model of Family Functioning. *Canadian Journal of Psychiatry, 29,* 77–88.

Stiles, W. B. (1980). Comparison of dimensions derived from rating versus coding of dialogue. *Journal of Personality and Social Psychology, 38,* 359–428.

Stockford, L., & Bissell, H. W. (1949). Factors involved in establishing a merit-rating scale. *Personnel, 26,* 94–116.

Straus, M. A. (1979). Measuring intrafamily conflict and violence: The Conflict Tactics (CT) Scales. *Journal of Marriage and the Family, 41,* 75–88.

Straus, M. A., & Brown, B. W. (1978). *Family measurement techniques: Abstracts of published instruments, 1935–1974* (rev. ed.). Minneapolis: University of Minnesota Press.

Straus, M. A., Gelles, R. J., & Steinmetz, S. K. (1980). *Behind closed doors: Violence in the American family.* New York: Anchor Press.

Straus, M. A., & Tallman, I. (1971). SIMFAM: A technique for observational measurement and experimental study of families. In J. Aldous et al. (Eds.), *Family problem solving.* Hinsdale, IL: Dryden Press.

Strom, R. D. (1984). *Parent as a Teacher Inventory manual.* Bensenville, IL: Scholastic Testing Service.

Sullivan, H. S. (1953). *The interpersonal theory of psychiatry.* New York: Norton.

Thorndike, R. L., & Hagen, E. P. (1977). *Measurement and evaluation in psychology and education* (4th ed.). New York: Wiley.

Tolor, A. (1967). An evaluation of the Maryland Parent Attitude Survey. *Journal of Psychology, 67,* 69–74.

Trickett, P. K., & Kuczynski, L. (1986). Children's misbehaviors and parental discipline strategies in abusive and nonabusive families. *Developmental Psychology, 22,* 115–123.

Walters, L. H. (1982). Are families different from other groups? In L. H. Brown & J. H. Kidwell (Eds.), Methodology: The other side of caring [Special issue]. *Journal of Marriage and the Family, 44*(4), 841–850.

Waters, E., & Deane, K. E. (1985). Defining and assessing individual differences in attachment relationships: Q-methodology and the organization of behavior in infancy and early childhood. In I. Bretherton & E. Waters (Eds.), Growing points in attachment theory and research. *Monographs of the Society for Research in Child Development, 50*(1–2, Serial No. 209).

Wedemeyer, N. V., & Grotevant, H. D. (1982). Mapping the family system: A technique for teaching family systems theory concepts. *Family Relations, 31,* 185–193.

Weinrott, M. R., Jones, R. R., & Boler, G. R. (1981). Convergent and discriminant validity of five classroom observation systems: A secondary analysis. *Journal of Educational Psychology, 73,* 671–680.

Weiss, R. L., Hops, H., & Patterson, G. R. (1973). A framework for conceptualizing marital conflict: A technology for altering it, some data for evaluating it. In F. W. Clark & L. A. Hammerlynck (Eds.), *Critical issues in research and practice: Proceedings of the Fourth Banff Conference on Behavior Modification.* Champaign, IL: Research Press.

Weiss, R. L., & Summers, K. J. (1983). Marital Interaction Coding System: III. In E. E. Filsinger (Ed.), *Marriage and family assessment.* Beverly Hills, CA: Sage.

White, K. M., Speisman, J. C., & Costos, D. (1983). Young adults and their parents: Individuation to mutuality. In H. D. Grotevant & C. R. Cooper (Eds.), *Adolescent development in the family: New Directions for child development.* San Francisco: Jossey-Bass.

White, K. M., Speisman, J. C., & Costos, D. (1984). *Family Relationships scoring manual.* Unpublished manuscript, Boston University.

Williamson, D. S. (1981). Personal authority via termination of the intergenerational hierarchical boundary: A "new" stage in the family life cycle. *Journal of Marital and Family Therapy, 7,* 441–452.

Williamson, D. S. (1982a). Personal authority via termination of the intergenerational hierarchical boundary: Part II. The consultation process and the therapeutic method. *Journal of Marital and Family Therapy, 8,* 23–37.

Williamson, D. S. (1982b). Personal authority in family experience via termination of the intergenerational hierarchical boundary: Part III. Personal authority defined, and the power of play in the change process. *Journal of Marital and Family Therapy, 8,* 309–323.

Williamson, D. S. & Bray, J. H. (in press). Family development and change across the generations: An intergenerational perspective. In C. J. Falicov (Ed.), *Family transitions: Continuity and change over the life cycle.* New York: Guilford Press.

Wynne, L. C., Ryckoff, I. M., Day, J., & Hirsch, S. I. (1958). Pseudomutuality in the family relations of schizophrenics. *Psychiatry, 21,* 205–220.

Zuckerman, E., & Jacob, T. (1979). Task effects in family interaction. *Family Process, 18,* 47–53.

Zuckerman, M. (1958). Reversed scales to control acquiescence response set in the Parental Attitude Research Instrument. *Child Development, 30,* 523–532.

PART TWO

ABSTRACTS OF FAMILY ASSESSMENT MEASURES

Section IV
Abstracts of Interaction
Coding Schemes

I-1
Affective Style Measure

GENERAL INFORMATION

Date of publication: 1981.

Author: J. A. Doane.

Source/publisher: UCLA Family Project; published in *Family Process, 20* (1981), 337–349.

Brief description: This coding system is used for calculating the frequency and quality of verbal statements indicative of support, criticism, guilt induction, and intrusiveness. By building on the frequencies of these events for particular mothers and fathers, classifications of parents as individuals and as dyads and can be made as "benign," "mixed," or "negative." These categories were successfully used to predict young adult psychiatric status. A raw sum of all of the negative codes can also be used as a measure of change.

Purpose: The purpose of this system is to specify behaviors in family interaction that are useful for predicting adolescent psychiatric status upon follow-up in a high-risk sample. It has also been used as a measure of change in a treatment study of families of adult schizophrenics at risk for relapse and as a predictor of relapse in bipolar manics.

Theoretical base: Family systems theory.

PHYSICAL DESCRIPTION OF CODE

Task and setting used to elicit behavior: Families are observed in direct interaction situations where the participants are asked to discuss a problem that has been previously determined as a problem for that specific family. This is done in order to obtain affectively charged interaction. Participants are told to discuss the topic, express their respective feelings and ideas, and make some attempt to resolve the issue. They are left alone to interact for 10 minutes.

Unit of study: Mother–child, father–child, or triad.

Unit of coding/analysis: "A unit of analysis was defined as up to six consecutive lines of uninterrupted speech by a single speaker. The unit was ended when a second speaker either significantly interrupted the first or began a distinct reply" (p. 340). For each parental speech unit, only one code from each major category could be assigned, with the code with the greatest impact taking precedence. Each unit, therefore, could receive from 0 to 3 codes (i.e., the coding system was neither mutually exclusive nor exhaustive). Adolescent behavior was not coded.

Organization of negative codes:

    I. Criticism
        A. Personal Criticism
        B. Benign Criticism
   II. Guilt Induction
  III. Intrusiveness
        A. Critical Intrusiveness
        B. Neutral Intrusiveness

Manual: Manual written for use only in conjunction with supervised training; contact the author (see "Author's Response").

Standardization and norms: None presented.

Evaluation of physical description of code: *Strengths:* Code categories are carefully designed to capture critical incidents that are hypothesized on theoretical grounds to be predictive of schizophrenia spectrum disorders in adolescents. *Weaknesses:* Code categories are neither mutually exclusive nor exhaustive. Adolescent's behavior is not coded; however, codes could be used to code child's speech as well as parental speech. Despite a family systems orientation, this coding strategy implies a unidirectional parent-to-child model of the etiology of psychopathology.

ADMINISTRATIVE PROCEDURES

Description of equipment needed and observation system: Interaction sessions were audiotaped at the clinic.

Data transcription and reduction: Verbatim transcripts of each interaction were made from audiotape. Typed transcripts (without the tapes) were coded by two raters blind to the initial status of the family and the outcome status of the adolescent. No information given on coder training, qualifications, or monitoring.

Scoring procedures, including calculation of summary scores: Each parent was classified as either "Benign" or "Negative," based on the use of the negative codes (Benign = no use of Personal Criticism, Guilt Induction, Critical Intrusiveness, or Excessive Neutral Intrusiveness; Negative = at least one use of one of the above codes). In addition, each parent was classified as Consistently Benign (Benign in both dyadic and triadic situation), Consistently Negative (negative in both situations), or Inconsistent (Benign in one situation and Negative in the other). Finally, families were classified as Bilateral Benign (both parents consistently Benign), Unilateral Benign (one parent consistently Benign and the other not); Bilateral Inconsistent (both parents Benign in one setting and Negative in the other); Unilateral Negative (one parent consistently Negative and the other inconsistent); or Bilateral Negative (both parents consistently Negative).

Evaluation of administrative procedures: *Strengths:* Verbatim transcripts enhance accuracy of coding; scoring system for critical events seems simple enough to be useful yet still theoretically meaningful. *Weaknesses:* Coders apparently work from transcripts alone, whereas using tapes as well might help clarify the affective connotation of certain utterances. Little information is available on coder training, qualifications, monitoring, and so forth.

EVALUATION OF CODE

Reliability: Because all codes occurred with low frequency, agreements on nonoccurrence were not included in calculating reliability. Cohen's kappa was applied to those instances in which one or both raters believed one of the codes to be applicable (kappa = .78, $p < .001$).

Validity: Predictive validity was established with a sample of families who came to the UCLA clinic for help with an adolescent. Coded family interaction at the time of initial assessment was used to predict diagnoses of the adolescents 5 years later. When an individual parent's classification in only one assessment situation was used, many errors in prediction occurred. However, when cross-situational classifications were used for each parent and the marital classifications described above were used, predictions of the severity of the young adult's problems were quite accurate. Concurrent validity studies using measures of expressed emotion have provided evidence for the validity of the codes.

Clinical utility: This code could be very useful to clinicians because it points to the salience of certain "critical events" in family interaction. The importance of cross-situational stability demonstrated in this study is an important lesson for both clinicians and researchers.

Research utility: The utility of this code in predicting severity of psychopathology in young adults was clearly demonstrated in this study. The usefulness of this code for studying normal families remains to be established. It has also been found useful in predicting relapse in adult schizophrenics and bipolar manics and as a measure of change in a family versus individual therapy treatment study.

SUMMARY EVALUATION

This code appears to be very useful for the purpose of predicting the course of psychiatric disturbance in adolescents and young adults. The demonstration of the usefulness of looking across situations and of computing higher-order scores is very important. The system could be made more consistent with its theoretical orientation by including the adolescent's contribution to family interaction. In addition, tapes as well as transcripts should be used in coding in order to make judgments about the affective connotation of critical events.

REFERENCES

Asarnow, J., Lewis, J. M., Doane, J. A., Goldstein, M. J., & Rodnick, E. H. (1982). Family interaction and the course of adolescent psychopathology: An analysis of adolescent and parent effects. *Journal of Abnormal Child Psychology, 10,* 427–442.

Doane, J. A., Goldstein, M. J., Falloon, I. R. H., & Mintz, J. (1985). Parental affective style and the treatment of schizophrenia: Predicting course of illness and social functioning. *Archives of General Psychiatry, 42,* 34–42.

Doane, J. A., Goldstein, M. J., Miklowitz, D., & Falloon, I. R. H. (1986). The impact of individual and family treatment on the affective climate of families of schizophrenics. *British Journal of Psychiatry, 148,* 279–287.

Doane, J. A., Goldstein, M. J., & Rodnick, E. H. (1981). Parental patterns of affective style and the development of schizophrenia spectrum disorders. *Family Process, 20,* 337–349.

Doane, J.A., West, K., Goldstein, M., Rodnick, E., & Jones, J. E. (1981). Parental communication deviance and affective style: Predictors of subsequent schizophrenia spectrum disorders in vulnerable adolescents. *Archives of General Psychiatry, 38,* 679–685.

Miklowitz, D. J., Goldstein, M. J., Falloon, I. R. H., & Doane, J. A. (1984). Interactional correlates of expressed emotion in the families of schizophrenics. *British Journal of Psychiatry, 144,* 482–487.

Miklowitz, D. J., Goldstein, M. J., Neuchterlein, K. H., Snyder, K. S., & Doane, J. A. (1986). Expressed emotion, affective style, lithium compliance, and relapse in recent onset mania. *Psychopharmacology Bulletin, 22,* 628–632.

Strachan, A. M., Leff, J. P., Goldstein, M. J., Doane, J. A., & Burtt, C. (1986). Emotional attitudes and direct communication in the families of schizophrenics: A cross-national replication. *British Journal of Psychiatry, 149,* 279–287.

Valone, K., Goldstein, M. J., Norton, J., & Doane, J. A. (1983). Parental expressed emotion and affective style in an adolescent sample at risk for schizophrenia-spectrum disorders. *Journal of Abnormal Psychology, 92,* 399–407.

AUTHOR'S RESPONSE

A detailed coding manual has been prepared, but it is used in conjunction with extensive training in coding of affective style. Since a high degree of inference is involved in making coding decisions, the manual is not available without additional training. Inquiries regarding training may be directed to Jeri A. Doane, PhD, Yale Psychiatric Institute, P.O. Box 12-A, Yale Station, New Haven, CT 06520. It should be noted that the use of tapes makes coding more difficult. Reliability was poor when two channels of input (audio and visual-verbal) were used.

I-2
Defensive and Supportive
Communication Interaction System

GENERAL INFORMATION

Date of publication: Unpublished manual not dated.

Author: James F. Alexander.

Additional contributors: Cole Barton, Holly Waldron, Charles W. Turner, Janet R. Warburton.

Source/publisher: James F. Alexander, PhD, Dept. of Psychology, SBS 502, University of Utah, Salt Lake City, UT 84112.

Availability: Available from author without cost.

Brief description: This is a coding system for scoring defensive and supportive communication in family interaction, family therapy, and marriage therapy.

Purpose: To compare frequencies and reciprocity of defensive and supportive communication or latencies between such communications within interactions as an indicator of adaptive process, relationship quality, and intervention efficacy.

Theoretical base: (1) Small-group research (Gibb, 1961); (2) systems theory (Haley, 1971).

PHYSICAL DESCRIPTION OF CODE

Task and setting used to elicit behavior: *For family interaction:* An experimental room with family members seated (father, adolescent, mother) at a long table facing a video camera 8 feet in front of them. Family members complete a family opinion questionnaire and then perform a 10-minute discussion task from a list of potential questions (e.g., "What are good parents?") and a 15-minute resolution of differences task based on revealed differences obtained from the questionnaire (Alexander, 1973a). *Also for family interaction:* A structured task, such as playing a modified game of Scrabble (Barton, Alexander, Waldron, Warburton & Turner, 1983), in an experimental context similar to the above. *For marriage and family therapy:* Naturally occurring family and marriage therapy sessions, which are recorded on video- and/or audiotapes using inconspicuous equipment in corners of the room.

Unit of study: *For family interaction:* Mother, father, and adolescent children. *For family and marriage therapy:* The family unit or marital dyad in addition to the therapist.

Unit of coding/analysis: *Time-sample approach:* A behavior is coded every 12 seconds for each family member, with 6 seconds devoted to observing and 6 seconds to recording. *For naturally occurring speech units:* Entire speeches (verbalizations of one participant bounded by verbalizations of other participants) are examined from transcripts for the occurrence of at least one defensive statement. If defensiveness is not present, the speech is examined for supportiveness and so rated if present. *For "meaning units":* Thought units (Gottman, 1979) are unitized and then coded for the occurrence of defensiveness or supportiveness.

Organization of code: Code is divided into two categories: Defensive and Supportive. Within each category are four behavior types. Behaviors within the categories are not mutually exclusive or exhaustive. Directions are not provided in the manual for scoring overlapping or multiple responses, since subcategories are generally used only as examplars for the purpose of training coders. The behaviors coded within each category follow:

Defensive: Judgmental-Dogmatism; Control & Strategy; Indifference; Superiority.

Supportive: Genuine Information Seeking/Giving; Spontaneous Problem Solving; Emphatic Understanding; Equality.

Manual: A coding manual has been compiled by the author that describes the code and the rationale and provides scoring guidelines and examples. Information on scoring, sample protocols, decisions for overlapping categories are not provided in manual. Some of this information is available in published articles.

Standardization and norms: None indicated.

Evaluation of physical description of code: Strengths: (1) Code is simple and appears to be easily mastered. (2) Clear definitions and examples of codes are provided in manual. *Limitations:* (1) Manual acknowledges that overlapping coding is possible but provides no remedy for this problem, which can be a problem when subcategories are conceptualized as independent phenomena. (2)

Manual would benefit from inclusion of decision rules, scoring procedures, and additional research on psychometric properties.

ADMINISTRATIVE PROCEDURES

Description of equipment needed and observation system: *For family interaction:* Experimental room equipped for video and audiotaping, chairs and a table for family members. *For marriage and family therapy:* Therapy rooms with appropriate furnishings and high-quality audiotape and/or videotape systems.

Data transcription and reduction: Little information is provided. Coders are reportedly trained to a criterion of 90% effective percentage agreement on subcategories (Waldron, Turner, Barton, Alexander, & Szykula, 1984) or only on the two major categories (Alexander, Barton, Schiavo, & Parsons, 1976; Barton et al., 1983). One rater is assigned to score each family member (and the therapist in the case of therapy studies). Coding can be performed directly from audio- and videotapes rather than from typed transcripts. When transcripts are used, the unit of analysis can be the speech, the thought unit, or a time interval superimposed on the transcript (Barton et al., 1983). The coding system can also be used by independent judges to assign summary scores for 5-minute intervals of interaction based on a 5-point Likert scale (Alexander et al., 1976).

Scoring procedures: In general, summary scores of the frequency of defensive and supportive behaviors summed across subcategories (when subcategories are coded) and summed across units to derive a defensive score and a supportive score are calculated for each participant. When videotapes are used, the source and object of a behavior can also be coded (Warburton, Alexander, & Barton, 1980). For sequential analyses (with temporally defined units as well as thought units and speeches) data are evaluated for frequencies, latencies (lags), and conditional probabilities across units (Barton et al., 1983).

Evaluation of administrative procedures: *Strengths:* (1) Coding system and procedures appear to be highly feasible. (2) The system has been successfully applied to a number of interaction contexts. *Limitations:* (1) Data collection procedure may be sufficiently intrusive to threaten ecological validity. This would seem to be more problematic in the family interaction studies, since many therapies generally include tape recording as a matter of course. (2) Information on data transcription, data reduction, training of coders is not provided in detail in the manual, though such descriptions are available in several of the cited research articles.

EVALUATION OF CODE

Reliability: Reliability has been assessed, with effective percentage agreements (Alexander, 1973a, 1973b) derived by dividing the number of scoring units of agreement between raters on the presence of each scoring category by the number of items on which either one of the two raters recorded the presence of that content. Forty-seven reliability checks were made, with effective percentage agreement averaging .94 for Supportiveness, .85 for Defensiveness, and .81 for Object of Communication. Later replications evaluated reliability with Cohen's kappa and produced indices of agreement ranging from .72 to 1.00, with a mean of .85 (Warburton et al., 1980), .76 to .92 (Barton et al., 1983).

Validity: An assessment of the convergent and discriminant validity of the coding scheme is currently in progress, with preliminary findings indicating, as expected, intercorrelations among the subcategories and negative correlations between the two categories. A discriminant function analysis revealed that all subcategories, except Equality, significantly differentiated adaptive and delinquent families (Waldron, Turner, Alexander, & Barton, in progress). The molar categories of Defensiveness and Supportiveness have been previously found to discriminate delinquent from nondelinquent adolescent families (Alexander, 1973a, 1973b; Barton et al., 1983). For both delinquent and nondelinquent families, they have also been found to discriminate between experimentally induced conditions of conflict and cooperation (Barton et al., 1983) as well as between more and less successful therapeutic interventions (Alexander et al., 1976; Barton et al., 1983; Waldron et al., 1984).

Clinical utility: The coding scheme does appear to have clinical utility both as a diagnostic tool and as a guide to intervention strategies with families.

Research utility: The coding scheme appears to be a useful and feasible research tool in a variety of contexts when the questions of interest center on the role of defensive and supportive communication. The procedures used to code and analyze defensive and supportive communications can be modified (e.g., coding latencies vs. frequencies) to target specific theoretical questions. The publication of a more thorough manual as well as recent assessments of the coding scheme's psychometric properties will be helpful.

SUMMARY EVALUATION

The Defensive and Supportive Communication Interaction System can be used as a time-sampling or content-unitized procedure for assessing these two communication styles within family and family–therapist systems. Strengths of the system include its feasibility, evidence of its discriminative validity, its clinical utility, and its versatility. Limitations include significant omissions in the manual and code organizational problems. Reported findings on the psychometric properties of the system appear promising, but specific data are not reported, making conclusions tenuous at this time.

REFERENCES

Alexander, James F. (with contributions by Cole Barton, Holly Waldron, Charles Turner, and Janet Warburton). *Defensive and Supportive Communication Interaction manual.* Unpublished research coding manual, University of Utah.

Alexander, J. F. (1973a). Defensive and supportive communication in normal and deviant families. *Journal of Consulting and Clinical Psychology, 40,* 223–231.

Alexander, J. F. (1973b). Defensive and supportive communications in family systems. *Journal of Marriage and the Family, 35,* 613–617.

Alexander, J. F., Barton, C., Schiavo, R. S., & Parsons, B. Y. (1976). Behavioral intervention with families of delinquents: Therapist characteristics and outcome. *Journal of Consulting and Clinical Psychology, 44*(4), 656–664.

Barton, C., Alexander, J. F., Waldron, H., Warburton, J., & Turner, C. W. (1983, December). *Family intervention, alternatives, and seriously delinquent youth: A program evaluation study.* Poster session presented at the World Congress on Behavior Therapy/Association for the Advancement of Behavior Therapy, Washington, DC.

Gibb, J. R. (1961). Defensive communications. *Journal of Communication, 3,* 141–148.

Gottman, J. M. (1979). *Marital interaction: Experimental investigations.* New York: Academic Press.

Haley, J. (Ed.). (1971). *Changing families: A family therapy reader.* New York: Grune & Stratton.

Waldron, H., Turner, C. W., Alexander, J. F., & Barton, C. (in progress). *Subcategories of supportive and defensive communications: Interdependence and discriminant ability.*

Waldron, H. Turner, C. W., Alexander, J. F., & Cole, B. (in progress). *Subcategories of supportive and defensive communications: Interdependence and discriminant ability.*

Waldron, H., Turner, C. W., Barton, C., Alexander, J. F., & Szykula, S. (1984, November). *The contributions of therapist defensiveness to marital therapy process and outcome: A path analytic approach.* Poster session presented at the Annual Meeting of the Association for the Advancement of Behavior Therapy, Philadelphia.

Warburton, J., Alexander, J. F., & Barton, C. (1980, August). *Sex of client and sex of therapist: Variables in a family process study.* Paper presented at the Annual Convention of the American Psychological Association, Montreal.

AUTHOR'S RESPONSE

Abstract revised to reflect author comments.

I-3
Developmental Environments Coding System (DECS)

General Information

Date of publication: 1982.

Author: Sally I. Powers.

Source/publisher: Powers, S. I. (1982). *Family interaction and parental moral development as a context for adolescent moral development.* Unpublished doctoral dissertation, Harvard University.

Availability: Available from the author at Department of Psychology, University of Massachusetts, Amherst, MA 01003. Dissertation available through University Microfilms International (#8308501).

Brief description: The DECS codes interaction variables elicited in a family interaction task. The microanalytic code consists of 24 types of behavior, grouped into eight conceptual categories. The codes indicate cognitively stimulating behaviors, cognitively inhibiting behaviors, and affective support and conflict. The codes assess the function of each speech in the discussion. Six additional codes indicate the content of each speech, who said the speech, to whom the speech was directed, and to whom the speech referred.

Purpose: The purpose of the code is to assess those familial variables predicted by structural-developmental theory to affect ego development, moral development, and related constructs such as defense mechanisms and adaptive coping processes.

Theoretical base: The code is strongly based on structural-developmental theory, most clearly exemplified by Piaget and Kohlberg. The coding system of Berkowitz and Gibbs (1979) for dyadic discussions of moral dilemmas was used as a model.

PHYSICAL DESCRIPTION OF CODE

Task and setting used to elicit behavior: Strodtbeck's revealed differences procedure was used to elicit family interaction. Each parent and one adolescent responded individually to Kohlberg's Moral Judgment Interview. Family members were then brought together and the differences in their solutions were revealed. Family members were asked to explain their individual positions and to attempt to reach a consensus that would represent the entire family. Each family discussed at least three differences (father and child vs. mother; mother and child vs. father; mother and father vs. child). (*Note:* Powers used the same data base as described for Hauser's Family Constraining and Enabling Coding System.)

Unit of study: Whole-family and individual interactions are studied, but analyses for particular dyads are possible.

Unit of coding/analysis: The largest possible unit of analysis was the speech: "all the words spoken by a single speaker from the time when he or she started to speak to the time when he or she stopped" (Powers et al., 1983, p. 11). Most frequently, however, the unit of analysis was a single, coherent thought within the speech. The key events studied were the adolescent's speeches and "a consistent amount of speeches surrounding each adolescent speech within the unit" (p. 11). Rather than coding only speeches within a standardized "key event unit," it is possible to use the DECS to code every speech (or a designated number of speeches) uttered in a family discussion. This is recommended by the author to save the time and expense of unitizing transcripts into key event segments and of obtaining reliability on this process. Not unitizing by key events is also recommended if analyses of speech sequences are planned.

Organization of code:

I. Functional Definition
  A. Focusing (Stimulating/Cognitive)
    1. Paraphrase
    2. Comprehension Check
    3. Intent for Closure
  B. Competitive Challenging (Stimulating/Cognitive)
    4. Competitive clarification
    5. Critique
    6. Competitive request
    7. Counter consideration
    8. Refinement/concession
    9. Competitive opinion statement
    10. Request for change
    11. Simple disagreement
  C. Noncompetitive Sharing of Perspectives (Stimulating/Cognitive)
    12. Opinion statement
    13. Clarification
    14. Request

        15. Simple agreement
- D. Avoidance (Interfering/Cognitive)
  - 16. Distracting
- E. Rejection of the task (Interfering/Cognitive)
  - 17. Refusal to do request or task
  - 18. Quit/devalue task
- F. Distortion (Interfering/Cognitive)
  - 19. Distortion
- G. Support (Stimulating/Affective)
  - 20. Encouragement
  - 21. Noncompetitive humor
  - 22. Listening responses
- H. Affective conflict (Interfering/Affective)
  - 23. Actively resist or threaten
  - 24. Devalue/hostility
- I. Other
  - 25. Interrupted/incomplete statements
  - 26. Unclear

II. Mode
- A. Competitive
- B. Noncompetitive
- C. Conflictual

III. Transactive or Nontransactive

IV. Content
- A. Speech concerned with reasoning about the solution to the dilemma
- B. Speech concerned with defining or commenting on the task
- C. Speech concerned with commenting on the interpersonal process

V. Direction
- A. Who said the statement
- B. To whom it was directed
- C. To whom it referred

Manual: Included as an appendix to Powers's dissertation.

Standardization and norms: No formal norms available. Published data are available for the first year of the Hauser/Powers longitudinal study.

Evaluation of physical description of code: *Strengths:* Code is strongly based in theory. *Weaknesses:* Coding manual not published and not easily available.

ADMINISTRATIVE PROCEDURES

Description of equipment needed and observation system: Family conversations are audiotaped. The experimenter presents the family's differences to them and then leaves the room. Psychiatric patient adolescents and their families were seen in the hospital; nonpatient families were seen at their adolescent's school.

Data transcription and reduction: Tapes of family interaction are transcribed and the typed transcripts, divided into units according to the presence of key events in the interaction, become the data base for interaction analysis. The "key event" used for unitizing is any intelligible speech expressed by the adolescent. A "section" of interaction is then specified for coding: a section begins with the two speeches immediately preceding the adolescent's speech and ends with the second adolescent speech. All speeches contained within each section are coded. Coders are blind to the group assignment of the family (psychiatric vs. nonpatient), sex of child, and ego stage of all family members. Coders work from typed transcripts without listening to audiotapes. It is also possible for coders to listen to the audiotapes while they code. According to the author, this does take more time, but it may be especially useful, although not necessary, in coding affective support and conflict.

Scoring procedures, including calculation of summary scores: Interaction scores for each category are computed for each individual and for the whole family. Because the total number of codes given to a discussion varied, interaction scores for each person and family were standardized by using the ratio of the frequency of codes given in a particular category to the frequency of total codes given.

Evaluation of administrative procedures: *Strengths:* Coding is done from carefully prepared transcripts. *Weaknesses:* Families were seen in psychiatric hospitals or in schools rather than in their own homes, raising concern about the ecological validity of the family observation. Coders worked only from typed transcripts, losing other interpretive cues (tone of voice, etc.) provided by audiotapes.

EVALUATION OF CODE

Reliability: Interrater reliability was calculated in three ways on a sample of 11 discussions with 2,178 coded responses. For the eight major categories of functional definitions, Pearson correlations ranged from .85 to .98, with an average of .94. Percentage agreement ranged from .84 to .98, with an average of .94. Cohen's kappa ranged from .63 to .73, with an average of .69 (Powers et al., 1983). Reliabilities on specific scales are published in Powers (1982).

Validity: *Criterion-related:* Cluster analyses of family patterns revealed very plausible associations between whole-family and individual family members' interaction and adolescent and parent ego and moral development (Powers et al., 1983; Powers, 1982; Powers et al., 1982a, 1982b). Adolescent and parent ego and moral development were most advanced when families presented high amounts of noncompetitive sharing of perspectives or competitive challenging within the context of high support or low affective conflict. Correlational analyses show that mothers', fathers', and adolescents' family interaction behaviors are significantly related to adolescents' use of defense mechanisms and adaptive coping processes when the adolescents are age 14 and age 16. The family behaviors that are related to adolescent boys' mature defenses and adaptive functioning, however, are different from the family behaviors that are related to adolescent girls' mature defenses and adaptive functioning (Powers et al., 1986; Powers, Jacobson, & Noam, 1987).

Clinical utility: This coding system is intended primarily as a research instrument. However, because of the authors' interests in both psychiatric and non-patient populations, they would likely feel that it could be clinically revealing. Because of the time-consuming and expensive nature of data reduction, however, it is doubtful that this coding scheme would be useful in everyday clinical practice.

Research utility: Although the code is cumbersome to use, it has demonstrated properties of reliability and validity that make it worthy of consideration for researchers studying similar issues within a structural-developmental framework.

SUMMARY EVALUATION

The coding system is strongly tied to a theoretical perspective and has clearly demonstrated reliability and criterion-related validity. The code's usefulness is limited, however, in that it is complex, time-consuming, and expensive to use.

REFERENCES

Berkowitz, M. W., & Gibbs, J. C. (1979). *A preliminary manual for coding transactive features of dyadic discussion.* Unpublished manuscript, Marquette University.

Powers, S. I. (1982). *Family interaction and parental moral development as a context for adolescent moral development.* Unpublished doctoral dissertation, Harvard University.

Powers, S. I., Beardslee, W., Jacobson, A. M., Hauser, S. T., Noam, G. G., Hopfenbeck, J., & Macias, E. (1986, December). *Family influences on the development of adolescent coping processes.* Paper presented at the Family Systems and Life-span Development Conference, Max Planck Institute for Human Development and Education, Berlin.

Powers, S. I., Hauser, S. T., Schwartz, J., Noam, G.G., & Jacobson, A. M.
    (1982a, August). *Adolescent ego development and family interaction.*
    In H. D. Grotevant and C. R. Cooper (Co-Chairs), Symposium on Sup-
    port and Conflict within Families and Adolescent Development: Mutual
    Effects. Paper presented at the meeting of the American Psychological
    Association, Washington, DC.
Powers, S. I., Hauser, S. T., Schwartz, J., Noam, G. G., & Jacobson, A. M.
    (1982b, October). *The family context of adolescent ego development: A
    social cognitive developmental perspective.* Paper presented at the An-
    nual Meeting of the National Council on Family Relations, Washington,
    DC.
Powers, S. I., Hauser, S. T., Schwartz, J. M., Noam, G. G., & Jacobson,
    A. M. (1983). Adolescent ego development and family interaction: A
    structural-developmental perspective. In H. D. Grotevant & C. R. Cooper
    (Eds.), *Adolescent development in the family: New directions for child
    development.* San Francisco: Jossey-Bass.
Powers, S. I., Jacobson, A. M., & Noam, G.G. (1987, April). *Parental influ-
    ences on the development of adolescent coping processes.* In W. A.
    Collins (Chair), *Parental Factors in Family Relations in Adolescence.*
    Symposium conducted at the Biennial Meeting of the Society for Re-
    search in Child Development, Baltimore.

AUTHOR'S RESPONSE

Current analyses not yet reported in publications include the examination of the
association of family, adolescent, mother and father behaviors (as measured by
the DECS) with the adolescent's use of 11 defense mechanisms and 15 adaptive
coping strengths. To understand why some teenagers can cope better with the
stresses of adolescence, it is important to examine the family's role in supporting or facilitating adolescent coping strengths. We are examining ways in which
support or inhibition of coping strengths might be communicated through the
family's verbal interactions. Preliminary analyses indicate that each of the cognitive and affective categories of the DECS are significantly related to adolescent coping.

I-4
Family Conflict and Dominance Codes: 3 Variations

GENERAL INFORMATION

Date of publication: (1) 1971; (b) 1974; (c) 1980.

Authors: (a) Hetherington, Stouwie, & Ridberg; (b) Jacob; (c) Henggeler & Tavormina.

Source/publisher: Coding information published in journal articles (see References).

Availability: Available in journal articles (see References).

Brief description: These variations on a coding system were designed to be process measures of dominance and conflict in family interaction. Using an unrevealed differences task to elicit family interaction, instances of specific behaviors indicative of conflict and dominance were tallied and developed into individual, dyadic, and family scores.

Purpose: The purpose of the code is to assess dominance and conflict in family interaction through a coding of family process.

Theoretical base: Based on psychiatric theories of the etiology of schizophrenia in family interaction (see Farina & Dunham, 1963).

PHYSICAL DESCRIPTION OF CODE

Task and setting used to elicit behavior:

Hetherington, Stouwie, & Ridberg (1971): In the structured family interaction task, each family member was individually presented with seven hypothetical situations involving problem behavior in adolescents. After each person had given an individual response as to how the situation should be handled, they were brought together to reach a mutually agreeable solution. Discussion continued until consensus was reached.

Jacob (1974): Jacob used a modified version of Bodin's unrevealed differences task. The family members (both parents and one child) were first placed in separate rooms and asked to complete a questionnaire in terms of "your own view of your family." They were each given eight questions, with five alternatives each, to be ranked from 1 ("most true or most like my family") to 5 ("least true or least like my family"). The content of the questionnaire was designed "to tap attitudes toward emotionally charged family concerns." After members completed the questionnaire (untimed), they were reunited and told the following:

> Each of you filled out the same questionnaire separately and so your individual questionnaires indicate how each of you view your family. I would now like you to fill out the questionnaire together. [One blank questionnaire and a pencil were placed on the table.] That is, I want you to discuss the questions and alternatives among yourselves and to fill out the questionnaire so as to represent the family's opinion or view.

The experimenter left the room and did not return until the family had completed the questionnaire.

Henggeler & Tavormina (1980): Each family member completed the unrevealed differences questionnaire, which was a modified version of that used by Jacob (1974). It included two tasks of four questions each; one task addressed expressive/internal family issues (e.g., "The best thing about our family is how we . . ."); the other addressed instrumental/external issues (e.g., "Where should the family go on its next vacation?"). Members were then brought together to discuss and complete the unrevealed differences questionnaire jointly. The assistant was not present during the audiotaped discussion.

Unit of study: Scores were calculated for individual family members, dyads, and for the family as a whole (see details below).

Unit of coding/analysis: Varies by type of behavior (see details below).

Organization of code:

Hetherington, Stouwie, & Ridberg (1971) variation:

Conflict
  Total words spoken per family
  Interruptions-ratio of number of interruptions of one person by another divided by total number of words spoken by the object of the interruptions (for each dyad)
  Simultaneous speech (for each dyad)
  Disagreements and aggressions (for each dyad)
  Failure to agree (number of times a family pair could not agree)

Dominance
  Speaks first (number of times each family member spoke first in seven inter-
    action situations)
  Speaks last (number of times each person made the final comment when it
    was not simply acceptance of someone else's idea)
  Percentage of total words spoken (for each person)
  Passive acceptance of the solution (frequency for each person)
  Percentage of successful interruptions (ratio of successful to total attempted
    interruptions)
  Degree of yielding (amount of shift from initial individual solution to final
    joint solution)

Jacob (1974) variation:
Conflict
  Attempted interruptions (both successful and unsuccessful; scored for each
    family member and the whole family during the first 8 minutes of inter-
    action)
Dominance
  Talking time (in seconds for each family member and for the whole family
    during the family's first 8 minutes of discussion)
  Successful interruptions (for each family member and for entire family dur-
    ing first 8 minutes of discussion)

Henggeler & Tavormina (1980) variation:
Conflict
  Attempted interruptions
  Simultaneous speech
  Initial disagreement
Dominance
  Talking time
  Sum of speaks first and speaks last
  Successful interruptions of second dyad member by first
  Successful interruptions of first dyad member by second
  Choice fulfillment

1984 coding manual additionally included the following:

  Total silent time
  Explicit informational units
  Aggressive communication (including disagreements)
  Defensive communication (Alexander code)
  Supportive communication (Alexander code)
  Rating scales for conflict, affect, and dominance

Manual: Coding details appear in published articles; no manuals are known to be available.

Standardization and norms: No normative data available, since each investigator used a variant of the methodology. Both Jacob (1974) and Hetherington, Stouwie, and Ridberg (1971) published means in their journal articles.

Evaluation of physical description of code: *Strengths:* Operational definitions are usually clearly presented in articles. *Weaknesses:* Each investigator used slightly different tasks and a different set of variables to measure conflict and dominance, leading to questionable comparability of results across studies.

ADMINISTRATIVE PROCEDURES

Description of equipment needed and observation system: Family interaction is audiotaped.

Data transcription and reduction: Hetherington et al. (1971) transcribed tapes to score latter. Jacob recorded talking times from listening to the tapes themselves. Henggeler and Tavormina appear to have counted or timed variables directly from audiotape onto a tally sheet.

Scoring procedures, including calculation of summary scores: Each of the indices listed in "Organization of code" above was measured as follows:

Hetherington, Stouwie, & Ridberg: Scores include simple frequency counts, lengths of time, and ratios of various behavioral indicators of conflict and dominance for each dyad. No "overall" conflict and dominance scores were computed.

Jacob: Attempted and successful interruptions were simple frequency counts made for each family member and the whole family; talking time was recorded in seconds for each family member and for the family as a whole during the first 8 minutes of the interaction.

Henggeler & Tavormina: Scores included simple frequency counts, lengths of time, and ratios of various behavioral indicators for individuals and dyads. No "overall" conflict and dominance scores were computed.

Evaluation of administrative procedures: Since transcribing and coding procedures are not fully explicated, we are not assured of comparability across studies. Full details about how variables were computed are not always available.

EVALUATION OF CODE

Reliability:

Hetherington et al.: Calculated percentage agreement between two advanced clinical psychology graduate students. Agreement ranged from 94% to 100%.

Jacob: Three trained undergraduate raters listened to tapes simultaneously. *Talk time:* When two scores were separated by more than 20 seconds, the tape was rerated and the mean of the two ratings was used. *Interruptions:* Two raters listened simultaneously and decided upon presence and whether successful or not. When they disagreed about success (4% of cases), a third rater decided.

Henggeler & Tavormina: Interrater reliability was calculated by Pearson correlation between initial scoring and second calculation for 20 families. Attempted interruptions, $r = .73$; simultaneous speech, $r = .87$; talk time, $r = .93$; sum of speaks first and speaks last, $r = .95$; successful interruption of first by second person, $r = .73$; others not given.

Validity:

Hetherington et al.: Criterion-related validity: Process measures revealed interpretable differences among four groups: nondelinquent, neurotic delinquent, psychopathic delinquent, and social delinquent. *Construct:* Behavioral measures did not correlate with self-report measures of parental behavior at a level greater than expected by chance.

Jacob: Criterion-related: Process measures of conflict and dominance (taken, as indicated above, from the family interaction task) and outcome measures of conflict and dominance (scores of agreement on the unrevealed differences questionnaires) were predicted by age of adolescent (11 vs. 16 years old) and social class (lower vs. middle). The results described shifts in family influence patterns as a function of child age and social class.

Clinical utility: These coding systems do not appear suited to in vivo clinical work, since they require the use of tapes or transcripts. They could be useful to clinicians to the degree that the theory on which the systems are based accurately describes differences between normal and pathological families.

Research utility: These schemes are somewhat easier to use than more complex discourse-oriented codes that focus more on function than on form of utterances. Because of the poor research showing of the conflict and dominance model of the development of family psychopathology, these schemes should probably not be used unless the researcher is interested in studying conflict and dominance for their own sake.

SUMMARY EVALUATION

Use of these coding systems is predicated on the importance of conflict and dominance as interaction patterns distinguishing normal from schizophrenic families—an outdated model. Studies measured the same constructs with different tasks and different utterance types, thus reducing comparability of results across studies. The coding of interruptions seemed particularly problematic: codes assumed that interruptions are indicators of conflict or dominance, when in fact they may perform different functions, depending on context. (For example, they may be indicators of family health and spontaneity in certain contexts.) Across these three coding systems, there was not always agreement about the assignment of interruptions as a measure of either conflict or dominance.

REFERENCES

Farina, A., & Dunham, R. M. (1963). Measurement of family relationships and their effects. *Archives of General Psychiatry, 9,* 64–73.

Hanson, C. L., Henggeler, S. W., Haefele, W. F., & Rodick, J. D. (1984). Demographic, individual, and family relationship correlates of serious and repeated crime among adolescents and their siblings. *Journal of Consulting and Clinical Psychology, 52,* 528–538.

Henggeler, S. W., Borduin, C. M., Rodick, J. D., & Tavormina, J. B. (1979). Importance of task content for family interaction research. *Developmental Psychology, 15,* 660–661.

Henggeler, S. W., & Tavormina, J. B. (1980). Social class and race differences in family interaction: Pathological, normative, or confounding methodological factors? *Journal of Genetic Psychology, 137,* 211–222.

Hetherington, E. M., Stouwie, R. J., & Ridberg, E. H. (1971). Patterns of family interaction and child-rearing attitudes related to three dimensions of juvenile delinquency. *Journal of Abnormal Psychology, 78,* 160–176.

Jacob, T. (1974). Patterns of family conflict and dominance as a function of child age and social class. *Developmental Psychology, 10,* 1–12.

I-5
Family Constraining and Enabling
Coding System (CECS)

GENERAL INFORMATION

Date of publication: 1987 (revised ed.; initially pub. 1983).

Authors: Stuart T. Hauser, Sally I. Powers, Bedonna Weiss-Perry, Donna Follansbee, Daranee C. Rajapark, & Wendy M. Greene.

Source/publisher: Unpublished manuscript; to be published in *Family Interiors of Adolescent Development,* by S. Hauser, with S. Powers, A. Jacobson, & G. Noam (in preparation for Free Press).

Availability: Available from Dr. Stuart Hauser, Adolescent and Family Development Project, Harvard Medical School, 74 Fenwood Rd., Boston, MA 02115.

Brief description: The CECS is a microanalytic scheme for coding family communication. Parent and adolescent speeches are coded for affective and cognitive constraining categories and for affective and cognitive enabling categories.

Purpose: This system is used to analyze transactions in family communication. Coding permits analysis of frequencies of communication events as well as communication sequences.

Theoretical base: The CECS is based on the psychoanalytically oriented theoretical work of H. Stierlin, who addressed how family members respond to adolescents who are attempting to individuate from the family.

PHYSICAL DESCRIPTION OF CODE

Task and setting used to elicit behavior: Two parents and the target adolescent engage in a revealed differences task, using members' responses to the Kohlberg Moral Judgment Interview as the material to discuss. Differences are presented to the family so that the following order of coalitions is standardized:

mother and child vs. father, father and child vs. mother, and mother and father vs. child. Family members are given 10 minutes for each set of differences and are asked to defend their individual positions and then come to consensus.

Unit of study: Whole-family interaction is studied, but analyses for particular dyads or individuals are possible.

Unit of coding/analysis: "The unit of analysis is a single numbered speech in a transcript. A speech is defined as a lengthy statement, phrase, fragment or utterance initiated by a family member" (Hauser, Powers, et al., 1987, p. 3). In lengthy speeches, scoring involves consideration of the intensity and specificity of the various constraining and/or enabling elements present in the speech.

Organization of code: Scales within each category are mutually exclusive and hierarchical.

Constraining Categories—Interactions in which parents actively resist differentiation of adolescent children:

Cognitive Constraining:
  Distracting
  Withholding
  Judgmental/Dogmatic
Affective Constraining:
  Indifference
  Gratifying/Affective Excess
  Devaluing

Enabling Categories—Interaction styles that assist and facilitate adolescent ego development by encouraging and supporting expression of independent thoughts and perceptions:

Cognitive Enabling:
  Explaining/Declaring
  Focusing
  Problem Solving
  Curiosity
Affective Enabling:
  Acceptance
  Active Understanding/Empathy

Discourse Change—Refers to how the individual family member shifts along the lines of contribution to discussion and complexity of expression between successive speeches. When the speech pertains to the same topic of conversation, the following mutually exclusive codes are applied:

Direction of Change—Regression
Direction of Change—Progression
Direction of Change—Foreclosure

When the focus of conversation shifts within the speech pair, the following mutually exclusive codes are applicable:

Topic Change—Regression
Topic Change—Progression
Topic Change—Foreclosure

Manual: A comprehensive manual is available from Hauser; it includes detailed definitions and examples of each coding category and also includes a sample coding sheet.

Standardization and norms: No formal norms are available. Published data are available for the first year of Hauser's longitudinal study.

Evaluation of physical description of code: *Strengths:* (1) A detailed coding manual is available. (2) Constructs are theoretically derived. (3) Categories are mutually exclusive and hierarchical. (4) The task used to elicit conflict in family interaction seems appropriate for the research issues under investigation. *Weaknesses:* A speech is a large unit of discourse and may include more than one function.

ADMINISTRATIVE PROCEDURES

Description of equipment needed and observation system: Family conversations are audiotaped. The experimenter presents the family's differences to them and then leaves the room. Psychiatric patient adolescents and their families were seen in the hospital; nonpatient "normal" families were seen at the adolescent's school.

Data transcription and reduction: Audiotapes are transcribed verbatim, preserving interruptions, simultaneous speech, laughter, and selected nonverbal signals. Entire transcripts are analyzed in order to perform sequential analyses (conditional and unconditional probabilities). Family members' raw scores are used in the final data analyses; these analyses control for number of speeches to permit interfamily comparisons. Coders are blind to the study's hypotheses, to the family members' ego development levels, and to the subsample source (psychiatric or high school).

Scoring procedures, including calculation of summary scores: All speeches may (but are not required to) receive a score on one scale from each of the

Constraining Categories (Affective and Cognitive) and on one scale from each of the Enabling Categories (Affective and Cognitive). The coder first makes a judgment about which of the scales of each of the four categories (Cognitive Constraining, Affective Constraining, Cognitive Enabling, Affective Enabling) applies to the speech and whether it is at a low level (minimal to somewhat evident presence) or a high level (moderate to extensive presence). In cases when two or more scales within a single category (e.g., Affective Constraining) are present, the scale that is present in greater intensity is scored. If two or more scales within the category are present on an equal level, the scale that is defined as the most specific according to the hierarchy of differentiated scales is scored. No more than one scale from a single category can be scored for any particular speech. Each speech is also coded for discourse change and for source and object (who-to-whom).

Evaluation of administrative procedures: *Strengths:* A careful transcription process was used. *Weaknesses:* Families were seen in the psychiatric hospital or in the adolescent's school rather than at home, raising concerns about the ecological validity of the family observation. Coders relied on transcripts only, losing information they might have gained from listening to the tapes.

EVALUATION OF CODE

Reliability: Reliabilities for the constraining and enabling codes have been calculated both in terms of percentage exact agreement (range: 84%–99%) and Cohen's kappa [range: .42 ($p < .05$) to .93 ($p < .001$)]. Reliabilities for discourse change codes range from 95%–98% agreement and from kappa = .45 ($p < .01$) to .73 ($p < .001$). During the course of Hauser's studies, intermittent reliability checks are made for observer drift.

Validity: *Criterion-related:* In one study (Hauser et al., 1980), family processes in two families with children at contrasting levels of ego development were compared. Parents of the preconformist adolescent had considerably higher levels of both cognitive and affective constraining interactions than the postconformist parents. The postconformist parents also showed many more empathy responses than the preconformist parents. In a second study of three diabetic families (Hauser et al., 1982), families of low-ego-development adolescents were found to express more constraining interactions than those of the postconformist adolescent. In addition, family acceptance scores increased with increasing ego levels of the adolescent. In a third study that included the families of 27 psychiatric patient adolescents and 34 nonpatient high school subjects (Hauser et al., 1984), ego development was predictably associated with family interactions. For example, adolescents higher in ego development expressed more cognitively enabling utterances and adolescents lower in ego development expressed more constraining utterances. The most recent study using sequential analyses of "macro" CECS categories (e.g., mutual enabling), reports significant discriminations between psychiatric and nonpatient families along theoretically expected lines (Hauser et al., in press). *Construct-related:* Because of the predictable associations between family interaction and ego development, Hauser (Hauser et al., 1984) has interpreted these data as supportive of Loevinger's ego development construct.

Clinical utility: The investigators make no claim for the usefulness of this coding system in the clinical setting because it is so time-consuming and costly to use. Because of their interest in both psychiatric and nonpatient families, however, they would view the coding system as containing relevant information for the functioning of families from a clinical perspective.

Research utility: The primary purpose of the coding system is to enable the researcher to characterize family patterns that are predictive of adolescent ego development and of progressions or regressions in ego development.

SUMMARY EVALUATION

This code has been carefully developed and carefully documented; satisfactory reliability and validity data have demonstrated its usefulness in research. The code has a strong theoretical base. The authors acknowledge the possibility of complex directions of influence in development and plan to investigate these by using both sequential analyses within family conversations and longitudinal analyses of family interaction across a 4-year period. Despite these strengths, the code is expensive and time-consuming to use.

REFERENCES

Hauser, S. T., Book, B. K., Houlihan, J., Powers, S., Weiss-Perry, B., Follansbee, D., Jacobson, A. M., & Noam, G. G. (1987). Sex differences within the family: Studies of adolescent and parent family interactions. *Journal of Youth and Adolescence, 16,* 199–219.

Hauser, S. T., Houlihan, J., Powers, S., Jacobson, A. M., Noam, G., Weiss-Perry, B., & Follansbee, D. (in press). Interaction sequences in families of psychiatrically hospitalized and non-patient adolescents. *Psychiatry.*

Hauser, S. T., Jacobson, A. M., Wertlieb, D., Weiss-Perry, B., Follansbee, D., Wolfsdorf, J. I., Herskowitz, R. D., Houlihan, J., Rajapark, D. C. (1986). Children with recently diagnosed diabetes: Interactions within their families. *Health Psychology, 5,* 273–296.

Hauser, S. T., Powers, S., Jacobson, A. M., Schwartz, J., & Noam, G. (1982). Family interactions and ego development in diabetic adolescents. *Pediatric and Adolescent Endocrinology, 10,* 69–76.

Hauser, S. T., Powers, S. I., Noam, G. G., Jacobson, A. M., Weiss, B., & Follansbee, D. J. (1984). Familial contexts of adolescent ego development. *Child Development, 55,* 195–213.

Hauser, S. T., Powers, S. I., Schwartz, J., Jacobson, A., & Noam, G. (1980, October). *Familial contexts of adolescent development.* Paper presented at the Theory Construction and Methodology Workshop at the meeting of the National Council on Family Relations, Portland, OR.

Hauser, S. T., Powers, S. I., Weiss-Perry, B., Follansbee, D., Rajapark, D. C., & Greene, W. M. (1987). *Family Constraining and Enabling Coding System (CECS) manual.* Unpublished manuscript, Harvard Medical School, Adolescent and Family Development Project.

AUTHOR'S RESPONSE

Although one of the strengths of the Family Constraining and Enabling Coding System (CECS) is its precision and thoroughness, this very exactness can also be a limitation. The CECS is applied to every speech in a transcript. At times, however, a speech does not fall neatly into one of the 12 subcategories, so a "forced-fit" process occurs, and the code is placed within the most appropriate category. Most often, the code will fall under one of the more general codes, and the cumulative effect of this process may be a blurring of the definitions of these codes (i.e., explaining). In addition, the CECS system is labor-intensive and requires a lengthy training period. As a microanalytic coding system, an important strength of the CECS is the specificity of the coding categories, which capture the subtleties of family interaction that can be lost using more global coding schemes. The CECS is applied to a small unit of analysis, and the coding categories are described in an explicit coding manual, which contains many examples. These factors combine to increase the level of objectivity as chances to infer meaning into phrases are decreased. In terms of its usefulness, the CECS is a reliable coding system for family interactions, and its theoretical validity has been empirically demonstrated. It is able to discriminate between functional and dysfunctional adolescents and between contrasting stages of ego development. While providing insight into individual development and changing family processes, the CECS allows a close examination of family influences on development.

I-6
Family Interaction Code

GENERAL INFORMATION

Date of publication: 1968.

Authors: E. G. Mishler & N. E. Waxler.

Source/publisher: Mishler, E. G., & Waxler, N. E. (1968). *Interaction in families: An experimental study of family processes and schizophrenia.* New York: Wiley.

Availability: Book available at most libraries or from publisher.

Brief description: The interaction code is a microanalytic coding scheme designed to examine the interaction of families with a schizophrenic member. It is composed of 10 code categories and 79 interaction index scores derived from the code categories.

Purpose: The code is designed to provide reliable and objective indicators of family interaction related to theory and clinical observations and to allow for enough flexibility in the analysis for new and unpredicted patterns to occur.

Theoretical base: (1) Family interaction as etiology of schizophrenia; (2) small-group research.

PHYSICAL DESCRIPTION OF CODE

Task setting used to elicit behavior: Family members were administered a 38-item revealed differences questionnaire developed by combining items from previously administered questionnaires of this type. Families were asked to try to come to a consensus on disagreed items. An optimum of 10 minutes was suggested for discussion of each item. The number of items discussed was manipulated in order to obtain 50 minutes of family discussion. Family discussions occurred in a hospital setting for both schizophrenic and normal families.

Unit of study: Whole family.

Unit of coding/analysis: The unit is a complete sentence, with one subject and one predicate, or a complete idea. Coding units may include more than one act.

Organization of code: Each of the interaction codes is applied to every marked act or unit. The code is composed of the interaction process analysis code developed for small-group process research (Bales, 1951) plus additional code categories of theoretical significance derived primarily from clinical literature. The interaction process analysis codes are:

  (1) Shows Solidarity (helps, rewards, gives status to others)
  (2) Tension Release
  (3) Agreement
  (4) Gives Suggestion
  (5) Gives Opinion
  (6) Gives Orientation
  (7) Asks for Orientation
  (8) Asks for Opinion
  (9) Asks for Suggestion
 (10) Disagreement
 (11) Shows Tension
 (12) Antagonism
  (0) Not Ascertainable

Additional code categories include:

  (1) Acknowledgment Stimulus/Acknowledgment Response (complete acknowledge to nonacknowledge to fragmented speech continuum)
  (2) Affect (positive–negative continuum)
  (3) Fragments (includes incomplete phrases, incomplete sentences, repetitions, laughter, and number of fragments in one act)
  (4) Interruptions (both successful and unsuccessful; interrupting and being interrupted)
  (5) Pause (occurrence of silence in the family interaction)
  (6) To Whom
  (7) Metacommunication (communication about a situation, about communication, about roles, or qualifications of communication)
  (8) Negation/Retraction (measures negative grammatical constructions)
  (9) Subject/Object (classifies subject/object into internal–external cells)
 (10) Tension (incomplete sentences, repetitions, fragments, laughter, number of tension indicators per act)

Manual: Information on training of coders, unitizing and coding data, data analysis, and code reliability is comprehensively presented in Mishler and Waxler (1968).

Standardization and norms: Means and percentages are provided.

Evaluation of physical description of code: *Strengths:* Code and coding procedures are well explicated in the manual, permitting replication. The code is comprehensive in scope and utilizes code categories of hypothesized theoretical significance regarding the etiology of schizophrenia in disturbed family communication. *Limitations:* The code is complex, with multiple codes to master. The code is not hierarchical, and categories are not mutually exclusive.

ADMINISTRATIVE PROCEDURES

Description of equipment needed and observation system: All family sessions were tape-recorded using a four-channel recorder; three microphones were used by the three family members and the fourth channel was used by the observer. An observer behind a one-way mirror recorded "who speaks to whom." Eye movements of the speaker, rather than probable speech intent, were used to determine to whom speech was directed. Tapes were transcribed using a four-channel transcriber.

Data transcription and reduction: Typed transcripts were made from the tape-recorded family sessions. Typescripts were then checked by another person for accuracy. Following the checking operation, interaction was broken into "units" and numbered sequentially. With the exception of the interaction process analysis codes and the Pause codes, all coding was done directly from the typescript while the coder listened to the tape. Coders coded typescripts by group of codes rather than applying the entire coding scheme at once. Each "unit" or "act" was placed on a separate IBM card, along with all the code numbers for that act as well as identifying information such as family number, item discussed, session number.

Coder training: Coders were women with bachelor's degrees, but not necessarily in psychology or related fields. Coders were trained to a criterion of 85% act-by-act agreement. Training required from 2 to 3 days to 3 to 4 weeks, depending on the complexity of the code category. A running reliability check was kept on all complex codes, with retraining if reliability fell below 85%.

Scoring procedures: To reduce the number of variables, behavior code categories were combined to form interaction index scores. The combining of code categories was determined primarily by theoretical interest; however, empirical distribution of code frequencies was also considered, with low-frequency codes ordinarily combined. To control for the variance across families in total speech "acts," frequencies are converted to index scores in the form of a percentage, which provides a standard score, allowing meaningful comparisons across families and family members.

Evaluation of administrative procedures: *Strengths:* Optimal procedures are delineated to assure accurate transcription and coding of data. Data formatting permits flexibility of data analysis. Conversion of data into standard scores is appropriate. *Limitations:* The derivation of index scores suffers from a lack of empirical validity. The use of factor analysis, as well as frequency distribution, of codes would give greater validity to derived constructs.

EVALUATION OF CODE

Reliability: All reliability measures were obtained from act-by-act comparisons between two coders. Reliability of selected codes, using Cohen's kappa statistic, ranged from .59 to .87. Using a percentage agreement approach, mean interrater agreement ranged from 64% to 97%. Codes were not included in the reliability analysis (e.g., negations, repetitions) when coding disagreements were likely due only to clerical error. Reliability was also obtained for the interaction indices. The mean percentage agreement between two coders ranged from 81% to 100%. Specifically, interrater reliability fell below 85% for the interaction process analysis and Acknowledgment Response codes.

Validity: *Concurrent validity:* Families with a schizophrenic member were significantly differentiated from nonpsychiatric control families on four indices reflecting composites of the individual codes: expressiveness (including affect); strategies of attention and personal control; speech disruption; and responsiveness (Mishler & Waxler, 1968).

Clinical utility: The Family Interaction Code has demonstrated clinical utility in differentiating families with a schizophrenic member from nonpsychiatric families; however, the complexity of the code, as well as the lack of empirical validity in code reduction, limits clinical use.

Research utility: Research utility is limited by the complexity and number of microanalytic code categories and by the failure to use empirical methods to derive composite indices.

SUMMARY EVALUATION

The Family Interaction Code provided an important standard to the field of family interaction study and has been influential in the development of coding schemes. The current usefulness of the code is limited, however, by the number of microanalytic code categories and by the failure to empirically derive the more easily utilized composite indices.

REFERENCES

Bales, R. F. (1951). *Interaction process analysis.*Cambridge: Addison-Wesley.
Mishler, E. G., & Waxler, N. E. (1968). *Interaction in families: An experimental study of family processes and schizophrenia.* New York: Wiley.

I-7
Family Interaction Coding System (FICS)

GENERAL INFORMATION

Date of publication: 1969 (revised).

Authors: G. R. Patterson, R. S. Ray, D. A. Shaw, & J. A. Cobb

Source/publisher: (1) *Manual for coding family interactions.* (1969). New York: Microfiche Publications. (2) J. B. Reid, (Ed.). (1978). *A social learning approach to family intervention: Vol. 2. Observation in home settings.* Eugene, OR: Castalia.

Availability: Available from Castalia Publishing Co., P.O. Box 1587, Eugene, OR 97440.

Brief description: The FICS is a microanalytic code that was designed to describe the aggressive behaviors of parents and children and their associated antecedents and consequences within a field setting. The code consists of 29 categories, with approximately half describing aversive behaviors and half describing prosocial behaviors.

Purpose: The FICS is designed (1) to provide an assessment methodology that accurately measures changes in family interaction, particularly changes resulting from intervention; (2) to provide data to support the development and validity of a theory of coercion and social aggression.

Theoretical base: Social learning theory.

PHYSICAL DESCRIPTION OF CODE

Task and setting used to elicit behavior: Data are collected in *semistructured* home settings, either prior to lunch or prior to dinner. The observation setting is structured by a set of formal rules, which include: everyone must be present; no guests; limited to two rooms; no telephone calls out and brief responses to incoming calls; no TV; no talking to observers. Observations are conducted for a minimum of 70 minutes and sampled in 5-minute blocks.

Unit of study: Dyads within the whole family (e.g., target and reactant). Each family member rotates as target for observation. The target's behavior and the consequent behavior by another family member (reactant) are recorded for a specified time period.

Unit of coding/analysis: Discrete units of behavior as it occurs. If required, several subject numbers and code categories may be used to describe a single interaction.

Organization of code: The FICS is composed of 29 code categories: Approval; Attention; Command; Command Negative; Compliance; Cry; Disapproval; Dependency; Destructiveness; High Rate; Humiliate; Ignore; Indulgence; Laugh; Noncompliance; Negativism; Normative; No Response; Play; Physical Negative; Physical Positive; Receive; Self-Stimulate; Talk; Tease; Touch; Whine; Work; Yell. Codes are not mutually exclusive; therefore, a hierarchy of first- and second-order behaviors has been imposed. First-order behaviors take precedence in coding, based on their presumed clinical and theoretical relevance. Double coding remains a possibility, however.

Manual: A comprehensive guide to the FICS is available (Reid, 1978). It includes not only a description of the code and examples for utilization but also information regarding code development, theoretical base, methodological issues, psychometric data, and observer training.

Standardization and norms: Mean behavior rates of each FICS code category are provided for normal and clinic boys, girls, sibs, and parents (Reid, 1978). A compilation of research data using the FICS is reported in Patterson (1982). Updated tables incorporating recent research studies are not provided in the 1982 publication.

Evaluation of physical description of code: *Strengths:* (1) Careful code development is based on 3 years of empirical investigation. (2) There is a comprehensive manual. (3) It is designed for field-setting use. (4) Normative data are available for certain ages and clinical groups. *Limitations:* (1) Time-sampling methodology and observation focus on one person at a time, limiting the utility of the code for family systems frameworks. (2) A lack of mutually exclusive and hierarchical categories unnecessarily increases the complexity of code. (3) Imposition of structure into the home environment attenuates the naturalness of the setting—a problem acknowledged by the code developers but defended as a means of maximizing occurrence of events of interest.

ADMINISTRATIVE PROCEDURES

Description of equipment needed and observation system: Before arrival at the family's home, observers must prepare rating sheets. One rating sheet is used for each family member for each 5-minute period. Rating sheets per member are placed in random order, but the sequence is maintained across the observation period. During the observation, the coder alternately codes, in sequence, the behavior of the subject and then the person(s) with whom the subject interacts. Data are recorded continuously. Observers receive an auditory signal (built into the clipboard) every 30 seconds, cuing them to shift to the next line of the observation sheet. On the average, observers record five interaction units (both members of a dyad) every 30 seconds. On the bottom of each behavior rating sheet, observers briefly describe the situation occuring during that period of observation.

Observer training: Observers are trained prior to field experience for approximately 15 to 20 hours with videotapes. Trainees also attend weekly meetings to clarify coding questions. Reliability is checked at various intervals throughout training. After a reliability of 80% is achieved on at least two 5-minute coding sheets, the trainee begins training in the home setting. Interobserver agreement of 75% must be achieved in the home setting on two consecutive observations before the observer is considered "reliable." Several home experiences are required to attain the criterion. No information is provided on the total time necessary to train observers.

Data transcription and reduction: Immediately following the observation, data from the behavior rating sheets are keypunched according to a described format. Data analysis techniques have been numerous and varied, with most recent research involving sequential analyses of data for both intrasubject and intersubject dependencies.

Scoring procedures: Scoring procedures are not clearly described and appear to vary with the research questions under investigation. Individual behavior codes provide one set of scored data. A common procedure is to sum the aggressive behavior codes (e.g., Tease, Whine, Yell, Cry) into a total aggressive behavior (TABs) score for statistical analyses. In addition, the following summary scores have been used: total deviant behavior, hostility, and social aggression (Reid, 1978). Many variables are expressed as "rates per minute."

Evaluation of administrative procedures: *Strengths:* Code categories and recording procedures are carefully described, permitting replication. *Limitations:* Data reduction techniques are less clearly articulated. Observer training is costly and time-consuming.

EVALUATION OF CODE

Reliability: Reliability of the FICS was established by Jones et al. (1975), utilizing generalizability theory. Results indicated that 60 to 100 minutes of observation data provide a reasonably stable estimate of behavior across a 2-week period with two-thirds of the behavior codes significantly correlated ($p < .01$). Reliability for low base rate events could not be determined. Analysis of variance of five high-frequency Behavior Codes × Subjects × Raters × Situation found 96 to 97% of behavior variance attributable to Subject and Subject × Occasion, with virtually no variance attributable to raters or to occasions, supporting the reliability of the code as evidenced by observer agreement and stability across time. Percentage agreement for interrater reliability on the 29 categories ranged from .30 to .96, with 14 categories below .70. Interrater correlations ranged from .59 to 1.00, with five categories below .70 (Reid, 1978, app. 13).

Validity: *Criterion-related:* The FICS has significantly differentiated families of normal children from families of children identified as antisocial, with the latter consistently found to be more coercive than comparable members of normal families (Patterson, 1976, 1980; Reid et al., 1981; Snyder, 1977; Conger & Burgess, 1978). Social aggressors were significantly differentiated from hyperactives using factor scores derived from the FICS (Carlson, 1981a, 1981b). The TAB (total aggressive behavior) score derived from the FICS has significantly differentiated stealers, social aggressors, and normals (Patterson, 1982). *Construct-related:* The FICS is significantly correlated with an alternative measure of family coercion, the Parent Daily Report (PDR) (Patterson, 1976; Chamberlain, 1980). Support for a bilateral coercive influence process has been obtained through multiple regression analyses using the TAB score (Patterson, 1981).

Clinical utility: The FICS was designed to be both a theoretically and clinically relevant measure. It has demonstrated clinical utility in differentiating types of socially aggressive family interactions and in documenting pre- and posttreatment changes. Although designed for clinical use, the complexity and cost of utilizing the FICS, as any microanalytic code, is prohibitive except in a well-funded research context. Provision of baseline frequency data is likely to be useful to clinicians for normative purposes.

Research utility: The FICS is highly suitable to research investigations that focus on aggressive behavior within a group context. Limitations to the use of the FICS are its complexity and microanalytic focus, and therefore high cost for data collection, reduction, and analysis.

SUMMARY EVALUATION

The FICS is a carefully constructed, theoretically sound microanalytic coding system with a substantial research data base to support it. It has demonstrated reliability and validity for both clinical and research purposes. Limitations to its use center on the high cost of observer training, data collection, and analysis.

REFERENCES

Carlson, W. (1981a). *Factor generated response class scaling.* Unpublished manuscript. (Available from Humboldt State University, Arcata, CA 95521)

Carlson, W. (1981b). *Hyperactive, conduct disordered, and normal children observed in their natural home environments.* Unpublished manuscript. (available from Humboldt State University, Arcata, CA 95521)

Chamberlain, P. (1980). *Standardization of a parent report measure.* Unpublished doctoral dissertation, University of Oregon.

Conger, R. D., & Burgess, R. (1978). *Reciprocity: Equity system stability.* Unpublished manuscript. (Available from University of Georgia, Athens, GA)

Jones, R. R., Reid, J. B., & Patterson, G. R. (1975). Naturalistic observations in clinical assessment. In P. McReynolds, (Ed.), *Advances in psychological assessment* (Vol. 3). San Francisco: Jossey-Bass.

Patterson, G. R. (1976). The aggressive child: Victim and architect of a coercive system. In L. A. Hamerlynck, L. C. Handy, & E. J. Mash (Eds.), *Behavior modification and families: Theory and research* (Vol. 1). New York: Brunner/Mazel.

Patterson, G. R. (1980). Mothers: The unacknowledged victims. *Monographs of the Society for Research in Child Development, 45* (5, Serial No. 186), 1–64.

Patterson, G. R. (1982). *A social learning approach to family intervention: Vol. 3. Coercive family process,* Eugene, OR: Castalia.

Reid, J. B. (Ed.). (1978). *A social learning approach to family intervention: Vol. 2. Observation in home settings.* Eugene, OR: Castalia.

Reid, J. B., Taplin, P. S., & Lober, R. (1981). A social-interactional approach to the treatment of abusive families. In R. Stuart (Ed.), *Violent behavior: Social learning approaches to prediction, management, and treatment.* New York: Brunner/Mazel.

Snyder, J. J. (1977). A reinforcement analysis of interaction in problem and nonproblem families. *Journal of Abnormal Psychology, 86*(5), 528–535.

I-8
Family Interaction Scales (FIS)

GENERAL INFORMATION

Date of publication: 1969.

Authors: Jules Riskin and Elaine E. Faunce.

Source/publisher: Mental Research Institute (MRI), 555 Middlefield Rd., Palo Alto, CA 94301.

Availability: Available from MRI.

Brief description: This microanalytic coding system is designed to observe whole-family interaction by using more objective, operational methodologies for assessing family interaction than impressionistic clinical observations.

Purpose: The purpose of this method is to contribute to the understanding of individual personality development by examining the family context in which the child's personality develops.

Theoretical base: The theoretical base comes from family therapy theory of Jackson and Satir.

> We view the family as providing the basic environment in which the child's personality develops. The parents influence the children by direct interaction with them. Also, the parental interaction in itself serves as a model for the children to observe and identify with and/or react against. Each child in turn influences his parents and siblings, and, thus, a mutually interactive process goes on. (Riskin & Faunce, 1970a, p. 505)

PHYSICAL DESCRIPTION OF CODE

Task and setting used to elicit behavior: The family was instructed: "Plan something you could all do together as a family; all of you please participate in the planning." Families were interviewed in a room with microphones and a one-way mirror at the Mental Research Institute.

Unit of study: Whole family.

Unit of coding/analysis: The unit of analysis was the speech: "all the sounds one person uttered until someone else made a sound, verbal or simply vocal but without distinguishable words" (Riskin & Faunce, 1970a, p. 508).

Organization of code: Each speech was coded on six major dimensions in the following order:

Agree/Disagree: measures the amount of agreement and disagreement among family members (coded as agreement or disagreement)

Clarity: measures whether or not the family members speak clearly—that is, (1) their words are clear and (2) their affect fits the idea or feeling that the words express (coded as clear or unclear).

Topic: measures whether or not the family members stay on the same topic and how they change topics (coded as same topic; different topic—appropriate change; different topic—inappropriate change).

Commitment: measures whether or not the family members take clear, definite stands—that is, commit themselves to ideas, suggestions, issues, and so forth (coded as spontaneous commitment, request for commitment, commitment made in response to request for commitment, avoidance of commitment after request for commitment).

Intensity: measures the relative amount of affective or emotional intensity that the family members show in their speech (rated on a 5-point scale from very low to very high).

Relationship: measures the amount of friendliness or attacking that occurs between family members (rated on a 5-point scale ranging from strongly negative to strongly positive).

Manual: The manual (Riskin & Faunce, 1969) is very comprehensive, providing detailed instructions for coding each category, typing instructions, and sample transcripts.

Standardization and norms: Norms are not presented in the manual; rank orders of frequencies for five different groups under investigation are presented in Faunce & Riskin (1970).

Evaluation of physical description of code: *Strengths:* Clear instructions for coding; categories mutually exclusive. Detailed information on calculation of the large number of variables may be found in Faunce and Riskin (1970). *Weaknesses:* Unit of coding (speech) may be too large for coding when the speech is long.

ADMINISTRATIVE PROCEDURES

Description of equipment needed and observation system: In the major study of 44 white, intact, middle-class families, families were observed by an "experienced interviewer'' at the MRI in a room with microphones and a one-way mirror; the family discussion was audiotaped through two systems: an overhead mike recorded the whole family on a mono tape recorder, and individual lavaliere mikes were connected to the two channels of a stereo tape recorder. Two observers watched the family through the mirror to keep notes on who spoke to whom. After giving instructions, the interviewer left the room and allowed the family 10 minutes to complete the task.

Data transcription and reduction: Highly accurate transcripts were prepared, taking at least 15 hours to prepare 4 to 5 minutes of the taped plan-something-together task. Transcribers had no knowledge of the families except the name, age, and sex of each person. The first 80 speeches and the third block of 80 speeches (representing minutes 1–2 and 5–6 of the tape) were scored. The written transcript alone was used to score agreement; tape plus transcript were used for all other categories. Coding of 160 speeches requires 3 to 4 hours. Coders were trained to 80% to 85% reliability on all scales, with ongoing interrater reliability checks made throughout the 6-month data reduction period.

Scoring procedures, including calculation of summary scores: Each transcript was scored for eight scales: (1) Speaker and Spoken To; (2) Interruptions; (3) Clarity; (4) Topic; (5) Commitment; (6) Agreement; (7) Intensity; (8) Relationship. The scoring options for each scale require low inference on the part of the coder. A total of 125 variables were computed, consisting of ratings along individual dimensions, combinations of ratings from two or more dimensions, ratios that compared two categories from one rating dimension (e.g., number of unclear speeches divided by the number of clear speeches), and complex ratios that compared ratings along one dimension with ratings along a second dimension.

Evaluation of administrative procedures: *Strengths:* Standardization of data collection situation; preservation of detailed information about the family's interaction. *Weaknesses:* No empirical justification for the choice of utterances to score; sequential analyses not performed; time-consuming data reduction.

EVALUATION OF CODE

Reliability: Three types were calculated, all percentage agreement:

Scale	Ongoing Interrater	Interrater Over Time	Intrarater Over Time
Clarity	94.5	95.0	96.6
Topic	85.3	87.4	90.7
Commitment	80.6	80.3	89.8
Agree/Disagree	89.1	88.6	94.5

Validity: *Criterion-related:* Families in the sample of 44 were divided into five groups on the basis of home interviews with a clinician: (1) multiproblem families ($N = 10$); (2) constricted families ($N = 5$); (3) families with child-labeled problems ($N = 12$); (4) families with nondiagnosed problems ($N = 8$); (5) "nonlabeled" families ($N = 9$). The 125 variables calculated allowed plausible distinctions to be made among these five groups of families. In general, those variables that were composed of ratios discriminated better than the simpler variables. The clearest discriminations were obtained with the Clarity, Commitment, and Relationship scales. Variables measuring topic continuity, agreement, intensity, interruptions, and who-speaks-to-whom did not discriminate between groups.

Lewis, Beavers, Gossett, and Phillips (1976) provided additional evidence for the validity of aspects of the FIS. Eleven of the 125 FIS variables that met the criteria of simple frequencies, whole-family variables, and statistical significance were selected for investigation. Twelve nonlabeled families engaged in a videotaped family evaluation consisting of several tasks, including a plan-something-together task. Frequencies of identified variables were obtained and used to rank-order families from most to least healthy. Total ranking was significantly correlated with clinical ranking, as were individual variables of clarity and high intensity. Several variables were combined to reflect theoretically derived constructs of family systems theory with similar results. Individual variable combinations had relatively weak discriminative power (exception: clarity), but the sum of variables provided a statistically significant correlation with the clinical ranking.

Clinical utility: The FIS would be very cumbersome to use in a clinical setting. It probably would not be useful, although it could be useful in clinical research because of the success with which some of the variables discriminated among family types.

Research utility: The FIS could be useful in research, as a number of the variables did make predicted discriminations, but it is very time-consuming and expensive to use. Riskin (1982) has dropped the use of this microanalytic code for a macroanalytic set of rating scales.

SUMMARY EVALUATION

The FIS captures aspects of family interaction that discriminate among family types. Detailed coding procedures are carefully documented and could be replicated by others. On the other hand, too many variables were derived. (Riskin said they should be pared down to a smaller number.) Riskin has dropped these scales in favor of a macro code, but no research has yet compared the relative validity of the two systems. Little research other than with the initial 44 families has used this coding system, which is time-consuming to learn and use.

REFERENCES

Faunce, E. E., & Riskin, J. (1970). Family Interaction Scales II. Data analysis and findings. *Archives of General Psychiatry, 22,* 513–526.

Jackson, D. D., Riskin, J., & Satir, V. (1961). A method of analysis of a family interview. *Archives of General Psychiatry, 5,* 29–45.

Lewis, J., Beavers, W., Gossett, J., & Phillips, V. (1976). *No single thread: Psychological health in family systems.* New York: Brunner/Mazel.

Riskin, J. (1964). Family Interaction Scales: A preliminary report. *Archives of General Psychiatry, 11,* 484–494.

Riskin, J. (1982). Research on ''nonlabeled'' families: A longitudinal study. In F. Walsh (Ed.), *Normal family processes.* New York: Guilford Press.

Riskin, J., & Faunce, E. E. (1969). *Family Interaction Scales scoring manual.* Palo Alto, CA: Mental Research Institute.

Riskin, J., & Faunce, E. E. (1970a). Family Interaction Scales I. Theoretical framework and method. *Archives of General Psychiatry, 22,* 504–512.

Riskin, J. & Faunce, E. E. (1970b). Family Interaction Scales III. Discussion of methodology and substantive findings. *Archives of General Psychiatry, 22,* 527–537.

AUTHOR'S RESPONSE

These scales were developed before present computer technology was available. Although the original procedure was extremely cumbersome, currently available technology would facilitate the scoring and data analysis tremendously. In addition, sequential analysis, which could yield valuable information—especially about important, though subtle, family interactional patterns—could be done quite easily with computer assistance.

I-9
Family Task

GENERAL INFORMATION

Date of publication: 1978.

Author: B. L. Rosman.

Source/publisher: Philadelphia Child Guidance Clinic.

Availability: Available from Bernice L. Rosman, PhD, Director of Research & Evaluation, Philadelphia Child Guidance Clinic, Two Children's Center, 34th St. & Civic Center Blvd., Philadelphia, PA 19104.

Brief description: The Family Task is a series of family interactive tasks that family members administer, structure, and carry out by themselves, plus coding procedures to analyze patterns of interaction specific to each task.

Purpose: The purpose of the Family Task is analysis of family interaction patterns to compare family functioning in psychosomatic and normal families.

Theoretical base: Structural family theory (Minuchin, 1974).

PHYSICAL DESCRIPTION OF CODE

Task and setting used to elicit behavior: Family members are provided with tape-recorded instructions for five tasks: planning a menu, discussing a family argument, describing pleasing and displeasing qualities of other family members, making up stories about family pictures, and putting together color-forms designs. Data are collected in a laboratory (clinic) setting; family interaction is videotaped (with audio collected via microphone) and observed through a one-way mirror.

Unit of study: Whole family unit (maximum two adults and three children). Some constructs (such as enmeshment) are scored at the level of the family, the subsystem, and the individual-interpersonal.

Unit of coding/analysis: Not clearly specified in manual. Every time a family member speaks, it appears to be coded as a unit.

Organization of code: The code varies for each task. The code is mutually exclusive and exhaustive. No hierarchy of code categories is indicated. Behavioral categories that are coded include (1) *Transactional* behavior (Executive leadership, control, guidance); Request for Executive Activity; Task Opinion; Agree; Disagree; Affectionate; Aggressive; Refusal to Answer; Unscorable; Inaudible); (2) *Enmeshment* behavior (Blurring of separate identities—mindreading, personal control, mediating; Distance; Reactivity); (3) *Alliances* (Support, Oppose, Join, Recruitment, Appeal, Disaffiliation, Alliance Shift, Alliances around executive behavior); (4) *Conflict* behavior (No Conflict, Conflict checked via numerous explicated strategies); (5) *Protectiveness* (concern with hunger, well-being, pacification, etc.).

Manual: The coding manual that has been compiled by the author is confusing and poorly articulated.

Standardization and norms: None provided.

Evaluation of physical description of code: *Strengths:* The code appears to have face content validity as an effort to behaviorally operationalize structural family theory. *Limitations:* The coding system is so poorly explicated in the manual that it is impossible to use without considerable personal communication with the author.

ADMINISTRATIVE PROCEDURES

Description of equipment needed and observation system: Family members seat themselves as they wish in an interview room with a microphone, around a table upon which are a tape recorder with the Family Task cassette, a folder with picture cards, and a folder with color-forms model pieces in envelopes. Videotaping of the process occurs through a one-way mirror.

Data transcription and reduction: No information available.

Scoring procedures: Scoring procedures are poorly articulated in the manual and appear to vary across tasks. A behavioral category is assigned to each designated speech unit. Alliance codes are scored only when there is a conflict situation. The Enmeshment subcategories of *Distance* and *Reactivity* are not used in the final scoring but rather are qualitative categories of clinical interest. In addition to the microanalytic behavioral code, scoring critera for a global rating of family conflict behavior are provided. Who speaks to whom and the content of the verbalization are recorded. Information for deriving final scores from coding instructions is not specified in the manual.

Evaluation of administrative procedures: *Strengths:* Use of multiple tasks to elicit family interaction. *Limitations:* Data transcription, reduction, and analysis procedures are not explicated, making it impossible for this coding procedure to be replicated.

EVALUATION OF CODE

Reliability: No information is provided. Minuchin, Rosman, and Baker (1978) state that reliability has been established and is to be reported in a publication in preparation.

Validity: No detailed information is provided. Minuchin et al. (1978) refer the reader to a report in preparation. Validity of the constructs is sought through comparing anorectic families with two other psychosomatic groups (asthmatic and diabetic) and with normal families.

Clinical utility: Constructs permit the differentiation of diagnostic categories of families; however, it is not clear whether the data used are derived from the microanalytic coding or from more global clinical analyses.

Research utility: The research utility of this task and code is currently limited by poor documentation of methods and procedures and by the lack of a mutually exclusive, exhaustive, hierarchically designed code.

SUMMARY EVALUATION

Although Minuchin et al. (1978) claim that the constructs assessed in the Family Task make useful clinical distinctions based on structural family theory, evaluation of this interaction assessment must await the publication of the data on which these claims rest.

REFERENCES

Minuchin, S. (1974). *Families and family therapy*. Cambridge: Harvard University Press.

Minuchin, S., Rosman, B. L. & Baker, L. (1978). *Psychomatic families: Anorexia nervosa in context*. Cambridge: Harvard University Press.

Rosman, B. L. (1978). *Philadelphia Child Guidance Clinic Family Task and scoring*. (Available from Bernice L. Rosman, PhD, Director of Research & Evaluation, Two Children's Center, 34th St. & Civic Blvd., Philadelphia, PA 19104)

I-10
Individuation Code

GENERAL INFORMATION

Date of publication: 1984.

Authors: Sherri L. Condon, Catherine R. Cooper, and Harold D. Grotevant.

Source/publisher: *Psychological Documents, 14* (1984), 8 (Ms. No. 2616).

Availability: *Manual for the Analysis of Family Discourse* is available from Select Press, P.O. Box 9838, San Rafael, CA 94912.

Brief description: This is a microanalytic code of family verbal interaction designed to capture *individuation*—the interplay of individuality and connectedness—in family relationships.

Purpose: The purpose is to code family discourse around a plan-something-together task.

Theoretical base: The role of individuation in development and mental health; family systems theory; conversational analysis and speech act theory.

PHYSICAL DESCRIPTION OF CODE

Task and setting used to elicit behavior: Family members, within their homes, are asked to engage in a family interaction task (FIT)—specifically, a plan-something-together task. Family members are seated around a table and are told they will have 2 weeks and unlimited funds for a vacation. Their task is to plan an itinerary in 20 minutes.

Unit of study: Whole family and dyads within the family.

Unit of coding/analysis: The unit is the utterance, defined as ''an independent clause together with any dependent clauses that are connected to it'' (Condon, Cooper, & Grotevant, 1984, p. 13). Independent clauses connected by *and* or *but* are separated.

Organization of code: The Individuation Code is organized into two mutually exclusive and exhaustive categories (MOVE and RESPONSE), to acknowledge that all speech units represent both a response to previous conversation and a direction for subsequent discourse. Each speech unit is coded in both categories. A hierarchical organization is also imposed to resolve the problem of speech units that have more than one MOVE or RESPONSE function. Code categories are arranged with "stronger functions spatially higher and receiving precedence in coding." The coding categories have been validated with factor analyses of the data on two samples. The resulting constructs and their behavioral indices for a sample of high school seniors were (Grotevant & Cooper, 1985):

Self-assertion: awareness of own point of view and clear communication of it (includes Suggests Action Directly).
Permeability: responsiveness to others' views (includes Acknowledgment, Requests Information/Validation, Agrees/Incorporates, Relevant Comments, Complies).
Mutuality: sensitivity to other's views (includes Indirect Suggestion, Compromise, States Other's Feelings, Answers Request for Information.
Separateness: expression of distinctiveness of self and others (includes Direct Disagreement, Indirect Disagreement, Requests Action, Irrelevant Comment).

The resulting constructs and behavioral indices for a sample of sixth-graders were (Cooper & Carlson, 1987):

Individuality: expression of distinctiveness from others (includes Direct Disagreement, Indirect Disagreement, Direct Suggestion, Requests Action, and Complies).
Connectedness: expression of sensitivity and responsiveness to other's views (includes Agrees/Incorporates, Indirect Suggestion, Acknowledgment, Requests Information/Validation, Answers, Relevant Comment).

Manual: A detailed coding manual has been compiled by the authors. It includes detailed coding conventions, examples, sample protocols, sample scoring, theoretical rationale, and reliability and validity data.

Standardization and norms: Normative data are not presented in the manual; research publications include sample means.

Evaluation of physical description of code: *Strengths:* (1) The coding system is well-explicated in the manual. (2) The code is organized into mutually exclusive and hierarchically ordered categories ideal for statistical analysis. (3) The code is carefully and explicitly grounded in theory. (4) The coding categories have been validated empirically through factor analysis. (5) The task to elicit behavior is congruent with theoretical constructs hypothesized and conducted within the home setting in order to maximize ecological validity. *Limitations:* (1) Although the coding categories are relatively straightforward, the instructions to coders are quite complex and appear time-consuming to master. (2) There is a lack of normative data.

ADMINISTRATIVE PROCEDURES

Description of equipment needed and observation system: Family interaction is audiotaped. Coding is done from written transcript and audiotape.

Data transcription and reduction: Coders are trained for approximately 20 hours in group meetings, then tested for reliability and allowed to begin coding under close supervision. Reliability is assessed 2 weeks later, and supervision is decreased with adequate performance. Reliability is assessed at a third unannounced time. Supervision, both group and individual, continues throughout coding. The coding process for 300 utterances takes 4 to 6 hours for experienced coders and up to 10 hours for complete transcripts (up to 1,000 utterances).

Scoring procedures: Each coded category is summed into totals for each participant in the interaction. Communication behaviors that are directed from one person to another (e.g., disagreements) are summed with respect to the source and object of the utterance.

Evaluation of administrative procedures: *Strengths:* (1) Utilization of written transcripts, although laborious, enhances reliability. (2) Coders are carefully trained and supervised. *Limitations:* (1) The coding, training, and supervision required by the code are demanding and time-consuming.

EVALUATION OF CODE

Reliability: Interrater reliability, assessed by the combination of reliability tests for coders, ranges from 52% to 100%. (All but three categories had percentage agreement $> 75\%$).

Validity: Content validity of the code has been established with two separate factor analyses of the 14 coded categories, resulting in four independent factors with eigenvalues greater than 1.0, which accounted for 51.3% of the variance in one sample of adolescents (Grotevant & Cooper, 1985), and two independent factors with eigenvalues greater than 1.0, which accounted for 81.8% of the variance in a second sample of young adolescents (Cooper & Carlson, 1987). The validity of the code as a measure of the theoretical construct of individuation has been demonstrated in research with adolescent identity exploration and role-taking, predicted by family interaction variables (Cooper & Grotevant, 1987; Cooper, Grotevant, & Condon, 1983; Cooper, Grotevant, Moore, & Condon, 1984; Grotevant & Cooper, 1985).

Clinical utility: The coding procedure is impractical for clinical use.

Research utility: The code appears to be highly relevant for investigations of family and peer interaction, particularly when the research question concerns the role of individuation within the family. Utility of the code as a measure of the individuation construct is so far limited to adolescent samples; its applicability to other developmental stages has yet to be determined.

SUMMARY EVALUATION

The Individuation Code is a microanalytic coding scheme for whole-family units that is designed to measure the theoretical construct of individuation in family relationships. The strength of the code is its clearly delineated theoretical base and strong evidence of construct validity. In addition, a carefully explicated manual of coding procedures is available. The code is limited in its clinical and research utility by the time required for data collection and transcription, as is typical of microanalytic coding systems, and by the lack of normative data. Research utility beyond families with adolescents has yet to be determined.

REFERENCES

Condon, S. L., Cooper, C. R., & Grotevant, H. D. (1984). Manual for the analysis of family discourse. *Psychological Documents, 14,* 8 (Ms. No. 2616)

Cooper, C., & Carlson, C. (1987). *Construct validation of individuation in family relationships during adolescence.* Unpublished manuscript.

Cooper, C. R., & Grotevant, H. D. (1987). Gender issues in the interface of family experience and adolescents' friendship and dating identity. *Journal of Youth and Adolescence, 16,* 247–264.

Cooper, C., Grotevant, H., & Condon, S. (1982). Methodological challenges of selectivity in family interaction: Assessing temporal patterns of individuation. *Journal of Marriage and the Family, 44,* 749–754.

Cooper, C. R., Grotevant, H. D., & Condon, S. M. (1983). Individuality and connectedness in the family as a context for adolescent identity formation and role taking skill. In H. D. Grotevant & C. R. Cooper (Eds.), *Adolescent development in the family: New directions for child development.* San Francisco: Jossey-Bass.

Cooper, C. R., Grotevant, H. D., Moore, M. S., & Condon, S. M. (1984).

Predicting adolescent role taking and identity exploration from family communication patterns: A comparison of one- and two-child families. in T. Falbo (Ed.), *The single child family*. New York: Guilford Press.

Grotevant, H. D., & Cooper, C. R. (1985). Patterns of interaction in family relationships and the development of identity exploration in adolescence. *Child Development, 56*, 415–428.

Grotevant, H. D., & Cooper, C. R. (1986). Individuation in family relationships: A perspective on individual differences in the development of identity and role taking skill in adolescence. *Human Development, 29*, 82–100.

AUTHOR'S COMMENT

In addition to the work reviewed above, the Individuation Code is also appropriate for the analysis of social interaction in other close relationships, such as friendships. Current work with the code involves the use of sequential analysis and log-linear analysis to explore the contingencies between partners in their expressions of individuality and connectedness.

I-11
Interaction Process Coding Scheme
(IPCS)

GENERAL INFORMATION

Date of publication: 1982.

Authors: David C. Bell, Linda G. Bell, and Connie Cornwell.

Source/publisher: Available from the authors at University of Houston at Clear Lake City, 2700 Bay Area Blvd., Houston, TX 77058. Also available through ERIC (Document No. ED 248 420).

Availability: See "Source/publisher," above.

Brief description: This is a microanalytic coding scheme for use with audio- or videotaped marital or family interaction. Five scales are coded: Topic, Orientation, Focus, Support, and Acknowledgment.

Purpose: The purpose is to code marital and family interaction in both clinical and nonclinical populations. It has been used primarily to code interaction around a revealed differences task.

Theoretical base: Family systems theory, with secondary emphases on family communication theory (Wynne) and individuation within the family (Bowen). The Acknowledgment scale is based heavily on that of Mishler and Waxler (1968). Parts of other scales were originally derived from Riskin and Faunce (1969). A major focus is on how participants share the floor.

PHYSICAL DESCRIPTION OF CODE

Task and setting used to elicit behavior: Family members were given the Moos Family Environment Scale individually and then were asked to discuss items on which they disagreed in order to reach a consensus. They were given 6 to 10 slips of paper, in an envelope, to discuss and had about 20 minutes for the task. When the coding scheme is used for discussion other than a revealed differences task, changes have to be made in the Topic scale.

Unit of Study: The task is used with both marital dyads and whole families (up to two parents and three children).

Unit of coding/analysis: Coded "speech units": "A speech unit is the shortest sequence of sounds that has independent meaning in an interpersonal context. Thus a complete sentence with a single independent clause and one or more dependent clauses is the largest unit we identify" (Bell, Bell, & Cornwell, 1982, p. 2). All independent clauses and speech fragments are coded; dependent clauses are coded with their independent clauses as one speech unit unless they change the direction of the thought. Utterances that have no content, such as laughter, and nonverbal behavior, such as shuffling papers, are also unitized as speech units, since the authors believe that this paraverbal communication conveys a critical relationship control message.

Organization of code: The five IPCS scales are designed to be representative of different aspects of the communication process:

Topic: The function of the speech unit in relation to the task:
Not codable for content
Interruptions
Active avoidance of the task
Metatask
Task
Nontask
Floor Control
Orientation: Speaker's point of view as indicated by subject and verb (includes questions, compliance demands, assertion of fact and opinion, and coding of verb tense)
Focus: Reference to behavior, feelings, or ideas, as indicated in the object of the subject–verb; includes feelings, attitudes, thinking process, behaviors, condition, possessions, location.
Support: Level of acceptance or rejection revealed in tone of voice; ranges on a 7-point scale from very supportive to very nonsupportive; two subordinate codes may be paired with the main nonsupport codes to indicate sadness or anxiety.
Acknowledgment: Response to others' contributions; includes no response, explicit invalidation, explicit refusal to respond, recognition, response to focus or intent or both.

Manual: A detailed coding manual has been compiled by the authors. It includes detailed coding conventions, many examples, sample protocols, and sample computer coding sheets.

Standardization and norms: Little published work is available as of yet; consequently, norms are not available. No data are presented in the manual itself.

Evaluation of physical description of code: *Strengths:* The coding manual is very detailed and provides excellent guidance for training. *Weaknesses:* (1) The code is very complex and operates at several levels simultaneously. (2) It takes a very long time to master, as coders require approximately 20 to 30 hours of training to code one scale. (3) No normative data are available. (4) The code organization is weakly integrated with the theoretical base; therefore, actual utility must await availability of multiple investigations.

ADMINISTRATIVE PROCEDURES

Description of equipment needed and observation system: Behavior is audiotaped. Family members wear individual clip-on mikes, and similar-sounding voices are recorded on different channels. Coding is done using the audiotape and typed transcript simultaneously.

Data transcription and reduction: Learning the code requires careful attention to detail. Coders in the Bells' studies were graduate students in behavioral science who had had at least one course in family therapy. Time estimates from manual are 3 to 6 hours for each of the following functions: typing, unitizing, coding each set of scales. (There were four codings: Topic, Orientation and Focus, Acknowledgment, Support.) Coding took approximately 25 hours for a marital transcript and 35 hours for a family transcript. Training requires about 20 to 30 hours per coder. Coders begin work after they have reached a criterion of 70% reliability. A segment of every fifth transcript is checked.

Scoring procedures, including calculation of summary scores: Not discussed in manual; presumably, scores are simple sums. A program for sequential analysis (INTERACT) has also been developed, but it is not discussed in detail in the coding manual.

Evaluation of administrative procedures: *Strengths:* (1) Use of written transcripts enhances reliability. (2) Attention to audiotaping on separate channels increases accuracy of transcripts. *Weaknesses:* Coding is extremely tedious and time-consuming, as is training and supervision of coding. Coders' sophistication (background in family therapy) may interfere with their ability to code without "reading in" inferences that more naive coders might have missed.

EVALUATION OF CODE

Reliability: Interrater reliabilities (percentage agreement) ranged from 71% to 97%, depending on the scale.

Validity: None reported in manual.

Clinical utility: The IPCS might be useful in a diagnostic sense for a clinician, but the coding procedure is totally impractical for clinical use.

Research utility: The coding system allows the researcher to develop scores for system-level constructs. However, it is not clear how the code works to differentiate whole-family from subsystem functioning. The IPCS allows for the creation of a wide variety of theoretically derived variables (see ''Author's Response,'' below). Whether it provides a way to measure the variables important in any particular study must be evaluated on a case-by-case basis.

SUMMARY EVALUATION

Strengths: The data reduction procedure allows for precise preservation of the family's interaction. The coding manual is detailed and provides many examples for coders. The code seems to improve on work by Riskin and Faunce by analyzing speech units that are more like utterances than speeches. *Weaknesses:* The code is very cumbersome and time-consuming to use. It is not clear that the categories of behavior coded would be the pertinent ones for a particular study. As far as we know, the code has been applied only to the authors' samples of 100 families of adolescent girls, collected in 1974, and a sample of child abuse couples collected in 1979–80.

REFERENCES

Bell, D. C., & Bell, L. G. (1981). *Patterns of verbal communication in strong families.* Paper presented at the meeting of the American Psychological Association, Los Angeles. Available from ERIC (Document No. ED 216 280).

Bell, D. C., & Bell, L. G. (1982). *Power and support processes in dual-career marriages.* Paper presented at the meeting of the Texas Council on Family Relations, San Antonio. Available from the authors.

Bell, D. C., & Bell, L. G. (1983). Parental validation and support in the development of adolescent daughters. In H. D. Grotevant and C. R. Cooper (eds.), *Adolescent development in the family: New directions for child development.* San Francisco: Jossey-Bass.

Bell, D. C., Bell, L. G., & Cornwell, C. (1982). *Interaction Process Coding Scheme.* Houston: University of Houston at Clear Lake City.

Bell, L. G., & Bell, D. C. (1979). *The influence of family climate and family process on child development.* Paper presented at the meetings of the International Council of Psychologists, Princeton. Available from ERIC (Document No. ED 178 177).

Mishler, E. G., & Waxler, N. E. (1968). *Interaction in families: An experimental study of family processes and schizophrenia.* New York: Wiley.

Riskin, J. & Faunce, E. E. (1969). *Family Interaction Scales scoring manual.* Palo Alto, CA: Mental Research Institute.

AUTHOR'S RESPONSE

We are presently involved in creating and evaluating reliability for summary variables derived from the IPCS. This includes variables such as "average level of support when father speaks to daughter." Since all codes (except Acknowledgment) are coded on each speech unit, scales can be combined to create particular complex variables. For instance, "husband makes a clear statement of opinion in a neutral tone of voice" involves the combination of codes from three scales: Speaker (husband), Orientation (assertion of fact), and Support (neutral). Or "mother asks a question of her son about his behavior in a negative tone of voice," involves Speaker, Person Addressed, Orientation, Focus, and Support. There are a very large number of such potential variables (for instance, "father makes a statement of fact to the daughter about her emotions in a negative tone of voice" is one such variable that involves the combination of codes from six scales). Thus, it is important that variables be created to serve particular theoretical needs.

I-12
Parent–Adolescent Interaction
Coding System (PAICS)

GENERAL INFORMATION

Date of publication: 1979.

Authors: Arthur Robin and Mary Fox.

Source/publisher: Unpublished *PAICS Training and Reference Manual for Coders*.

Availability: Available from Dr. Arthur Robin, Dept. of Psychology, Children's Hospital of Michigan, Detroit Medical Center, 3901 Beaubien Blvd., Detroit, MI 48201.

Brief description: This is a microanalytic code, based on the Marital Interaction Coding System (MICS) (Weiss, Hops, & Patterson, 1973), that is used "to record objectively all verbal behaviors emitted by parents and adolescents during attempts to solve their problems" (Robin & Fox, 1979, p. 3). The code contains 15 behaviors (7 positive, 5 negative, 3 neutral); one code is given for each "behavior unit."

Purpose: The purpose is "to record objectively all verbal behaviors emitted by parents and adolescents during attempts to solve their problems" (Robin & Fox, 1979, p. 3)

Theoretical base: Social learning theory.

PHYSICAL DESCRIPTION OF CODE

Task and setting used to elicit behavior: Prior to the family interaction session, both parents and the adolescent complete the Issues Checklist, which requires them to recall disagreements about 44 specific issues (smoking, curfew, etc.) Each item checked is also rated for degree of negative affect and frequency of discussing the topic. The topics with highest weighted frequency by anger-intensity scores on the checklists are used to elicit parent–adolescent communication. Families are then asked to discuss and attempt to resolve two problems for 10 minutes each.

Unit of study: Father–mother–adolescent triads in some studies; parent–adolescent dyads in other studies.

Unit of coding/analysis: The "behavior unit":

> A behavior unit is a verbal response which is homogeneous in content without regard to its duration or its arbitrary syntactical properties, such as division into words or sentences. Homogeneity of content is judged with reference to the 15 PAICS categories. In most cases one sentence will be considered one behavior unit. . . . A coder must learn to discriminate behavior units by attending to changes in content only, and then learn to categorize each behavior unit within the 15 behavior categories. (Robin & Fox, 1979, p. 3)

A 30-second timing block is used to facilitate coding; each block is coded at least once and may include many codes, depending on the number of shifts in behavior units.

Organization of code:

Positive Behaviors
  Agree-Assent
  Appraisal
  Consequential Thinking
  Facilitation
  Humor
  Problem Solution
  Specification of the Problem
Negative Behaviors
  Command
  Complain
  Defensive Behavior
  Interrupt
  Put Down
Neutral Behaviors
  No Response
  Problem Description
  Talk

Manual: A training and reference manual is available from the authors. It includes descriptions of coding procedures, definitions of each behavior, and conventions for distinguishing among the different codes.

Standardization and norms: None published.

Evaluation of physical descriptions of code: *Strengths:* The task seems appropriately chosen for eliciting parent–adolescent conflict and discussion over affectively charged issues. The behaviors coded are clearly defined in the manual, as are the coding procedures. *Weaknesses:* The combination of time sampling (30-second intervals) and event sampling seems to be cumbersome; however, it enables coders to code directly from tapes rather than from typed transcripts.

ADMINISTRATIVE PROCEDURES

Description of equipment needed and observation system: Family discussions are audiotaped; coders require tape recorders and beepers that emit a signal every 30 seconds.

Data transcription and reduction: Coding is done from audiotapes without the use of transcripts. A modified time-sampling technique (begin new coding segment every 30 seconds) is used to enhance reliability and pace the coding. A new behavior unit is coded every time the content of the verbal behavior changes and at the beginning of every 30-second interval.

Scoring procedures, including calculation of summary scores: Frequencies of behaviors are summed across the two 10-minute interaction segments. In some studies, frequencies of each behavior for each person are computed. In other studies, behaviors are summed into Positive, Negative, and Neutral categories. Proportions of positive and negative communication behavior for each family member can be computed as well.

Evaluation of administrative procedures: *Strengths:* Audiotapes are used in coding to permit judgments on the basis of tone of voice and other cues. *Weaknesses:* Since transcripts are not used, coders must make on-the-spot judgments of changes in content in order to know when to assign a new code.

EVALUATION OF CODE

Reliability: In one study (Robin, 1981), average product-moment correlations for six pairings of four coders were $r = .92$ for positive parent behavior; $r = .73$ for negative parent behavior; $r = .88$ for positive adolescent behavior; and $r = .87$ for negative adolescent behavior. In the same study, percentage agreement on coding the 15 specific behaviors ranged from 51% to 81% (average $= 64\%$).

Validity: The code has been used to evaluate changes in parent–adolescent communication following problem-solving communication training, alternative family therapy, or no treatment. The group trained in communication skills improved on composite indices measuring problem solving and communication;

the family therapy group improved slightly on communication behavior; the no-treatment group worsened or remained unchanged (Robin, 1981). Using an earlier version of the code (a 23-code version adapted more directly from the Marital Interaction Coding System), 14 distressed and 14 nondistressed mother–adolescent son dyads were compared on the 23 behaviors. The code distinguished between the two groups in predictable ways on 12 of the 23 behaviors (Robin & Weiss, 1980). Concurrent validity of the modified MICS code mentioned above was also established by comparing the results of coding with global ratings of tapes made by family members and mental health professionals. Ratings of conflict, effectiveness of problem solving, and positiveness of communication were correlated $r = .81$, $r = .90$, and $r = .89$, respectively, with the MICS problem-solving composite score (Robin & Canter, 1984).

Clinical utility: The clinical utility of the PAICS seems limited because of the time-consuming nature of the coding process; however, the modified time-sampling technique of this method makes it less time-consuming than many other codes. The content of the coding scheme seems well suited to clinical issues, as there is demonstrated evidence of its effectiveness in differentiating distressed from nondistressed families with adolescents.

Research utility: The coding system seems very accessible to researchers who are interested in issues dealing with communication difficulties in families with adolescents. The system seems particularly well suited to intervention studies that involve communication skill training. Further investigations should be conducted concerning the effect of the training on the parent–adolescent relationship.

SUMMARY EVALUATION

The PAICS seems to be a very useful code for examining parent–adolescent communication around difficult issues. The code, based on a carefully developed marital code, is strongly grounded in social learning theory, is clearly articulated in terms of procedures, and has accrued a fair-sized body of evidence documenting its reliability, validity, and use in intervention programs.

REFERENCES

Robin, A. (1981). A controlled evaluation of problem-solving communication training with parent–adolescent conflict. *Behavior Therapy, 12,* 593–609.
Robin, A. L., & Canter, W. (1984). A comparison of the Marital Interaction Coding System and community ratings for assessing mother–adolescent problem-solving. *Behavioral Assessment, 6,* 303–313.

Robin, A., & Fox, M. (1979). *Parent–Adolescent Interaction Coding System: Training and Reference Manual for Coders.* Unpublished manual. (Available from Arthur Robin)

Robin, A., & Koepke, T. (1982, August). *Global-inferential versus frequency codes for recording parent–adolescent interactions.* Paper presented at the meeting of the American Psychological Association, Washington, DC.

Robin, A. L., & Weiss, J. G. (1980). Criterion-related validity of behavioral and self-report measures of problem-solving communication skills in distressed and non-distressed parent–adolescent dyads. *Behavioral Assessment, 2,* 339–352.

Weiss, R. L., Hops, H., & Patterson, G. R. (1973). A framework for conceptualizing marital conflict: A technology for altering it, some data for evaluating it. In F. W. Clark & L. A. Hammerlynck (Eds.), *Critical issues in research and practice: Proceedings of the Fourth Banff International Conference on Behavior Modification.* Champaign, IL: Research Press.

AUTHOR'S RESPONSE

It should be noted that adequate reliability can be difficult to achieve with this code. Although transcripts of tapes were not used in my research, they are highly recommended whenever possible. The selection of coders is also important. Users of the system need to screen potential coders for interpersonal sensitivity. Older women who have raised children of their own make the most sensitive coders in our experience. We have recently completed a revision of the PAICS, reducing it to six categories, eliminating the 30-second intervals, and simplifying coding procedures. Early trials of the revised PAICS have proved promising.

I-13
Structural Analysis
of Social Behavior (SASB)

GENERAL INFORMATION

Date of publication: 1979.

Author: L. S. Benjamin.

Source/publisher: Benjamin, L. S. (1979). Use of Structural Analysis of Social Behavior and Markov chains to study dyadic interactions. *Journal of Abnormal Psychology, 88,* 303–319.

Availability: A manual with details of the scoring system and software for studying sequences are available upon request from Lorna Smith Benjamin, University of Wisconsin Hospital & Clinics, Dept. of Psychiatry, 600 Highland Ave., Madison, WI 53792.

Brief description: The SASB is a circumplex model of interpersonal relations and their intrapsychic representations. The model proposes that a full array of systemic, interpersonal, and intrapsychic events can be described by the three focuses of attention (other, self, and intrapsychic) and two orthogonal dimensions of affiliation and interdependence. One methodology developed for the SASB is a microanalytic coding process that classifies social interactions and intrapsychic events. (Questionnaires and rating scales are also available.) The SASB model is designed for clinicians to provide reliable and valid diagnosis for psychosocial as well as medical treatment. While applicable to the variety of psychotherapeutic contexts, the SASB has been used to examine pathological family interaction.

Purpose: To provide a methodology for coding observed interactions in the psychotherapeutic context with the goal of rendering psychotherapy process and the study of distressed families scientific.

Theoretical base: Directly related to object relations theory, the personality theories of Murray (1938) and Sullivan (1953) and the interpersonal circumplex model of Leary (1957). The model also has biological roots in ethology, as it is "built on primate behaviors thought to be basic to the evolutionary process".

The SASB is considered to be compatible with structural and communication theories of family therapy and useful in the validation of a variety of theories regarding the familial components of individual dysfunction.

PHYSICAL DESCRIPTION OF CODE

Task and setting used to elicit behavior: No specific task is essential to the use of the SASB. However, because the coding process is microscopic and expensive, the authors recommend using the SASB for relatively brief but intense or "loaded" family process. Examples of tasks that elicit "loaded" process are (1) ask family to reach consensus on how much listening behavior is directed toward the identified patient; (2) ask family to conduct a time-limited, free-flowing discussion on a subject over which there has been a recent disagreement; (3) select critical points during therapy (Benjamin, Giat, & Estroff, 1982, p. 2). Interactions of at least 10 minutes' duration are necessary to the coding process in order to perform sequential analyses of the data. The setting for the SASB has been inpatient clinical population. Interactions are either video- or audiotaped. Videotaping is recommended.

Unit of study: The code is applicable to a range of units. Up to seven "referents" may be assigned to each session. Referents may be individuals, coalitions, the family group, absent family members, abstract forces, or society.

Unit of coding/analysis: The primary unit of coding/analysis is the *"element,"* defined as "a complete thought" or "psychologically meaningful interaction." A given unit or individual speech utterance may have several elements.

Organization of code: Each element is coded for

1. Who Speaks to Whom
2. Process (here and now transaction)
3. Content (what is being talked about)
4. Focus (other, self, introjection)
5. Affiliation (very friendly to very unfriendly)
6. Interdependence (very autonomous to very submissive)

The Focus, Affiliation, and Interdependence codings are combined into a final (Topic) clinical code for the *element* that represents one of the cluster classification categories of the circumplex model. A recent revision (1984) of the SASB utilizes an 18-point versus a 5-point Affiliation–Interdependence coding.

Manual: An unpublished manual is available from the author. Coding procedures and examples, training of coders, data transcription and reduction, and reliability are described. Description of the SASB model requires use of additional sources.

Evaluation of physical description of code: *Strengths:* The code is designed to be broadly applicable for use in family research and in clinical settings to examine the psychotherapeutic process. *Limitations:* The SASB model and accompanying coding process are complex and require considerable clinical skill or time to master. Use of a circumplex model for the final codes used in the SASB requires multiple inference decisions by the coder, thus increasing the probability of error with each decision. The circumplex model also makes differentiation of adjacent code classifications difficult.

ADMINISTRATIVE PROCEDURES

Description of equipment needed and observation system: Interactive behavior to be coded is audio- or video-recorded. Videotapes are preferred because the nonverbal behavior and context of a speech are used to make coding decisions. Field recorders have not been used successfully with the SASB coding process.

Data transcription and reduction: Typescripts of the recorded interaction are prepared to define units of speech. Trained coders first examine the recorded interaction as a whole to "get a feel" for the interaction but then code from the typescript. Finally, coders review the recorded interaction to be sure that what they have coded really fits what is on the tape. Coders rate the speech unit of analysis on Focus, Affiliation, and Interdependence and then, following the logic of the SASB model, generate a cluster judgment. The cluster judgment is the primary code of data analysis interest, although the coding system is flexible in its ability to generate various constructs of interest. Data are analyzed using sequential analysis. Computer programs have been developed by the authors for use with the coding schema.

Considerable discussion is provided regarding the training of coders. The SASB is a complex, microscopic system that is expensive and requires fairly extensive coder training. A trial period of 6 training hours is provided to screen coders for their responsiveness to learning the code. Basic coder training takes 60 to 80 hours, with training sessions of 2 hours each and approximately 2 hours of homework prior to each session. Clinically inexperienced students may take 60 to 100 hours to train, plus "hundreds of hours of training and coding" to become "experts." Expert clinicians have mastered SASB coding in 12 to 15 hours. An outline of the training program is provided in the manual.

Scoring procedures: After rating Focus, Affiliation, and Interdependence, the SASB model is used to generate a cluster judgment that best fits the element of speech. This is followed by a clinical judgment by the coder, using paralinguistic cues and context to decide among alternative codings. Computer programs are used to summarize variables and to perform sequential analyses.

Evaluation of administrative procedures: *Strengths:* Utilization of both recorded and typescript methods for coding decisions. *Limitations:* The SASB model and coding process require extensive coder training and/or high entry-level skill. Coders are required to make high-level inferences about family interaction.

EVALUATION OF CODE

Reliability: Reliability of the SASB code is determined using Cohen's weighted kappa. Benjamin et al. (1984) reported kappas for process codes ranging from .65 to .78 and .62 to .86 for content ratings. Kappas were shown to improve with additional training (process code range: .74 to .91; content mean: .89) The kappa tends to be a conservative estimate of reliability but essential for sequentially analyzed data.

Validity: *Construct:* The SASB code was compared with the modified Marital Interaction Coding System and was found to provide a better explanation of clinical phenomena (Humphrey, Apple, & Kirschenbaum, 1986). (*Note:* The constructs of the SASB model have been carefully validated with the questionnaire methodology (see Humphrey & Benjamin, 1986). *Criterion-related:* The SASB differentiated bulimic-anorexic from normal families (Humphrey, Apple, & Kirschenbaum, 1986).

Clinical utility: The SASB model and coding process are designed for clinical use; therefore, unlike many coding systems with a singular research orientation, this system emphasizes constructs of interest to clinicians. Although the expense of coder training might discourage clinical use, learning the SASB enhances clinical skill, according to the author (L. S. Benjamin, personal communication, November 30, 1984).

Research utility: A strength of the SASB is its potential usefulness in research with any theoretical model of psychotherapy or family functioning (Humphrey & Benjamin, 1986). On the other hand, the initial complexity of the SASB system, and the cost of coder training, may discourage broad application.

SUMMARY EVALUATION

The SASB represents a unique model and parallel multitrait, multimethod assessment for classifying interpersonal transactions. It is one of the few coding schemes oriented toward research investigations of family process in psychotherapy. As such, the SASB represents an important contribution to both clinical and social science research. Limitations of the SASB coding scheme are (1) considerable coder training is necessary to gain adequate reliability with the highly inferential coding process and the complex theoretical system; and (2) although the validity of the SASB model is well established, published validity in studies of the SASB coding system applied to family interaction is limited. Revisions of the coding scheme are in progress and are expected to improve reliability.

REFERENCES

Benjamin, L. S. (1974). Structural analysis of social behavior. *Psychological Review, 81,* 392–425.

Benjamin, L. S. (1979). Use of Structural Analysis of Social Behavior and Markov chains to study dyadic interactions. *Journal of Abnormal Psychology, 88,* 303–319.

Benjamin, L. S. (1984). Principles of prediction using Structural Analysis of Social Behavior (SASB). In R. A. Zucker, J. Aronoff and A. J. Robin (Eds.), *Personality and the prediction of behavior.* New York: Academic Press.

Benjamin, L. S. (1986). Operational definition and measurement of dynamics shown in the stream of free associations. *Psychiatry, 49,* 104–130.

Benjamin, L. S., Foster, S. W., Giat-Roberto, L., & Estroff, S. E. (1984). Breaking the family code: Analyzing videotapes of family interactions by Structural Analysis of Social Behavior. In L. Greenberg & W. Pinsoff (Eds.), *Psychotherapeutic process: A research handbook.* New York: Guilford Press.

Benjamin, L. S., Giat, L., & Estroff, S. E. (1981). *Manual for coding social interactions in terms of Structural Analysis of Social Behavior (SASB).* Unpublished manuscript, University of Wisconsin.

Humphrey, L. L., Apple, R. F., & Kirschenbaum, D. S. (1986). Differentiating bulimic-anorexic from normal families using interpersonal and behavioral observation systems. *Journal of Consulting and Clinical Psychology, 54,* 190–195.

Humphrey, L. L., & Benjamin, L. S. (1986). Using Structural Analysis of Social Behavior to assess critical but elusive family processes: A new solution to an old problem. *American Psychologist, 41*(9), 979–989.

Leary, T. (1957). *Interpersonal diagnosis of personality: A functional theory and methodology for personality evaluation.* New York: Ronald Press.

Murray, H. A. (1938). *Explorations in personality.* New York: Oxford University Press.

Sullivan, H. S. (1953). *The interpersonal theory of psychiatry.* New York: Norton.

AUTHOR'S RESPONSE

Your repeated emphasis on the "high level of inference" required for SASB is your rightful opinion, but I would like you to know that it makes me think that I have not succeeded in communicating what SASB is. If I were to write about the strengths, I would say that by following a relatively simple three-step procedure, an infinite number of clinically important SASB codes can be reliably generated. Three not-very-inferential judgments about focus, affiliation, interdependence, generate codes of quite abstract concepts. Complex concepts like double bind, pseudo mutuality, internal conflict, can be identified at a very respectable level of reliability. Given the complexity of the task that is accomplished by this code, the level of inference is amazingly small. These judgments can reliably be made by expert clinicians with little training, or by unsophisticated college graduates with extensive training.

Section V
Abstracts of Rating Scales

R-1
Beavers-Timberlawn Family
Evaluation Scale (BTFES)

GENERAL INFORMATION

Date of publication: 1976.

Authors: J. M. Lewis, W. R. Beavers, J. T. Gossett, and V. A. Phillips

Source/publisher: Lewis, J. M., Beavers, W. R., Gossett, J. T., & Phillips, V. A. (1976). *No single thread.* New York: Brunner/Mazel.

Availability: The scale is printed in cited sources. A descriptive manual and additional psychometric information is available from the Southwest Family Institute, 12532 Nuestra, Dallas, TX 75230.

Brief description: The BTFES is a 13-subscale observational rating instrument designed to evaluate level of family functioning based on videotaped family interaction.

Purpose: The purpose of the Family Evaluation Scale is to provide a quantitative index of family health/pathology on continuums representing a family systems framework. It is designed to be used in conjunction with the Centripetal/Centrifugal Family Style Scale.

Theoretical base: Beavers Systems Model of Family Functioning

PHYSICAL DESCRIPTION OF RATING SCALE

Task and setting used to elicit behavior: Family interaction is videotaped in a clinical setting. Ratings of behavior are based on 10 to 15 minutes of interaction. The eliciting task for a clinical population is: "Discuss together what you would like to change about your family as a result of therapy."

Unit of study: Whole family.

Scales and dimensions: The Family Evaluation Scale consists of 13 subscales and a Global Health–Pathology scale. The 13 subscales are rated on 5-point scales, with nine anchor points provided by half-point gradations. Headings, subscales, and measured dimensions are:

I. Structure of Family: Subscales—Overt Power (chaos to egalitarian); Parental Coalition (parent–child to strong parental); Closeness (indistinct boundaries to close, distinct boundaries).
II. Mythology (very reality congruent to very reality incongruent)
III. Goal-Directed Negotiations (efficient to inefficient problem solving)
IV. Autonomy: Subscales—Clarity of Expression (clear to unclear expression of thoughts and feelings); Responsibility (regularly to rarely voice responsibility for actions); Invasiveness (members speaking for one another); Permeability (very open to unreceptive to statements of others).
V. Family Affect: Subscales—Range of Feelings (open, direct to no expression of feelings); Mood and Tone (warm, optimistic, humorous to cynical, hopeless, pessimistic); Unresolvable Conflict (severe to none); Empathy (consistent, empathic responsiveness to grossly inappropriate responses to feelings).
VI. Global Health/Competence (most healthy/competent to least healthy/ pathological)

The Beavers Systems Model of family assessment additionally integrates a second major dimension, Family Style. This dimension is assessed by means of the Centripetal/Centrifugal Family Style Scale, which is described separately (see next abstract).

Manual: Descriptions of appropriate theoretical and operational interpretations of each code category are provided.

Standardization and norms: In process; not currently available in literature.

Evaluation of physical description of rating scale: *Strengths:* Scales are consistent with theoretical framework. Although each of the nine anchor points is not defined, three to five gradations within the continuum are clarified with descriptions. This is particularly necessary, as many of the subscale dimensions do not represent a logical continuum (i.e. from less to more) but, rather, represent a health/pathology continuum, which may vary from a direct, linear progression. *Limitations:* (1) Subscales blend two or more construct continuums within the same rating dimension (e.g. the Overt Power subscale blends the dimensions of power with flexibility/rigidity; the Closeness subscale blends intimacy with boundary clarity; the Clarity of Expression subscale blends expression of thoughts with expression of feelings and blends expression with clarity; the Conflict subscale blends level of confict with impairment to group functioning). This can be expected to decrease reliability of ratings and to increase demands for observers to be highly familiar with the particular theoretical framework employed.

ADMINISTRATIVE PROCEDURES

Description of equipment needed: Ratings are based on videotaped family interaction; therefore, videotaping equipment and/or a one-way observation mirror is required.

Training: General familiarization with family systems theory and specific familiarity with the Beavers Systems Model of Family Functioning are helpful but not required.

Special issues for raters: There may be difficulty in rating the family as a whole when individuals or dyads within the family vary. Rater fatigue from extended rating periods may lead to reduced accuracy of ratings.

Scoring procedures: Each individual dimension is assigned a numerical value. To score the BTFES, first reverse identified subscales. Once reversals are taken into account, standardize the first 12 subscale scores, convert to a 10-point scaling (with a mean of 5 and a standard deviation of 1). Next, sum across all 13 subscales, and average. This score is compared with the Global subscale score as an "ecological check." The average subscale score can then be placed on the Beavers Model map for conceptual clarity.

Evaluation of administrative procedure: *Strengths:* Use of videotape allows the observer to replay the family interaction, which may increase rater reliability. *Limitations:* There is a lack of information on rater training and a lack of treatment of special issues for raters. It is expected, based on the theoretical embeddedness of these scales, that reliable rating would require mastery of family systems theory.

EVALUATION OF CONSTRUCTS MEASURED

Reliability: Interrater reliability is published for the Family Evaluation Scale only. Interrater reliability (correlations) on the scales (1) for two sets of two coders and (2) for subsequent evaluations (Y. F. Hulgus, personal communication, 1985):

	$N = 36$	$N = 12$	$N = 93-157$	
Overt Power	.45	.66	.66	141
Parental Coalitions	.20 (NS)	.67	.60	93
Closeness	.47	.60	.58	157
Mythology	.31	.60	—	
Goal-Directed Negotiations	.69	.65	.70	156
Clarity of expression	.41	.17 (NS)	.69	156

	$N=36$	$N=12$	$N=93-157$	
Responsibility	.30	.26 (NS)	.66	156
Invasiveness	.21 (NS)	.73	—	
Permeability	.17 (NS)	.71	.58	156
Range of Feelings	.25	.29	.67	156
Mood and Tone	.31	.82	.74	157
Unresolvable Conflict	.36	.65	.77	157
Empathy	.34	.57	.68	157
Global Health/Competence	—	—	.79	157
Sum of scales:	.45	.82	.84	93

The improving interrater correlations suggest that considerable training is necessary for reliable use of this measure; nevertheless, several dimensions remain unacceptably low in reliability.

With intensive training of experienced family therapists, by retaining a specific constellation of raters, and by eliminating troublesome items, Green, Kolevzon, and Vosler (1985) attained an average reliability of .90; however, unacceptably low interrater reliability was reported, consistent with the Timberlawn associates, for the subscales of Mythology (.54) and Invasiveness (.30).

Validity: The BTFES obtained significant correlations between all subscales and between all subscales and the Global Family Health Pathology Scale. *Criterion:* With few exceptions, the BTFES subscales significantly differentiated healthy and patient-containing families (Lewis et al., 1976). *Convergent:* Green et al. (1985) found minimal convergence between their version of the BTFES and the FACES. However, Beavers, Hampson, and Hulgus (1985) found moderate to high correlations between the Health factor of their self-report version of the BTFES (the SFI) and FACES II dimensions ($r=.64$ for Adaptability; $r=.82$ for Cohesion) but moderate to low correlations between the SFI and Green et al. 1985).

Clinical utility: As a measure based on family systems theory, the scales have considerable clinical potential. Limitations to clinical utility lie in (1) the failure to construct scale dimensions with clear continuums, (2) the blurring of several constructs within one scale, (3) unacceptable reliability of several scales, (4) high level of family therapy expertise and/or training required, and (5) the upper middle class bias inherent in some of the scales (e.g., egalitarian style of power viewed as most healthy).

Research utility: The BTFES was designed for research purposes and has demonstrated some utility in this area, particularly the Global Family Functioning Scale. Additional research is necessary to determine the research utility of the entire measure and its utility across socioeconomic groups.

SUMMARY EVALUATION

The primary strength of the BTFES lies in its theoretical integration with family systems theory. The primary weaknesses are (1) anchor points are poorly defined on some scales; (2) scales do not necessarily represent a logical continuum and a single construct and, in some cases, are socioculturally biased; (3) norms are not available; and (4) considerable clinical skill is required for raters.

REFERENCES

Beavers, J., Hampson, R. B., Hulgus, Y.F., & Beavers, W. R. (1986). Coping in families with a retarded child. *Family Process, 25,* 365–378.

Beavers, W. R., Hampson, R. B., & Hulgus, Y. F. (1985). Commentary: The Beavers Systems approach to family assessment. *Family Process, 24,* 398–405.

Beavers, W.R., & Voeller, M. N. (1983). Family models: Comparing and contrasting the Olson Circumplex Model with the Beavers Systems Model. *Family Process, 22,* 85–98.

Green, R. G., Kolevzon, M.S., & Vosler, N. R. (1985). The Beavers-Timberlawn Model of Family Competence and the Circumplex Model of Family Adaptability and Cohesion: Separate but equal? *Family Process, 24,* 385–398.

Hulgus, Y.F. (1982). *Beavers-Timberlawn Family Evaluation Scale and family style evaluation manual.* (Available from Southwest Family Institute, Dallas, TX)

Hulgus, Y.F. (1985). *Scoring guide for the Beavers-Timberlawn Family Evaluation Scale and the Centripetal/Centrifugal Family Style Scale.* (Available from Southwest Family Institute, Dallas, TX)

Lewis, J. M., Beavers, W. R., Gossett, J. T., and Phillips, Y. A. (1976). *No single thread: Psychological health in family systems.* New York: Brunner/Mazel.

AUTHOR'S RESPONSE

We are addressing several limitations described in this review of the Beavers-Timberlawn Family Evaluation Scale. We feel that some of the criticisms are not valid in light of the conceptual frame of the scale.

First, much psychometric evaluation of the scale is in progress, with publication dates expected in the coming year. Further, materials for rater training are in preparation. To date, however, all rater training is accomplished through seminars and practice. It is our experience that raters do not have to master family systems theory to become reliable, but a good working knowledge of systems theory and the Beavers Family Systems Model is most helpful. Second, the comments concerning the "blending" of constructs within subscales would be appropriate if the scales were purported to be unitary and orthogonal, which they are not. The notions contained in any subscale are highly interrelated under the Beavers Systems Model, and reflect systemic evaluation as opposed to assessing discrete bits of familial behavior. The subscales are designed to direct the rater's attention to the most salient aspects of family functioning, according to the Beavers Systems Model. Since the totality of the scale is what is most useful, and not any subscale in isolation, and since (1) the scale shows good internal consistency (Cronbach's alpha = .94) and (2) there is high interrater reliability for the average of the subscales, it is our opinion that lower individual subscale interrater reliabilities are not a major limitation. Finally, extensive experience has suggested to us that this scale works well with a wide variety of economic, racial, and cultural groups (J. Beavers, Hampson, Hulgus, and Beavers, 1986).

R-2
Centripetal/Centrifugal Family Style
Scale (CP/CF)

GENERAL INFORMATION

Date of publication: 1981.

Author(s): M. Kelsey-Smith and W. R. Beavers.

Source/publisher: Kelsey-Smith, M., & Beavers, W. R. (1981). Family assessment: Centripetal and Centrifugal family systems. *American Journal of Family Therapy, 9,* 3–12.

Availability: The scale is printed in cited sources. A descriptive manual and additional psychometric information are available from the Southwest Family Institute, 12532 Nuestra, Dallas, TX 75230.

Brief description: The Centripetal/Centrifugal Family Style Scale (CP/CF) is a nine-item rating scale designed to assess a family's style of "being" as a systemic unit.

Purpose: The purpose of the CP/CF is to rate family stylistic characteristics without bias regarding family health/competence. The scale is designed to be used in conjunction with the Beavers-Timberlawn Family Evaluation Scale.

Theoretical base: Beavers Systems Model of Family Functioning.

PHYSICAL DESCRIPTION OF RATING SCALE

Task and setting used to elicit behavior: Family interaction is videotaped in a clinical setting. Ratings of behavior are based on 10 to 15 minutes of interaction. The eliciting task for a clinical population is: "Discuss together what you would like to change about your family as a result of therapy."

Unit of study: Whole family.

Scales and dimensions: The CP/CF consists of nine subscales assessing the areas of Dependency Needs, Styles of Adult Conflict, Proximity, Social Presentation, Verbal Expression of Closeness, Aggressive/Assertive Behaviors, Expression of Positive/Negative Feelings, Internal Scapegoating, and a Global Family Style rating. The first eight subscales are rated on 5-point scales with appropriate descriptors along their continuums, with the Global rating providing half-point anchors.

The Beavers Systems Model of family assessment additionally integrates a second major dimension, Family Health/Competence. This dimension is assessed by means of the Beavers-Timberlawn Family Evaluation Scale, which is described separately (see preceding abstract).

Manual: Descriptions of appropriate theoretical and operational interpretation of each code category are provided.

Standardization and Norms: In process; not currently available in literature.

Evaluation of physical description of rating scale: The defined anchor points on this scale appear to be clear; typically, however, only three of five points are defined, leaving midpoint ratings difficult to evaluate. Moreover, several subscales require not only aggregate decisions by raters but also inferences regarding the interval states of family members, (e.g., ease of expression of positive feelings versus frequency of expression), which can be expected to reduce reliability.

ADMINISTRATIVE PROCEDURES

Description of equipment needed: Ratings are based on observation of family interactions; therefore, videotaping equipment and/or a one-way observation mirror is required.

Training: General familiarization with family systems theory and specific familiarity with the Beavers Systems Model of Family Functioning are helpful but not required.

Special issues for raters: There may be difficulty in rating the family as a whole when individuals or dyads within the family vary. Rater fatigue from extended rating periods may lead to reduced accuracy of ratings.

Scoring procedures: Each individual subscale is assigned a numerical value. To score the CP/CF, first reverse identified subscales. Once reversals are taken into account, sum across all subscales, and average. This score is compared to the Global subscale score as an "ecological check." The average subscale score can then be placed on the Beavers Model map for conceptual clarity.

Evaluation of administration procedure: *Strengths:* Use of videotape allows the observer to replay the family interaction, which may increase rater reliability. *Limitations:* There is a lack of information on rater training and a lack of treatment of special issues for raters. It is expected, based on the theoretical embeddedness of these scales, that reliable rating would require mastery of family systems theory and, of course, the Beavers Family System Model.

EVALUATION OF CONSTRUCTS MEASURED

Reliability: Kelsey-Smith and Beavers (1981) report significant (.05) interrater reliability on 11 of 12 subscales of the original version of the CP/CF scale ($N = 42$). Interrater reliability for the revised CP/CF yields (Hulgus, 1985):

	r	N
Social Presentation	.54	156
Verbal Expression of Closeness	.62	156
Positive Expression of Feelings	.63	156
Parental/Adult Conflict	.71	108
Parental Control—Clinging	.33	156
Parental Control—Aggressive	.39	156
Global Family Style	.63	108
Sum of subscales	.68	108

Reliability coefficients for three of the nine subscales are not provided: Dependency, Physical Spacing, and Scapegoating. Details regarding reliability are not provided. Reliability appears to be unacceptable for the Parental Control subscales.

Validity: *Construct:* Significant CP/CF differences were obtained in 6 of the 11 scales (original version), with 2 additional scales approaching significance in a sample of 42 families who were midrange in level of competence. CP families contrasted sharply with CF families in their marital descriptions, concern with social correctness, emphasis on family conflict, expression of positive feelings, and display of overt parental conflict. Less significantly, CP families were likely to scapegoat one family member and to discourage independent, aggressive behavior on the part of their children (Kelsey-Smith & Beavers, 1981). Based on this investigation, two subscales were dropped from the current CP/CF Scale.

Clinical utility: Preliminary investigation suggests that the CP/CF Scale may differentiate family style and thus provide guidance regarding appropriate intervention. However, additional research is necessary to confirm clinical utility. Limited documentation in published materials of rater expertise and training requirements currently constrains widespread utilization.

Research utility: Preliminary investigation (Kelsey-Smith & Beavers, 1981) indicates that the CP/CF Scale may differentiate family styles; however, the utility of this differentiation remains to be determined by subsequent research.

SUMMARY EVALUATION

The primary advantage of the CP/CF is its theoretical fit with the Beavers Systems Model of Family Functioning, thus providing the clinician or researcher with the ability to "map" or "locate" a family systematically within a conceptual framework. Additionally, the CP/CF subscales are relatively straightforward and comprehensible. The low reliability of the Parental Control scales begs for clarification: Is the task failing to elicit an adequate sample of this behavior, or is the construct being measured obscure? The clinical and research utility of the scale await further investigation of its merits.

REFERENCES

Beavers, W. R., Hampson, R. B., & Hulgus, Y. F. (1985). Commentary: The Beavers Systems approach to family assessment. *Family Process, 24,* 398–405.
Beavers, W. R., & Voeller, M. N. (1983). Family models: Comparing and contrasting the Olson Circumplex Model with the Beavers Systems Model. *Family Process, 22,* 85–98.
Hulgus, Y. F. (1982). *Beavers-Timberlawn Family Evaluation Scale and family style evaluation manual.* (Available from Southwest Family Institute, Dallas, TX)
Hulgus, Y.F. (1985). *Scoring guide for the Beavers-Timberlawn Family Evaluation Scale (BT) and the Centripetal/Centrifugal Family Style Scale (CP/CF).* (Available from Southwest Family Institute, Dallas, TX)
Kelsey-Smith, M., & Beavers, W. R. (1981). Family Assessment: Centripetal and centrifugal family systems. *American Journal of Family Therapy, 9,* 3–12.

AUTHOR'S RESPONSE

Several criticisms found in this review of the Centripetal/Centrifugal Family Style Scale are in the process of being addressed. Much psychometric evaluation of the scale is in progress, with publication dates expected in the coming year. Further, materials for rater training are in preparation. To date, however, all rater training is accomplished through seminars and practice. It is our experience that raters do not have to master family systems theory to become reliable, but a good working knowledge of systems theory and the Beavers Family Systems Model is most helpful.

It is important to note that the Beavers-Timberlawn Family Evaluation Scale and the Centripetal/Centrifugal Family Style Scale were reviewed separately, yet these instruments are integrated into a unified family assessment system. In fact, these instruments comprise the observational level of the system, with our Self-Report Family Inventory (Beavers, Hampson, and Hulgus, 1985) representing the self-report level of the assessment scheme. Given the fact that these instruments work together, the use of any of the three in isolation reduces the utility of the information obtained.

These instruments have been published separately, which may, therefore, be somewhat confusing. To correct this confusion, we have revised and integrated our observational scales into a single assessment scheme—the Beavers Observational Systems Scales. This is used in conjunction with our family self-report instrument, which was developed from the same conceptual framework. In doing so, we have addressed some of the limitations cited in the reviews of the BT and CP/CF. We expect that these revisions will lead to greater ease of use and an increased interrater reliability.

R-3
Clinical Rating Scale for the Circumplex Model of Marital and Family Systems

GENERAL INFORMATION

Date of publication: 1985.

Authors: David H. Olson and Elinor Killorin.

Source/publisher: Available from the author (see below).

Availability: Available from David H. Olson, Dept. of Family Social Science, University of Minnesota, 290 McNeal Hall, St. Paul, MN 55108.

Brief description: The Clinical Rating Scale allows a clinician to make global ratings of marital and family systems on the basis of a semistructured family interview. Following the interview, the clinician rates the family on subscales for three major dimensions: cohesion, adaptability, and communication. On the basis of the cohesion and adaptability ratings, families may be placed on the Circumplex Model grid.

Purpose: The purpose of the Clinical Rating Scale is to allow clinicians to describe the type of marital or family system being evaluated in order to identify what characteristics might be most useful to focus on in terms of intervention.

Theoretical base: Family systems theory; specifically, the Circumplex Model of Marital and Family Systems

PHYSICAL DESCRIPTION OF RATING SCALE

Task and setting used to elicit behavior: The semistructured clinical interview should be structured to elicit information about family cohesion, adaptability, and communication. No specific format is prescribed, although the authors recommend an interview that asks the family to engage in a discussion with one another about how they handle general family issues such as time, space, discipline, and so on. "Asking the family to describe what a typical week is like and how they handle their daily routines, decision-making, and conflict is often illuminating" (see manual).

Unit of study: May be used with couples or families.

Scales and dimensions: The three major constructs derive directly from the Circumplex Model and are all assessed by the Clinical Rating Scale. Anchor points for all dimensions are clearly specified in tables supplied with the scales. The psychological distance between scale points seems to be roughly equal. The dimensions assessed include the following:

1. *Cohesion.* Each dimension is rated on a scale of 1 (disengaged) to 8 (enmeshed):
   Emotional Bonding
   Family Involvement
   Marital Relationship
   Parent–Child Coalitions
   Internal Boundaries
   External Boundaries
2. *Adaptability.* Each dimension is rated on a scale of 1 (rigid) to 8 (chaotic):
   Leadership
   Discipline
   Negotiation
   Roles
   Rules
3. *Communication.* Each dimension is rated on a scale of 1 (low) to 6 (high):
   Continuity Tracking
   Respect and Regard
   Clarity
   Freedom of Expression
   Listener's Skills
   Speaker's Skills

Manual: A brief manual is available. It provides instructions for use and tables listing the criteria for the various ratings (available from Olson).

Standardization and norms: None.

Evaluation of physical description of rating scale: Although no formal manual is available, descriptions of the anchor points to be covered are provided. No standardized data collection procedure is specified; although this provides the therapist with flexibility in assessment, it makes standardization of the technique problematic.

ADMINISTRATIVE PROCEDURES

Description of equipment needed: Sessions can be videotaped or audiotaped.

Training: No training is required; instructions assume that the instrument will be used by therapists or family researchers.

Special issues for raters: None of these issues are directly addressed. It is assumed that the following biases could affect data collected with this instrument: halo effects, leniency/severity, error of central tendency, logical error, contrast error, proximity error. The amount of relevant contact with subjects is not standardized; clinicians who are very familiar with certain families may use information other than that contained in the interview to make judgments.

Scoring procedures: After the interview, the therapist rates each dimension on the appropriate scale. On the basis of *global* ratings (only one rating for each dimension), the family is placed on the Circumplex Model grid. The communication dimension does not play a role in the placement of the family on the grid; it is considered the "facilitating dimension."

Evaluation of administrative procedures: The technique for administering the rating scale is very flexible; however, this appears to be the authors' intent. Little attention has been paid to the special issues that rating scales must deal with (see above).

EVALUATION OF CONSTRUCTS MEASURED

Reliability: Using five raters in a study of 45 families, average interrater reliabilities of .88 for cohesion, .84 for adaptability, and .92 for communication were obtained. Agreement within 1 point on global ratings was 91% for cohesion, 89% for adaptability, and 94% for communication.

Validity: No studies available.

Clinical utility: The primary purpose of the scale is for clinical practice. No published studies have yet demonstrated its usefulness.

Research utility: No published studies have yet demonstrated research utility.

SUMMARY EVALUATION

The major strengths of this instrument seem to be its flexibility for use in a clinical setting with both families and couples and its clear ties to the Circumplex Model. Its major weaknesses include unknown qualities of reliability and validity, inattention to rating scale issues such as halo effects, and failure to utilize ratings on the third dimension of communication in any meaningful way.

REFERENCES

Olson, D. H. & Killorin, E. (1985). *Clinical Rating Scale for the Circumplex Model of Marital and Family Systems.* St. Paul: University of Minnesota, Department of Family Social Science.

Olson, D. H., Russell, C. S., & Sprenkle, D. H. (1983). Circumplex Model VI: Theoretical update. *Family Process, 22,* 69–83.

Olson, D. H., Sprenkle, D. H., & Russell, C. S. (1979). Circumplex Model of Marital and Family Systems: I. Cohesion and adaptability dimensions, family types, and clinical applications. *Family Process, 18,* 3–28.

AUTHOR'S RESPONSE

A large study of family interaction is currently being conducted, which will yield formal reliability and validity statistics for the scale. The Family Social Science Department has records of approximately 50 studies that have used or are using the CRS; these are available from the author for an additional charge.

R-4
FAM Clinical Rating Scale (FAM-CRS)

GENERAL INFORMATION

Date of publication: 1986.

Authors: Harvey A. Skinner and Paul D. Steinhauer.

Source/publisher: Addiction Research Foundation, Toronto, Ontario, Canada.

Availability: Available from Dr. Harvey Skinner, Addiction Research Foundation, 33 Russell St., Toronto, Ontario, Canada M5S2S1.

Brief description: The FAM-CRS rates family functioning according to the Process Model of Family Functioning. It is dimensionally consistent with the self-report Family Assessment Measure (FAM-III). The CRS is designed to be used with a structured clinical interview currently under development by the authors.

Purpose: To provide observational indices of family functioning in accordance with the Process Model of Family Functioning.

Theoretical base: Process Model of Family Functioning (Steinhauer, Santa-Barbara, & Skinner, 1984).

PHYSICAL DESCRIPTION OF RATING SCALE

Task and setting used to elicit behavior: The FAM-CRS is designed to be used in conjunction with a structured clinical interview.

Unit of study: Primarily whole family; dyadic relationships are rated in one item.

Scales and dimensions: The FAM-CRS consists of six subscales or dimensions: Task Accomplishment; Role Performance; Communication; Involvement; Control; and Values and Norms. Each subscale is rated on a 5-point Likert scale (1 = major strength, 5 = major weakness, or NA = not assessed/not appropriate) with all anchor points defined. Items within each subscale are differentiated into the categories of Essential Processes and Critical Aspects. All subscales correspond with a subscale on the self-report FAM-III; however, the Affective Expression subscale of the FAM-III is nested under Communication in the FAM-CRS.

Manual: None.

Standardization and norms: None.

Evaluation of physical description of rating scale: *Strengths:* (1) Theoretically derived; (2) dimensionally consistent with FAM-III self-report measure, permitting multimethod evaluation of family functioning; (3) all anchor points clearly defined; (4) quality of dyadic relationships within the family assessed in one subscale. *Limitations:* Because of recent development, lack of essential information for reliable use.

ADMINISTRATIVE PROCEDURES

Description of equipment needed: None.

Training: Training manual and videotapes are currently being developed.

Special issues for raters: Familiarity with the Process Model of Family Functioning is a specified prerequisite.

Scoring procedures: Simple addition of scores appears to be the scoring method.

Evaluation of administrative procedure: *Strengths:* None noted. *Limitations:* Because of recent development, lack of essential information for reliable administration and training of raters.

EVALUATION OF CONSTRUCTS MEASURED

Reliability: No published or unpublished data.

Validity: No published or unpublished data.

Clinical utility: The FAM-CRS would appear to have considerable clinical utility, depending on the adequacy of published resources for reliable administration, scoring, and interpretation.

Research utility: The FAM-CRS would appear to have potential research utility as a method of evaluating family interactive process that is theoretically based and that corresponds with a self-report measure of family functioning, the FAM-III. As noted, demonstrated research utility awaits publication of procedures and psychometric validation studies.

SUMMARY EVALUATION

Strengths of the FAM-CRS include its theoretical derivation, dimensional consistency with the self-report FAM-III, clearly written items, well-defined anchor points, and the assessment of dyadic relationships within at least one dimension. Because the FAM-CRS has been recently developed, information critical to the reliable use of the instrument is currently unavailable and empirical validation studies have not yet been conducted. A further consideration, noted by the authors, is the necessity of familiarity with the Process Model of Family Functioning for valid use.

REFERENCES

Skinner, H. A., & Steinhauer, P. D. (1986). *Family Assessment Measure Clinical Rating Scale*. Toronto: Addiction Research Foundation.
Skinner, H. A., Steinhauer, P.D., & Santa-Barbara, J. (1984). The Family Assessment Measure. *Canadian Journal of Community Mental Health,* 2(2), 91–105.
Steinhauer, P.D., Santa-Barbara, J., & Skinner, H. (1984). The Process Model of Family Functioning. *Canadian Journal of Psychiatry, 29,* 77–87.

AUTHOR'S RESPONSE

Presently, we are giving considerable attention to the development of a structured clinical interview, based on the Process Model, that can be used to stimulate sufficient information for completing the Clinical Rating Scale. Over the next year, we will be developing a comprehensive manual and training program for interviewer and raters, as well as conducting validation studies in which therapists' ratings using the Clinical Rating Scale will be compared with family self-reports using FAM. We believe that each assessment instrument will provide a useful complement to the other.

R-5
Family Interaction Q-Sort (FIQ)

GENERAL INFORMATION

Date of publication: 1981.

Authors: Per Gjerde, Jack Block, and Jeanne H. Block.

Source/publisher: See below.

Availability: Available from Per Gjerde, Department of Psychology, University of California at Berkeley, Berkeley, CA 94720.

Brief description: The Family Interaction Q-Sort is a 33-item technique that is designed to examine parent–child and parent–parent relationships.

Purpose: The FIQ was developed to provide a macroscopic assessment instrument for examining parent–child and parent–parent relationships in nonreferred, nonclinical families. The FIQ is designed to describe the parents' behavior toward the school-age child and the young adolescent as well as toward the second parent in both dyadic (parent–child) and triadic (mother–father–child) situations.

Theoretical base: The authors state that the times do not stem from any single theoretical framework. An effort was made to include items that represent a variety of theoretical frameworks.

PHYSICAL DESCRIPTION OF RATING SCALE

Task and setting used to elicit behavior: The manual clearly outlines six tasks used to elicit behavior:

1. Phenomenology of emotions (15 min.—dyadic)
2. Consequences test (6 min.—dyadic)
3. Lowenfield Mosaic test (5 min.—dyadic)
4. Description of ideal person (15 min.—triadic)
5. Strategies (6 min.—triadic)
6. Venn diagrams (5 min.—triadic)

Unit of study: Dyads or mother–father–adolescent triad.

Scales and dimensions: The FIQ consists of 33 items that are sorted into a forced-choice, nine-step distribution (ranging from "most uncharacteristic" to "most characteristic"). In one study, factor analysis was used to reduce the number of items to a more workable number of underlying dimensions. Four principal components were retained, accounting for 64% of the variance, and 13 residual FIQ items were excluded from further analysis. The factors included the following:

1. Self-Oriented, Competitive Disregard vs. Nurturant Appreciation
2. Tense Ambivalence vs. Relaxed Consistency
3. Affiliative Orientation vs. No Affiliative Orientation
4. Interpersonal Withdrawal vs. Interpersonal Engagement

Manual: The manual for the Family Interaction Q-Sort provides an introduction, information regarding how the scale was developed, the actual items and tasks, lists of materials, and instructions for each dimension assessed.

Standardization and norms: No information is provided regarding a normative sample.

Evaluation of physical description of rating scale: *Strengths:* Relatively quick assessment time; covers a broad range of family activities. Some items are anchored very clearly in behavioral terms ("A tends to be critical, hostile, and rejecting of B's ideas and suggestions"), whereas other items require much more subjective judgments ("A appears to be aware of, and to be comfortable with, B's sexuality"). *Weaknesses:* No explicit theoretical basis for the construction of the scale; hence, the comprehensiveness of the item coverage is impossible to evaluate. Ratings are made across time and tasks, therefore requiring global judgments when a variety of relevant behaviors have occurred.

ADMINISTRATIVE PROCEDURES

Description of equipment needed: Each task requires its own materials. These include Q-sort answer board; Q-sort cards; box with colored plastic pieces; five puzzle boards of increasing difficulty; plastic pieces of different shapes, colors, and sizes.

Training: Because the use of the FIQ involves making global integrative judgments of complex psychological dimensions, use of the Q-sort "requires considerable observational skill, extensive psychological knowledge, and experience in working with families" (manual, p. 2). In one study, judges were mostly graduate students or PhD level professionals and had had extensive experience in working with families in either clinical or research settings.

Special issues for raters: Issues such as halo effects, leniency/severity effects, error of central tendency appear to be negated because of the forced-choice format of the Q-sort. Ratings are made from videotapes, presumably by professionals otherwise unfamiliar with the family.

Scoring procedures, including calculation of summary scores: While observing the family interactions on videotape, the observers rate the family on each of the 33 items.

Evaluation of administrative procedures: *Strengths:* Families are assessed in multiple situations, thus reducing the possibility of situation-specific responding. Special issues peculiar to rating scales are reduced in importance because of the Q-sort format. *Weaknesses:* Successful use of the Q-sort requires highly experienced judges.

EVALUATION OF CONSTRUCTS MEASURED

Reliability: Because of the complexity of judgments required, studies typically involved multiple raters. In one sample, 18 heterogeneous judges assessed parental behavior using the FIQ. Different combinations of judges were systematically assigned to families, and each family was rated by more than one judge. "Thus, the resulting Q-sort formulations will possess a higher degree of generalizability and be relatively independent of private sets of theoretical preferences" (Morrison, Gjerde, & Block, 1983b, p. 2). When two judges were assigned to rate an interaction session, their independent evaluations were typically composited. In the approximately 10% of cases in which the two raters could not agree, a third judge was involved, and the two most consensual judgments were used. In Gjerde, Block, and Block (1985), reliability was calculated by two methods. First, average interrater correlations were computed for each family; the Spearman-Brown adjusted reliabilities ranged from .70 to .73. Second, Spearman-Brown reliabilities were computed for the 33 individual FIQ descriptions (average interrater correlation followed by application of the Spearman-Brown formula); the average reliability was .59 (range: .40 to .74). Low reliabilities tended to be associated with low-frequency events.

Validity: *Criterion-related:* FIQ scales have been found to discriminate successfully between mother–child and father–child interaction patterns in families characterized by high parental disagreement on child-rearing issues (Morrison, Gjerde, & Block, 1983b). FIQ dimensions assessed when children were ages 3 to 13 were found to predict the development of adolescent depression at age 14 successfully (Gjerde, 1985). Hypotheses derived from family systems theory concerning second-order effects in triadic family interaction were supported (Gjerde, 1986). The FIQ distinguished in predictable ways between mother–son and mother–daughter relationships in single-parent families (Block, Block, & Gjerde, in press).

Clinical utility: Although the instrument has been used primarily in research to date, it could be used by clinicians who videotape family sessions.

Research utility: The FIQ methodology has been used successfully in several research endeavors and promises to be useful in future work.

SUMMARY EVALUATION

The Family Interaction Q-Sort has shown itself to be a very useful way of characterizing family dynamics in different types of families. The Q-sort format avoids some of the pitfalls typically associated with rating scales. Because sorts require high degrees of inference, raters must be highly trained.

REFERENCES

Block, J., Block, J. H., & Gjerde, P. F. (in press). Parental functioning and the home environment in families of divorce: Prospective and concurrent analyses. *Journal of the Academy of Child Psychiatry.*

Gjerde, P. F. (1983, August). *Parent–adolescent interaction in family context: Importance of second-order effects.* Paper presented at the meeting of the American Psychological Association, Anaheim.

Gjerde, P. F. (1985, April). *Adolescent depression and parental socialization patterns: A prospective study.* Paper presented at the meeting of the Society for Research in Child Development, Toronto.

Gjerde, P. F. (1986). The interpersonal structure of family interaction settings: Parent–adolescent relations in dyads and triads. *Developmental Psychology, 22,* 297–304.

Gjerde, P. F., Block, J., & Block, J. H. (1985, April). *Parental interactive patterns in dyads and triads: Prospective relationships to adolescent personality characteristics.* Paper presented at the meeting of the Society for Research in Child Development, Toronto.

Morrison, A. L., Gjerde, P. F., & Block, J. H. (1983a, April). *A prospective study of divorce and its relationship to family functioning.* Paper presented at the meeting of the Society for Research in Child Development, Detroit.

Morrison, A. L., Gjerde, P. F., & Block, J. H. (1983b, August). *Interaction in families characterized by parental disagreement: Mother–father differences.* Paper presented at the meeting of the American Psychological Association, Anaheim.

AUTHOR'S RESPONSE

No additional comments.

R-6
Global Coding Scheme

GENERAL INFORMATION

Date of publication: 1985.

Authors: Linda G. Bell, Connie S. Cornwell, and David C. Bell.

Source/publisher: See below.

Availability: Available from ERIC Document Reproduction Services (Document No. ED 248 420); included in Bell, D. C., & Bell, L. G. (1981). *Family Research Project progress report*. Abstracted in *Resources in Education*, February 1983.

Brief description: The Global Coding Scheme is intended for macroanalysis of family interaction in a battery of three tasks: marital couple revealed differences, family revealed differences, and family paper sculpture.

Purpose: The purpose of the coding scheme is to operationalize theoretically derived variables for assessing aspects of family functioning.

Theoretical base: The Global Coding Scheme is based on family systems theory. The scales themselves were based on the Beavers-Timberlawn Family Evaluation Scale and the Family Behavioral Snapshot, developed by Meyerstein in 1979.

PHYSICAL DESCRIPTION OF RATING SCALE

Task and setting used to elicit behavior: These scales have been used to rate families who have participated in a three-part assessment battery: (1) an audiotaped sample of marital interaction around a revealed differences task based on items from the Moos Family Environment Scale about which the couple disagreed (20 minutes); (2) a similar sample of whole-family interaction (father, mother, adolescent daughter, and her siblings); and (3) audiotaped interaction of the family while it was preparing a family paper sculpture (L. G. Bell, 1987) representation of itself.

Unit of study: Some scales refer to the marital couple; others refer to the whole family.

Scales and dimensions: The coding scheme consists of six sections: Couple Interaction, Family Interaction, Family and Task, Family Affect, Paper Sculpture, and Summation. Seven scales have been developed by the authors: Interpersonal Boundary, Comfort with Differences, Ability to Resolve Differences, Covert Conflict, Warmth and Support, Depression, and Influence of Children. The total scale includes 55 items in addition to several opportunities for written descriptions by the observer. Scales typically are rated on 5- to 6-point scales from "almost always" to "almost never" or on a scale relevant to the item (e.g., "very vague" to "very clear"). Within each section, various items were combined to form scales; for example, Interpersonal Boundary was measured by two items—"Family members take responsibility for their own actions" (#34) and "Family members are not overly close, stuck, or overconnected" (#50). On all items, anchor points are explicitly stated. Since a detailed theoretical framework is not laid out in the manual, it is difficult to say whether the items comprehensively sample the domains considered important.

Manual: The manual includes a brief introduction to the background of the scales, their theoretical origins, data collection procedures, and information about scale reliability. It also includes a section of coding conventions and definitions of terms used in the rating scales in addition to the scales themselves.

Standardization and norms: Since the number of studies using the code is limited, no norms are available at this time.

Evaluation of physical description of rating scale: The items on the scale seem to be well constructed in terms of consistency and clarity of anchor points, although distinguishing between points could be very challenging (e.g., "somewhat clear" expression of ideas vs. "fairly clear"). Coding conventions provided in the manual are useful for clarifying potential issues that might make rating difficult. Since little validity work has been done, the degree to which the code adequately covers the theoretical domain is not clear. The manual is useful and should provide enough information for the code's use in a research setting.

ADMINISTRATIVE PROCEDURES

Description of equipment needed: The ratings are based on audiotaped marital and family interaction.

Training: The coders whose reliability data were presented in the manual were all advanced students in a master's level training program in family therapy.

All had completed most of their coursework as well as a practicum in family therapy. The ability to train coders with less clinical skill is unknown. The manual does not state how much training was required to achieve the level of reliability described.

Special issues for raters: Issues such as halo effects, leniency/severity effects, error of central tendency, logical error, contrast error, and proximity error are not addressed in the manual. The amount of relevant contact with subjects is controlled because ratings are made from audiotapes of families whom the coders have not seen in person.

Evaluation of administrative procedures: Strengths include ease of administration, which requires audiotaping only. Potential limitations of the administrative procedures include the extensive training to which the coders had been exposed and the lack of treatment of special issues for raters. The actual negative impact of these potential limitations is unknown until further studies are undertaken.

EVALUATION OF CONSTRUCTS MEASURED

Reliability: Interrater reliability (correlations) on composite scales for two coders assessing nine families:

Interpersonal Boundary: $r = .63$
Comfort with Differences: $r = .45$
Ability to Resolve Differences: $r = .81$
Covert Conflict: $r = .44$
Warmth and Support: $r = .75$
Depression: $r = .73$
Influence of Children: $r = .80$

Single-item reliability correlations were calculated for 15 items; r ranged from .51 to .90.

Validity: *Construct:* The Average Extremeness of Family Relationship Distances (as measured by Family Paper Sculpture) was positively correlated with Overt Conflict and Covert Conflict and negatively correlated with Personal Responsibility, Ability to Resolve Differences, and Warmth and Support (Bell, Ericksen, Cornwell, & Bell, 1984). *Criterion:* Several family variables (Accurate Interpersonal Perception, Comfort with Differences, and Positive Receptive Attitude) were predictive in theoretically meaningful ways of Differentiated Self-Awareness and Positive Self-Regard in adolescent females (D. C. Bell & Bell, 1983). The degree of emotional closeness among family members was predictive of the degree to which adolescents' friendship choices were reciprocated (Bell, Cornwell, & Bell, 1985).

Clinical utility: The code was designed for research purposes only and is not used diagnostically.

Research utility: Several items and scales have shown themselves to be useful as predictors of theoretically relevant outcomes. Although relatively little research has been published to date, the code appears to have potential for the investigation of family processes.

SUMMARY EVALUATION

The primary strengths of these scales lie in their theoretical foundation and promising validity evidence. The primary weaknesses concern the high degree of inference involved (and the extensive clinical training of the coders who have worked with the scales thus far) and the authors' lack of discussion about the breadth of the theoretical domain that the scales were intended to assess. Further work will be necessary to determine whether less highly skilled coders can achieve satisfactory reliability with the scales.

REFERENCES

Bell, D. C., & Bell, L. G. (1983). Parental validation and support in the development of adolescent daughters. In H. D. Grotevant & C. R. Cooper (Eds.), *Adolescent development in the family: New directions for child development.* San Francisco: Jossey-Bass.

Bell, L. G. (1987). Using the Family Paper Sculpture for education, therapy, and research. *Contemporary Family Therapy—An International Journal, 9.*

Bell, L. G., Cornwell, C. S., & Bell, D. C. (1985). *Peer relationships of adolescent daughters as a reflection of family relationship patterns: A family systems approach.* Manuscript submitted for publication.

Bell, L. G., Ericksen, L., Cornwell, C., & Bell, D. C. (1984, June). Experienced closeness and distance among family members. Paper presented at a meeting of the American Family Therapy Association.

AUTHOR'S RESPONSE

The Global Coding Scheme has proved useful for training clinicians. By using the scales to describe and discuss taped family interactions, students gain increased sensitivity to family system patterns. The Global Coding Scheme is still evolving. We are presently using it to evaluate videotaped interviews with Japanese families. This cross-cultural experience has led to modifications of the scale, primarily in the areas of nurturance (or mutual dependency) and the expression of feelings. From a Japanese perspective, the American version of the coding scheme did not adequately tap the ability of family members to depend on and to nurture each other. In addition to our original questions about the amount of feelings expressed and how directly and clearly these feelings are expressed, we are now giving attention to whether the feelings being expressed are surface/socially appropriate feelings or whether they are deep/personal feelings. In Japan, feelings are most frequently expressed nonverbally; there is more emphasis on the empathy of the listener, and the surface–depth distinction is highly salient.

R-7
Global Family Interaction Scales (FIS-II)

GENERAL INFORMATION

Date of publication: 1982.

Author: Jules Riskin.

Source/publisher: Jules Riskin, Mental Research Institute, 555 Middlefield Rd., Palo Alto, CA 94301.

Availability: Available from the author.

Brief description: This coding system represents a revision of the original microanalytic FIS into a macroanalytic rating of family interaction.

Purpose: Like the FIS-I, the FIS-II shares the goal of contributing to the understanding of the relationship between family functioning and personality development by examining family interaction with an objective, but cost-beneficial, methodology.

Theoretical base: (1) Interactional approach. (2) Developmental—that is, development of individual self-esteem, autonomy, and the individuality as relates to family interaction.

PHYSICAL DESCRIPTION OF RATING SCALE

Task and setting used to elicit behavior: One-hour family interviews were audiotaped and observed through a one-way mirror at the Mental Research Institute. Families were instructed to discuss a variety of topics designed to generate family interaction. Two of 18 interviews were conducted in the home setting and centered on the evening meal.

Unit of study: Whole family.

Unit of coding/analysis: Whole interview or any segment of it.

Scales and dimensions: There are 17 dimensions of family interaction, which are rated independently of each other. Each dimension is rated on a 5-point scale from 5 = high or very much to 1 = low or very little. Dimensions assessed include Clarity; Topic Continuity; Appropriate Topic Change; Commitment; Request for Commitment; Information Exchange; Agreement; Disagreement; Support; Attack; Intensity; Humor; Interruptions; Laughter; Who Speaks; Intrusiveness; Mind Reading.

Manual: Brief instructions are provided in published source (Riskin, 1982).

Standardization and norms: None available.

Evaluation of physical description of code: *Strengths:* Simplicity of code and easy of mastery. *Limitations:* (1) No empirical or theoretical evidence is provided for inclusion of coded dimensions. (2) Clarification of anchor points for ratings is not provided, making replication inconsistent. (3) Dimensions do not clearly represent constructs of theoretical significance. (4) Dimensions rated are taken directly from the FIS-I microanalytic system. Several (e.g., Clarity, Intensity, Request for Commitment) reflect individual behaviors and others reflect dyadic interactions (e.g., Topic Change, Disagreement) rather than whole-family characteristics. Clarity regarding the integration of individual, dyadic, and whole-system levels of rating is not provided.

ADMINISTRATIVE PROCEDURES

Description of equipment needed and observation system: Every family interview held at MRI was observed by two to six people behind a one-way mirror. Ratings were made on the basis of the live interview.

Training: Training of raters takes about 10 minutes, which includes clarification of the dimensions, scoring, and rules of rating. Raters need not be familiar with the original FIS. Of the 37 observers, 25 were clinicians with a wide range of orientation and 12 were nonclinicians but white, middle-class professionals.

Special issues for raters: Observers rated the families on the global form of the FIS immediately following the family interview and before any discussion of the family. Mean ratings were derived for each family on each interview by combining the scores of several raters, yielding a set of 18 mean ratings for each dimension.

Evaluation of administrative procedures: *Strengths:* Ease of utilization. *Limitations:* Lack of rigorous rater training; lack of clarity regarding necessary reliability before observers' ratings are included; lack of information on number of raters used to determine each mean dimension score; consequently, high susceptibility to all rater biases inherent in rating scales.

EVALUATION OF CODE

Reliability: The reliability of the global rating procedures was assessed by Kendall's coefficient of concordance *(W)*. Probabilities that the obtained ratings resulted from chance ordering were less than .01 for Commitment, Intensity, Humor, Laughter, and Interruptions; probabilities were less than .05 for Appropriate Topic Change, Disagreement, Support, and Intrusiveness, and less than .10 for Clarity, Information Exchange, and Attack. Scales that did not show adequate agreement among raters were Topic Continuity, Request for Commitment, Agreement, Who Speaks, and Mind Reading.

Validity: *Criterion-related:* Two Caucasian, middle-class, intact, nonlabeled families were observed over a 4- to 5-year period and rated on the global FIS. The two families were significantly differentiated on the scales of Commitment, Information Exchange, Disagreement, Attack, Intensity, Humor, Interruptions, and Laughter.

Clinical utility: The simplicity of the rating scale suggests the potential clinical utility of this instrument; however, the lack of theoretical basis for the selected rating scale dimensions, the difficulty of rating whole-family dimensions that were designed to capture individual speech, and the lack of criterion validity studies with clinical families limit its current applicability.

Research utility: The research utility of the global FIS is limited by the lack of either a strong empirical or theoretical basis for the selection of rating scale dimensions. Thus, researchers must await considerable use of the measure to determine its utility.

SUMMARY EVALUATION

The FIS-II was found to differentiate stylistically nonclinical families. Although interesting hypotheses regarding the normal range of family behavior have been developed, these have not been investigated. Thus, the clinical and research utility of the instrument remains uncertain and dependent on a considerable amount of subsequent descriptive research. Concerns that have emerged from preliminary data include the inadequate reliability of several dimensions and the failure of dimensions to clearly reflect constructs of theoretical significance.

REFERENCE

Riskin, J. (1982). Research on "nonlabeled" families: A longitudinal study. In F. Walsh (Ed.), *Normal family processes*. New York: Guilford Press.

AUTHOR'S RESPONSE

The macroanalytic form of the FIS has been used a few times, but only informally, since the 1982 article. The FIS do not reflect specific theoretical constructs because they were not intended to reflect or test any specific theory of family interaction. It was hoped they would be valid even though atheoretical. They were originally developed (around 1964) when there were many constructs at a high level of abstraction, but very few empirically based measures that were both operational and nontrivial. The scales were consistent with (can be used to assess) several constructs (e.g., power/hierarchy, cohesion, communication style, homeostasis/morphogenesis). The problem of the precise meaning of theoretical constructs, how to operationalize them, and how and if these constructs, as used by different authors, can be compared still remains unresolved today. For example, note the often contradictory findings on "cohesion" that appear in current family interaction literature. The matter is made more complex by attempting to compare data collected in different ways (e.g., self-report or observation) of family assessment.

R-8
McMaster Clinical Rating Scale

GENERAL INFORMATION

Date of publication: 1982.

Authors: N. B. Epstein, L. M. Baldwin, and D. S. Bishop.

Source/publisher: Brown/Butler Family Research Program, 345 Blackstone Blvd., Providence, RI 02906

Availability: Available from source (above).

Brief description: The scale assesses seven dimensions of family functioning: Problem Solving, Communication, Roles, Affective Responsiveness, Affective Involvement, Behavior Control, and Overall Family Functioning.

Purpose: The purpose is to identify families that need professional intervention.

Theoretical base: McMaster Model of Family Functioning.

PHYSICAL DESCRIPTION OF RATING SCALE

Task and setting used to elicit behavior: Clinicians complete the rating scale following a family clinical interview. Videotaped family sessions may also be utilized.

Unit of study: Whole family.

Scales and dimensions: The scale consists of seven dimensions of family functioning:

1. Problem Solving
2. Communication
3. Roles

4. Affective Responsiveness
5. Affective Involvement
6. Behavior Control
7. Overall Family Functioning

Each dimension is represented on a 7-point scale, from 1 = severely disturbed functioning to 7 = superior functioning.

Manual: The manual provides a detailed description of each of the rating dimensions, including definition of the concepts involved, a description of the family characteristics at three levels of functioning (severely disturbed, nonclinical, and superior), and principles for rating.

Standardization: None available.

Norms: A rating between 1 and 4 on any scale indicates a need for clinical help; however, these cutoff points do not appear to be empirically derived.

Evaluation of physical description of rating scale: *Strengths:* (1) Scale dimensions well-constructed along logical continuums, with anchor points for values 1, 5, and 7 clearly defined in the manual; (2) theoretically based. *Limitations:* (1) There is a lack of normative data. (2) Each scale is multidimensional and requires a high level of inference on the part of the rater. (3) The task used to elicit behavior may vary across families, leading to a lack of standardization.

ADMINISTRATIVE PROCEDURES

Description of equipment needed: None indicated.

Training: Familiarity with the McMaster Model and manual is essential; no additional training or education is needed.

Special issues for raters: None specified.

Scoring procedures: The score on each dimension equals the assigned anchor point. Ratings ranging from 1 to 4 indicate clinical functioning and from 5 to 7, healthy functioning.

Evaluation of administrative procedure: *Strengths:* Administrative procedures simple; scoring categories not empirically derived. *Limitations:* Rater education or training not clearly specified; no scoring procedure provided for Overall Family Functioning.

EVALUATION OF CONSTRUCTS MEASURED

Reliability: Interrater reliability coefficients for three raters with 37 videotapes of psychiatric inpatient family interaction:

Problem Solving: $r = .84$
Communication: $r = .83$
Roles: $r = .85$
Affective Responsiveness: $r - .68$
Affective Involvement: $r = .88$
Behavior Control: $r = .86$
Overall Family Functioning: $r = .87$

A high correlation was obtained between the dimension scales (average $r = .68$) (C. Little-Bert, personal communication, July 5, 1984); however, when the effects of overall functioning were partialled out, the correlations between scales decreased dramatically (average $r = .12$) (I. W. Miller, personal communication, October 28, 1986).

Validity: *Criterion-related:* The rating scale was compared with the Family Assessment Device, a self-report, objective measure based on the McMaster Model. A moderate correlation was obtained for all scales ($r = .45-.64$) except for the Affective Involvement and Behavior Control scales, which were somewhat less related ($r = .28, .31$, respectively). These correlations were based on a sample of 36 families with a member currently in a psychiatric hospital. Limited range may lower the correlations. Data analysis comparing the CRS and FAD with 200 families is in progress (I. W. Miller, personal communication, October 28, 1986).

Clinical utility: For the clinician operating within the McMaster Model, the rating scale is likely to be very useful in determining both the general need and specific target areas for family intervention. Although the face validity is promising, research is necessary to confirm utility.

Research utility: May be useful to investigations based on the McMaster theoretical model; however, confirmation awaits its use in research.

SUMMARY EVALUATION

The McMaster Clinical Rating Scale, based on the McMaster Model of Family Functioning, assesses the degree to which a family is in need of professional intervention, based on their functioning on six dimensions: Problem Solving, Communication, Roles, Affective Responsiveness, Affective Involvement, and Behavior Control. With the exception of Overall Family Functioning, rating scale dimensions are clearly constructed and anchor points defined. Reliability is good for five of the seven scales; criterion validity studies find good correspondence with a self-report measure based on the same theory for all dimensions except Problem Solving. The CRS demonstrates good clinical and research utility for the family functioning dimensions of Communication, Roles, Behavior Control. At this time, affective dimensions appear unreliably rated and the construct of Problem Solving varies when viewed from the insider and outsider perspectives.

REFERENCES

Epstein, N. B., Baldwin, L. M., & Bishop, D. S. (1982). *McMaster Clinical Rating Scale*. Unpublished manuscript, Brown/Butler Family Research Program, Providence, RI.

Epstein, N. B., & Bishop, D. S. (1981). Problem centered systems therapy of the family. In A. Gurman & D. Kniskern (Eds.), *Handbook of family therapy* (pp. 444–482). New York: Brunner/Mazel.

Epstein, N. B., Bishop, D. S., & Levin, S. (1978). The McMaster Model of Family Functioning; *Journal of Marriage and Family Counseling, 4,* 19–31.

AUTHOR'S RESPONSE

Regarding the relatively high correlations between scales when the effects of overall functioning are not partialled out, we have argued regarding a similar finding in our self-report measure, the Family Assessment Device, that the dimensions of the McMaster Model (or perhaps any dimensions of family functioning) are not expected to be independent. In developing the CRS as well as the Family Assessment Device, we attempted to maintain a balance between the psychometric demands for independence of scales and clinical reality of nonorthogonal dimensions.

We have recently developed a semistructured interview schedule that provides a specific interview format and questions to conduct a family interview assessing the McMaster Model dimensions. Completion of this interview should produce sufficient data to make a CRS rating. Validation of this interview is in progress (I. W. Miller, personal communication, October 28, 1986).

Section VI
Abstracts of Self-Report Questionnaires: Whole-Family Functioning

W-1
Children's Version of the Family Environment Scale (CVFES)

GENERAL INFORMATION

Date of publication: 1984.

Authors: Christopher Pino, Nancy Simons, and Mary Jane Slawinowski.

Source/publisher: Slosson Educational Publications, Inc.

Availability: Available from Slosson Educational Publications, Inc., P.O. Box 280, East Aurora, NY 14052. (Also available from Consulting Psychologist Press, Inc., and Psychological Assessment Resources.)

Brief description: The CVFES is a 30-item pictorial, multiple-choice measure designed to measure children's subjective perceptions of their family social environments.

Purpose: The purpose is to provide a conceptually equivalent children's version of the Family Environment Scale.

Theoretical base: Social-ecological-psychology theory; family systems theory.

PHYSICAL DESCRIPTION OF QUESTIONNAIRE

Physical features: The CVFES is a 30-item pictorial, multiple-choice measure. Each item has three equivalent pictures containing four cartoon figures that represent a son, daughter, father, and mother. Pictures are identical across each item except for the one feature that indicates the characteristic in question. The CVFES is developed for children ages 5 to 12.

Unit of study: Whole family.

Respondent: Individual child.

Scales and dimensions: Scales and dimensions are identical to those in the Family Environment Scale (Moos & Moos, 1986). See the FES abstract for further information.

Manual: A published manual is available. It includes the measure rationale and development, normative data, psychometric validation, test administration, scoring, and interpretation guidelines.

Standardization and norms: The CVFES was normed on 158 children in the Buffalo, New York, area. They were primarily low to middle socioeconomic status, in grades one through six (26 in each grade). An equal number of boys and girls was included. The sample was predominantly Roman Catholic. Means and standard deviations are provided in the manual. Further standardization work is in progress.

Evaluation of physical description of questionnaire: *Strengths:* Pictorial format; conceptual equivalence with the FES; available manual and normative data; standardization efforts completed and in progress. *Limitations:* To date, normative data are limited in number and in the generalizability of the sample. Possible ambiguity of the stimulus pictures is a concern.

ADMINISTRATIVE PROCEDURES

Directions: The CVFES can be administered in a group or individual situation. Individual administration is preferred and is considered essential for children under grade 3 or children with low reading levels. A test booklet and answer sheets are available to permit reuse of test booklets. Children are informed regarding the characters in the cartoons and are then instructed to choose a picture most like their family.

Ease of use: Directions for administration are straightforward; however, the cartoons appear difficult to differentiate and are expected to require help from the examiner. Attention to the advisability of individual administration is not discussed in the manual in the test administration section and is easily overlooked.

Training for administration and scoring: No training beyond reading the manual appears necessary for administration and scoring; however, no standardized guidance for explaining the pictures to the child is provided to the administrator. Familiarity with the FES is likely to facilitate administration and scoring.

Scoring procedures: Items are scored on a 3-point scale. A scoring key is provided. Each subscale score is summed. Raw scores are converted to standardized scores using the table of norms and then plotted on FES profile sheets.

Evaluation of administrative procedures: *Strengths:* Scoring and administration are simple, clearly explained, and consistent with the FES. *Limitations:* Concerns regarding administration decisions are addressed only minimally in the manual and are not supported with empirical data. Specifically, ability of children with low reading levels or below-average intelligence to differentiate the meaning of cartoons appears warranted.

EVALUATION OF CONSTRUCTS MEASURED

Reliability: Test–retest reliability over a 4-week period with the normative sample was adequate ($r = .80$). Internal consistency reliability of individual scales was not provided.

Validity: *Content:* In an evaluation of the structural pictoral properties, or "stimulus pull," of each cartoon, 56 children (26 third-graders and 30 seventh-graders) were asked to write out the meaning and intent of each of the pictures, in a single sentence, for all of the scales. Two expert raters (interrater reliability $= .84$) then evaluated whether the child's response matched the FES scale dimension. Z-values were calculated to determine the hit rate. All 10 scales were significantly correctly identified. Items within scales varied appreciably (.65 to .95) within two scales (#2 and #6). Differences by age were not statistically evaluated (Pino, 1985).

Clinical utility: The CVFES was designed for clinical use; however, the clinical utility of this measure has not yet been investigated.

Research utility: The CVFES is not explicitly designed for research; however, it is designed to be conceptually compatible with the FES and thus could be expected to have research as well as clinical utility. The conceptual compatibility of the two measures has not yet been investigated, however.

SUMMARY EVALUATION

The CVFES provides an important potential contribution to available self-report family assessment as the first measure available for use with elementary school–aged children. This pictorial downward extension of the FES, with its conceptual FES compatibility, promises significant clinical and research utility. Psychometric validation is very preliminary, however, and remains the major obstacle to widespread use. Possible ambiguity in interpretations of the pictures is a concern.

REFERENCES

Moos, R. H., & Moos, B. (1986). *Manual for the Family Environment Scale* (2nd ed.). Palo Alto, CA: Consulting Psychologists Press.

Pino, C. J. (1985). A content validity study of the Children's Version of the Family Environment Scale. *Child Study Journal, 14*(4), 311–316.

Pino, C. J., Simons, N., & Slawinowski, M. J., (1983). Development and application of the Children's Version of the Family Environment Scale. *Journal of Mental Imagery, 7*, 75–81.

Pino, C. J., Simons, N., & Slawinowski, M. J. (1984a). The Children's Family Environment Scale. *Family Therapy, 9*(1), 85–86.

Pino, C. J., Simons, N., & Slawinowski, M. J. (1984b). *The Children's Version of the Family Environment Scale manual.* East Aurora, NY: Slosson.

AUTHOR'S RESPONSE

The clinical utility of the CVFES will be discussed in a forthcoming book: C. J. Pino, *The CVFES Sourcebook: Imagery in Family Diagnosis and Therapy* (East Aurora, NY: United Educational Press).

W-2
Colorado Self-Report Measure
of Family Functioning

GENERAL INFORMATION

Date of publication: 1985.

Author: Bernard L. Bloom.

Source/publisher: Bloom, B. L. (1985). A factor analysis of self-report measures of family functioning. *Family Process, 24,* 225–239.

Availability: Available through the source (see above) or from the author: Bernard L. Bloom, Department of Psychology, Box 345, University of Colorado, Boulder, CO 80309.

Brief description: The Colorado Self-Report Measure of Family Functioning is a 75-item self-report measure with a four-choice format. It is based on four other well-known self-report measures: Moos's Family Environment Scale, van der Veen's Family Concept Test, Olson's Family Adaptability and Cohesion Evaluation Scales, and Skinner's Family Assessment Measure.

Purpose: The purpose of the measure is to provide a description of whole-family functioning along 15 dimensions under three general headings: relationship dimensions, personal growth or value dimensions, and system maintenance dimensions.

Theoretical base: The measure is based on dimensions from family systems and family development theories. The overriding theoretical approach could be described as structural family systems theory.

PHYSICAL DESCRIPTION OF QUESTIONNAIRE

Physical features: The measure is a 75-item self-report questionnaire that uses a four-choice format ("very true for my family," "fairly true for my family," "fairly untrue for my family," "very untrue for my family").

Unit of study: Whole family.

Respondent: Individual family member.

Scales and dimensions: The 15 family functioning scales are Cohesion, Expressiveness, Conflict, Intellectual-Cultural Orientation, Active-Recreational Orientation, Religious Emphasis, Organization, Family Sociability, External Locus of Control, Family Idealization, Disengagement, Democratic Family Style, Laissez-Faire Family Style, Authoritarian Family Style, and Enmeshment.

Manual: None.

Standardization and norms: Bloom (1985) reports means on the 15 scales for samples of adolescent subjects from intact and disrupted families. Supplementary tables (available from the author) include ranges, means, standard deviations, and 25th and 75th percentile scores on the 15 scales with several samples. Although descriptive data from several samples are reported, no formal norming procedure on a large representative sample has been accomplished. Minor item changes on four scales have recently been instituted (available from the author).

Evaluation of physical description of questionnaire: *Strengths:* The four-choice response is more acceptable than true–false formats (for psychometric reasons) or nine-item formats (for discrimination). The length of the instrument appears to be appropriate. The reading level required is modest, so most family members should be able to interpret the questions accurately. Measures from which the instrument is derived are appropriate for persons above age 11. *Limitations:* The normative sample is limited. The past-tense wording of the items invites ambiguous interpretations concerning the time frame in which the respondent is to consider the statement and limits the utility of the measure to retrospective studies. No manual is available.

ADMINISTRATIVE PROCEDURES

Directions: Not available.

Ease of use: Easy to administer, requiring only the items, answer sheet, and a pencil; can easily be computer-scored.

Training for administration and scoring: Could be administered and scored by nonprofessionals.

Scoring procedures, including calculation of summary scores: Scale scores are constructed by reversing the points allocated to reverse-scored items and then simply summing the points.

Evaluation of administrative procedures: *Strengths:* The instrument is easy to administer and score. *Limitations:* Respondent directions are not available in the published source.

EVALUATION OF CONSTRUCTS MEASURED

Reliability: Measures of reliability using the Cronbach alpha method ranged from .40 to .88 (mean = .71). Cronbach alphas on revised scales ranged from .59 to .86. No test–retest results are reported.

Validity: *Construct-related:* Factor analyses of item responses yielded 13 factors with eigenvalues exceeding 1.0 and closely matching the anticipated theoretical constructs (Bloom, 1985). *Criterion-related:* Significant differences emerged on 12 of the 15 scales in samples of adolescents whose parents were intact versus divorced (Bloom, 1985).

Clinical utility: Until more standardization data have been obtained from a wider range of subjects, it would appear that this measure has questionable clinical value in its present state. If further investigation is as promising as the author hopes, this measure may be of value in the clinical setting to help determine the influence of the family of origin on present functioning.

Research utility: At present, the research utility of the instrument remains to be established with further studies of validity. If such investigations are successful, this measure has great potential as a research tool, as it has been carefully developed from a psychometric perspective to date.

SUMMARY EVALUATION

Although derived from several well-known measures of current family functioning, the Colorado Self-Report Measure of Family Functioning, in its present form, is a retrospective measure. The instrument shows very promising psychometric qualities, but it is still largely untested. Any weaknesses noted are largely a function of the instrument's newness. Thanks to careful theoretical and psychometric development, the measure has the potential to be a valuable clinical and research tool.

REFERENCES

Bloom, B. L. (1985). A factor analysis of self-report measures of family functioning. *Family Process, 24,* 225–239.

Bloom, B. L., & Lipetz, M.E. (1987). *Revisions on the Self-Report Measure of Family Functioning*. Technical Report No. 2. University of Colorado, Department of Psychology, Center for Family Studies, Boulder, CO 80309.

AUTHOR'S RESPONSE

No additional comments.

W-3
Conflict Tactics Scale (CTS)

GENERAL INFORMATION

Date of publication: 1979.

Author: Murray A. Straus.

Source/publisher: Straus, M. A. (1979). Measuring intrafamily conflict and violence: The Conflict Tactics (C.T.) Scales. *Journal of Marriage and the Family, 41,* 75–88.

Availability: Available from the author: Dr. Murray A. Straus, Family Research Laboratory, University of New Hampshire, Durham, NH 03824.

Brief description: The original version (Form A) of the CTS consists of a list of 14 actions that a family member might take when in conflict with another family member. Respondents rate items according to frequency of occurrence within the past year on a 6-point Likert scale. Form N is similar, with 19 items. The CTS can be used to obtain conflict tactics scores for all dyads in the family.

Purpose: The purpose is to measure the use of reasoning, verbal aggression, and violence as modes of dealing with conflict in relationships within a family.

Theoretical base: The CTS is based on sociological conflict theory. Distinctions are made between conflicts of interest, tactics used for resolving such conflicts, and hostility, or feelings of dislike or antipathy for another. The CTS was constructed to investigate tactics used to resolve conflicts of interest.

PHYSICAL DESCRIPTION OF QUESTIONNAIRE

Physical features: Form A is composed of 14 possible responses to family conflict which are rated on a 6-point Likert scale according to frequency of occurrence within the past year (from 0 = never to 5 = more than once a month). Form N is similar, with 19 items and a 7-point response format (an "I don't know" option is also included). Reading requirements for form A seem to be at the high school level. Form N is designed to be administered as an interview and has a greater emphasis on tactics of violence.

Unit of study: Dyadic relationships: husband–wife, father–child, mother–child, and child–child (parent–child scores can also be calculated).

Respondent: Form A can be used with the husband, wife, or adolescent in the family. The interview (Form N) can be administered to younger children, but lower age limits are not given.

Scales and dimensions: The CTS is composed of three scales: the Reasoning scale, tapping the use of such tactics as rational discussion to resolve disputes; the Verbal Aggression scale, referring to the use of verbal and nonverbal acts to symbolically hurt the other; and the Violence scale, designed to measure the use of physical force against the other. Scores on the three scales can be computed for all possible family dyads. In construction of Form N, Reasoning scale items were deleted and Violence scale items were added.

Manual: None available.

Standardization and norms: The CTS (Form N) was standardized using a national probability sample of couples, and percentiles are available for use as national norms. Distributions of percentile norms are based on the following sample sizes: husband–wife, 2,105; wife–husband, 2,114; couple, 2,088; child–child, 899; father–child, 521; mother–child, 620 (Straus, 1979).

Evaluation of physical description of questionnaire: *Strengths:* Strengths include the availability of national norms and the dyadic relationship focus of the measure. Items are of comprehensible length, and the response format is clear, with an adequate range. Reading level is appropriate for adolescents and adults, and the behavioral focus of the items requires a low level of inference from respondents. *Limitations:* Explanations about how various scales are derived from the two forms of the CTS are not always clear. A manual would be useful. The normed version of the scale (From N) is available only as an interview.

ADMINISTRATIVE PROCEDURES

Directions: Clear directions are provided with the measure.

Ease of use: Form A is easily administered, requiring only the items and a pencil. Form N is designed to be administered as an interview, but although administration appears straightforward, clear directions are not given. Form N could easily be adapted to paper-and-pencil administration for adult or adolescent respondents. Adaptation for computer scoring is also an option.

Training for administration and scoring: Administration of From A is simple and should not require special training. Form N would require minimal training in the interview procedure. Once a scoring method is chosen, scoring should require very little training.

Scoring procedures, including calculation of summary scores: Several methods for scoring the CTS are at the user's disposal: (1) The simplest method is to add response category code values for the items that make up each of the scales. (2) Items from Form N can be weighted in accordance with frequencies indicated by response categories endorsed by the respondent. Points on the 0 to 6 scale are weighted 0, 1, 2, 4, 8, 15, and 25. (3) A percentage of the possible total score can be calculated by dividing each raw score by the maximum possible score, multiplying by 100, and rounding to an integer. (4) The national norm tables can be used to convert raw scores to percentile scores (Straus, 1979). (5) Overall violence indexes can be calculated for any of the dyads (e.g., husband-to-wife violence or mother-to-child violence) for a particular sample by finding the percentage of respondents who carried out one or more violent acts during the previous 12 months (endorsement of at least one of items k through r on Form N). (6) Severe violence indexes are calculated by finding the percentage of respondents endorsing at least one item referring to severe violence (items n through r) on Form N (Straus, Gelles, & Steinmetz, 1980). (7) Minor (or "ordinary") violence indexes are calculated in a similar manner by finding the percentage of respondents endorsing at least one item referring to minor violence (items k, l, or m) on Form N. (8) The "severity weighted index" is a score that takes into account the severity as well as the frequency of violence. A person's score consists of a sum of the items multiplied by both a weight for frequency (see previous frequency weights) and a weight for severity (e.g., weight for "kick" = 2, weight for "beat up" = 5). Note that this index refers to scores for individuals, whereas the previous "violence indexes" refer to incidence rates for a sample. (9) Straus also discusses the possibility of using the CTS as a Guttman scale (Straus, 1981).

Evaluation of administrative procedures: *Strengths:* Ease of administration; possibility of deriving several different types of scores; scoring can be adapted to research or clinical needs. *Limitations:* Although attempts were made to reduce reactivity in the construction of the CTS, inaccuracy due to socially desirable responding is likely because of the social undesirability of some questions (e.g., "pushed, grabbed or shoved her"). No attempts to discourage socially desirable responding are included in the instructions for Form A. Accurate responses to CTS items require accurate recall from the respondent. Another limitation is the lack of clarity in explaining the scoring procedures. A manual summarizing this information, which now must be gleaned from different sources, would be helpful.

EVALUATION OF CONSTRUCTS MEASURED

Reliability: For Form A, internal consistency reliability was examined by computing an item analysis to determine correlation of CTS items with the total score. Correlations ranged from .44 to .91 and were higher for items on the Violence scale (.79 to .88) than for items on the Reasoning and Verbal Aggression scales. For Form N, alpha coefficients were computed. Alphas were high for the Verbal Aggression (.77 to .88) and Violence (.62 to .88) scales and relatively low for the reasoning scale (.50 to .76) (Straus, 1979), a finding that was replicated by Schumm, Martin, Bollman and Jurich (1982).

Validity: *Criterion-related:* Concurrent validity was examined by comparing parent-report CTS scores with student-report CTS scores. Correlations for the Reasoning scale (− .12 to .19) were low. However, for the Verbal Aggression (.43 to .51) and Violence (.33 to .64) scales, they were relatively high. In a comparison of student and parent reports of incidence rates (overall violence indexes), student reports were higher than fathers' self-reports of their own violence but lower than mothers' self-reports ($N = 117$). A larger sample of students ($N = 385$) reported incidences of parental violence similar to parental self-reports in a national probability sample (Straus, 1979; Straus et al., 1980). Schumm et al. (1982) found significant correlations between adolescents' reports of parental violence on the CTS and responses to other items about their parents' verbal violence (correlations with CTS verbal items are higher, supporting discriminant validity). *Construct-related:* Straus (1979) cites the following evidence for construct validity: (1) Consistency has been demonstrated between findings using the CTS and other findings concerning the "catharsis" theory of aggression control. (2) High rates of occurrence of socially undesirable acts of verbal and physical aggression obtained using the CTS are consistent with previous in-depth interview studies. (3) Previous empirical findings and theory about the familial transmission of violent behavior support CTS data on correlations of patterns of violence from one generation to the next. (4) Numerous correlations between CTS scores and other variables are consistent with relevant theory—for example, negative correlations between socioeconomic status and family violence and high reported family violence in cases of extreme husband dominance or extreme wife dominance (Straus, 1979). Factor analyses were conducted on CTS husband-to-wife and wife-to-husband data, Forms A and N. Three factors corresponding to the theoretical scales were found for Form A. Analysis of Form N resulted in four factors, with items referring to extreme violence (threatening with or using a knife or gun, not on Form A) making up a separate factor (Straus, 1979). Factor analysis of a modified version of the CTS revealed three dimensions of spousal violence: psychological abuse (e.g., sulking, stomping out of the room), physical aggression (e.g., hitting, pushing), and life-threatening violence (composed of the beating up, threatening with a knife or gun, and using a knife or gun) (Hornung, McCullough, & Sugimoto, 1981). Factor analysis of items selected from several sources, including the CTS, resulted in three factors corresponding to the theoretical scales found by Straus for the CTS (Jorgensen, 1977). The CTS has been used in numerous studies, including Hornung et al. (1981); Jorgensen (1977); Schumm et al. (1982); Straus (1974, 1977–78, 1980a, 1980b); and Straus et al. (1980).

Clinical utility: There is evidence that the way in which the CTS is constructed facilitates accuracy in self-reports of family violence (Schumm et al. 1982; Straus, 1979, 1980a, 1980b). Scores of family members can be compared with national norms. Although the CTS was constructed for research purposes and the clinical utility of the instrument remains undetermined, it would appear to have considerable clinical utility in screening, in evaluation of treatment, and as a means of encouraging discussions about tactics used for resolving conflict in families.

Research utility: The CTS has proved useful in survey research about family violence. It is constructed in such a way as to encourage accurate reporting. The Verbal Aggression and Violence scales (which have been of most interest to researchers) have shown good internal consistency, and substantial evidence has supported the construct validity of the instrument. Further evidence of criterion-related validity would enhance the value of the CTS in research. The ease of administration of the instrument and its versatility (i.e., the possibility of deriving various scores for various dyads, different modes of administration) add to its usefulness.

SUMMARY EVALUATION

Although more evidence of criterion-related validity is needed and the internal consistency of the Reasoning scale is less than adequate, the psychometric properties of the CTS are generally good. The instrument is versatile and easy to use and has demonstrated usefulness in research about family violence. The instrument has good potential for use in a clinical setting as well.

REFERENCES

Hornung, C. A., McCullough, B. C., & Sugimoto, T. (1981). Status relationships in marriage: Risk factors in spouse abuse. *Journal of Marriage and the Family, 43,* 675–692.
Jorgensen, S. R. (1977). Social class heterogamy, status striving, and percep-

tion of marital conflict: A partial replication and revision of Pearlin's contingency hypothesis. *Journal of Marriage and the Family, 39,* 653–689.

Schumm, W. R., Martin, M. J., Bollman, S. R., & Jurich, A. P. (1982). Classifying family violence, whither the woozle? *Journal of Family Issues, 3,* 319–341.

Straus, M. A. (1974). Leveling, civility and violence in the family. *Journal of Marriage and the Family, 36,* 13–29.

Straus, M. A. (1977–78). Wife beating: How common and why? *Victimology, 2,* 443–458.

Straus, M. A. (1979). Measuring intrafamily conflict and violence: The Conflict Tactics (C.T.) Scales. *Journal of Marriage and the Family, 41,* 75–88.

Straus, M. A. (1980a). Social stress and marital violence. *Annals of the New York Academy of Sciences, 347,* 229–251.

Straus, M. A. (1980b). Stress and physical child abuse. *Child Abuse and Neglect, 4,* 75–88.

Straus, M. A. (1981, July). *A reevaluation of the Conflict Tactics Scale violence measures and some new measures.* Paper presented at the National Conference on Family Violence Research. Durham, NH.

Straus, M. A. (1983). Ordinary violence, child abuse, and wife-beating: What do they have in common? In D. Finkelhor, R. J. Gelles, G. T. Hotaling, & M. A. Straus (Eds.), *The dark side of families: Current family violence research* (pp. 213–234). Beverly Hills, CA: Sage.

Straus, M. A., Gelles, R. J., & Steinmetz, S. K. (1980). *Behind closed doors: Violence in the American family.* New York: Anchor Press.

AUTHOR'S RESPONSE

No additional comments.

W-4
Family Adaptability and Cohesion Evaluation Scales III (FACES III)

GENERAL INFORMATION

Date of publication: 1985.

Authors: David H. Olson, Joyce Portner, and Yoav Lavee.

Source/publisher: Department of Family Social Science, University of Minnesota.

Availability: Available from David H. Olson, Family Social Science, University of Minnesota, 290 McNeal Hall, St. Paul, MN 55108.

Brief description: The FACES III is a 20-item scale used to assess family cohesion and adaptability. Family members complete the instrument twice, once indicating the present perception of their family and once indicating how they would like their ideal family to be (optional).

Purpose: The instrument was designed to provide measures of family cohesion and adaptability as well as both perceived and ideal family functioning. The discrepancy between perceived and ideal functioning provides an inverse measure of family satisfaction.

Theoretical base: The Circumplex Model of Marital and Family Systems.

PHYSICAL DESCRIPTION OF QUESTIONNAIRE

Physical features: The questionnaire includes 20 perceived and 20 ideal items (10 items on each tapping cohesion and adaptability). Each item is responded to on a 5-point Likert scale, ranging from 1 = "almost never" to 5 = "almost always." The instrument is suitable for children as young as 9 years of age.

Unit of study: Whole family; a version is also available for couples without children living at home.

Respondent: Individual family member.

Scales and dimensions: The instrument yields four scores: Perceived Cohesion, Perceived Adaptability, Ideal Cohesion, and Ideal Adaptability. Although they are not scored as separate scales, cohesion items assess emotional bonding, supportiveness, family boundaries, time and friends, and interests and recreation. Family adaptability is assessed by leadership, control, discipline, and roles and rules. From scores on the two scales, family members may be placed on the circumplex grid, which allows their perception of family functioning to be classified into one of 16 types. Additional scores can be derived (see "Scoring Procedures").

Manual: A detailed manual is available from the author. It includes theoretical discussion and psychometric and normative data.

Standardization and norms: Norms and cutting points for classification into the 16 types have been developed for adults ($N=2,453$), families with adolescents ($N=1,315$), and young couples ($N=242$) (Olson, Portner, & Lavee, 1985).

Evaluation of physical description of questionnaire: *Strengths:* The instrument appears to be tapping two dimensions of family functioning that are persistently acknowledged in the literature to be important. It has a clear response format, adequate response range, comprehensible response length, norms and manual available, and appropriate reading level. *Limitations:* Item content reflects whole-family functioning, whereas perceptions of the family might vary for certain individuals or subsystems within the family. Scores are subject to a response bias, in that all items are scored in the positive direction.

ADMINISTRATIVE PROCEDURES

Directions: The instrument is easy to administer, in that individuals are simply asked to describe the frequency with which various events occur in their family.

Ease of use: The instrument is easy to complete, likely in 10 minutes or less.

Training for administration and scoring: Very little training is required. The measure can easily be hand-scored or computer-scored.

Scoring procedures: The sum of the responses to the odd-numbered items yields the cohesion score; the sum of the responses to the even-numbered items yields the adaptability score. Scores can be classified into a family system type by the Circumplex Model. A linear "distance from center" (DFC) score can be derived for use in research. Cutoff scores are available for clinical use.

Evaluation of administrative procedures: *Strengths:* The instrument is very easy to administer, complete, and score. A variety of derived scoring procedures enhances the utility of the measure. *Limitations:* The ease of use may be deceptive, in that complex family functioning variables are being assessed. As with other self-report measures, the following factors may influence responses: reactivity, the respondents' conceptualization of the questions, response sets, self-awareness, and accuracy of retrospective recall.

EVALUATION OF CONSTRUCTS MEASURED

Reliability: Internal consistency: Cronbach's alpha for cohesion = .77, for adaptability = .62. Test–retest reliability over a 4-week interval: cohesion = .83, adaptability = .80.

Validity: *Construct-related:* FACES III was developed in part to be an improvement over FACES II, in that cohesion and adaptability are uncorrelated (as specified in the Circumplex Model). Although there was considerable correlation between the two constructs in the FACES II ($r = .65$), the correlation was reduced to .03 in the FACES III (Olson, 1986). Factor analysis of the 20 items shows that when the results are limited to two factors, the cohesion and adaptability items load on the appropriate factors. The item-total correlations within each scale are also appropriately high (on cohesion, r ranges from .51 to .74; on adaptability, from .42 to .56: Olson, Portner, & Lavee, 1985).

Clinical utility: The FACES III has been used clinically to compare perceptions of family members on both perceived and ideal family functioning. The availability of clinical cutoff scores enhances its utility in diagnosis. The DFC score and real–ideal forms permit pre–post intervention evaluations. Olson (1986) views the measure as very useful clinically.

Research utility: Many studies are in progress. Given the conceptual model on which the instrument is based and the ease of administration, use, and scoring, the instrument will likely attract wide usage. The instrument seems most useful for assessing families with adolescents rather than infants or young children. A new version for children under 10 is being developed.

SUMMARY EVALUATION

The FACES III provides an easy assessment of current and ideal family functioning as perceived by various family members, consistent with Olson's Circumplex Model. However, the Circumplex Model is not universally accepted as the most useful way to view family functioning; thus, the instrument might not be considered useful by researchers or clinicians with other theoretical leanings. The ease of use may be deceptive: the instrument is attempting to measure complex family-level variables with 20 simple items and may not capture the richness or complexity of family life needed for clinical or research assessment.

REFERENCES

Olson, D. H., Portner, J., & Lavee, Y. (1985). *FACES III manual*. Unpublished manual. (Available from D. H. Olson, Family Social Science, University of Minnesota, 290 McNeal Hall, St. Paul, MN 55108.)

Olson, D. H., Sprenkle, D. H., & Russell, C. S. (1979). Circumplex Model of Marital and Family Systems I: Cohesion and adaptability dimensions, family types, and clinical applications. *Family Process, 18*, 3–28.

Olson, D. H. (1986). Circumplex model VII: Validation studies and FACES III. *Family Process, 25*, 337–351.

In addition, a bibliography of 41 publications relating to the FACES and the Circumplex Model may be found in the FACES III manual.

AUTHOR'S RESPONSE

The Family Social Science Department has records of more than 300 studies that have used or are using FACES III. These have been divided into several content areas. A list is available from the author.

W-5
Family APGAR

GENERAL INFORMATION

Date of publication: 1978.

Author: Gabriel Smilkstein.

Source/publisher: Smilkstein, G. (1978). The Family APGAR: A proposal for a family function test and its use by physicians. *Journal of Family Practice, 6,* 1231–1239.

Availability: Instrument instructions and reprints of validity studies are available from Gabriel Smilkstein, MD, William Ray Moore Professor, Department of Family Practice, School of Medicine, University of Louisville, Louisville, KY 40292-0001. The instrument may be reproduced without charge for clinical or research use.

Brief description: The Family APGAR is a five-item screening instrument designed to measure family members' satisfaction with five basic components of family functioning: adaptation, partnership, growth, affection, and resolve. The instrument has a second part that elicits qualitative information concerning social support from individual family members.

Purpose: The Family APGAR is a utilitarian screening instrument designed to give family physicians an overview of family functioning as perceived by the patient. The Family APGAR is designed for clinical and research use with single persons and nontraditional families as well as with traditional nuclear families.

Theoretical base: Family systems theory, stress and coping theory.

PHYSICAL DESCRIPTION OF QUESTIONNAIRE

Physical features: The Family APGAR consists of five questions about satisfaction with family life. Two response formats are available. The three-choice format (''almost always,'' ''some of the time,'' ''hardly ever'') is recommended for clinical use because it exhibits adequate reliability and is simple to use. The five-choice format ("never," "hardly ever," "some of the time," "almost always," "always") is recommended for research because it has slightly higher internal consistency reliability. The reading level is simple. Item content appears appropriate for individual respondents aged 10 and above (Smilkstein, Ashworth, & Montano, 1982).

Unit of study: Whole family.

Respondent: Individual family member.

Scales and dimensions: Each of the following components of family functioning is measured by a Family APGAR question: Adaptation, or family problem solving; Partnership, or sharing of responsibility and decision making; Growth; Affection; and Resolve, or commitment to share time, space, and material resources with other family members.

Manual: A short book of instructions is available that contains descriptions of constructs measured, scoring instructions, a list of situations in which the Family APGAR might be useful, and some case studies.

Standardization and norms: Although no formal standardization sample is available, several studies present data on the instrument. Means of small samples of graduate students ($n = 38$) and outpatient clinic subjects ($n = 20$) have been reported (Good, Smilkstein, Good, Shaffer, & Arons, 1979), as well as means, standard deviations, and score distributions for college freshmen and sophomores ($n = 527$) and new family practice patients ($n = 133$). Means and standard deviations were reported for large groups of "well-adjusted" ($n = 1,164$) and "maladjusted" ($n = 1,377$) 10- to 13-year-old Taiwanese children and for a group of 158 psychiatric outpatients divided into groups according to the type of class or number of individual therapy sessions attended (Smilkstein, et al., 1982).

Evaluation of physical description of questionnaire: *Strengths:* Strengths of the Family APGAR include the availability of two response formats, a manual, and norms for limited samples of certain groups (most notably, college students and clinic outpatients). The reading level is appropriate; items are of comprehensible length; response formats are clear; and the five-point format has adequate range. *Limitations:* Norms applying to a greater variety of people would be a welcome addition to data concerning the Family APGAR. Although this five-question screening instrument does appear to be a rough measure of global family functioning, it seems doubtful that different components of family functioning can be measured with such a short instrument. The relationship between item 1, "I am satisfied that I can turn to my family for help when something is troubling me," to the construct it is purported to measure—Adaptation, or resources for problem solving—seems particularly doubtful. In addition, al-though the items refer to whole-family functioning, perceptions of individual family members are likely to vary in response to the questionnaire.

ADMINISTRATIVE PROCEDURES

Directions: Clear directions for respondents are provided on the questionnaire.

Ease of use: The questionnaire is very easy to administer, requiring only the items and a pencil. It can easily be computer-scored.

Training for administration and scoring: Clear scoring and interpretation guidelines are provided in the instruction manual. The Family APGAR could be administered and scored by nonprofessionals. It was designed for the busy family physician who is unaccustomed to using family assessment instruments.

Scoring procedures, including calculation of summary scores: For the three-choice response format, the responses are weighted (0, 1, 2) and summed, yielding a maximum score of 10. A score of 8–10 is thought to suggest a highly functional family, with a score of 4–7 suggesting a moderately dysfunctional family, and a score of 0–3 suggesting a severely dysfunctional family. Enmeshed families, which are likely to score from 8 to 10, are exceptions to these scoring guidelines. Responses to the five-choice format are weighted 0 to 4, yielding a maximum score of 20.

Evaluation of administrative procedures: *Strengths:* The instrument is short and easy to administer, with a format explicitly designed for use by medical doctors. The instrument has been found to be of value in relating the perception the individual has of family functioning to behavioral and biomedical health outcomes. *Limitations:* The Family APGAR is not designed to measure within-family or whole-family functioning, Therefore, it cannot be used to diagnose complex family functioning variables, such as enmeshment.

EVALUATION OF CONSTRUCTS MEASURED

Reliability: The instrument exhibits moderate internal consistency. Interitem correlations given were .65 and .67 (Good et al., 1979; Dr. Gabriel Smilkstein, personal communication, July 22, 1987). Split-half reliability, calculated by correlating items 1, 3, and 5 with items 2 and 4 was .93 (Good et al., 1979). Two-week test–retest reliability was .83. Slightly better internal consistency reliability was demonstrated for the five-choice format (Cronbach's alpha = .86) than for the three-choice format (Cronbach's alpha = .80) (Smilkstein et al., 1982).

Validity: *Construct-related:* The correlation between the Family APGAR and the Pless-Satterwhite Family Functioning Index (FFI) was .80 for a group of 33 college students' families. The interspouse correlation for this group was .67, a correlation slightly higher than for the FFI scores ($r = .65$). A correlation of .64 was obtained between the Family APGAR and therapist ratings of family function for 20 community mental health center outpatients. *Criterion-related:* In the same study, there was a significant difference between total Family AP- GAR scores of clinic (presenting problems not necessarily family problems) and non-clinic families ($t = 3.43$, $p < .001$). Scores on the first four items of the instrument also showed significant differences. Item 5, reflecting satisfac- tion with amount of time spent with the family, failed to discriminate between the two groups, with the nonclinic families scoring slightly lower on this item. Item 5 was subsequently revised to reflect satisfaction with quality, rather than with quantity, of time spent with the family (Good et al., 1979).

In a study conducted at the National University of Taiwan, the Family AP- GAR scores of 1,377 "maladjusted" students were significantly lower than the scores of 1,164 "well-adjusted" students for individual items as well as for total score. The Family APGAR scores of adopted children were significantly lower than those of biological children, and students separated from their fam- ilies had significantly lower scores than those from intact families (Smilkstein et al., 1982). In another study, low Family APGAR scores predicted postpar- tum complications for mothers with high biomedical risk (Smilkstein, Helsper- Lucas, Ashworth, Montano, & Pagel, 1974).

Clinical utility: Although normative data are available for only small samples of predominantly college student and outpatient clinical groups, the Family APGAR has potential for use as a screening instrument for detecting an indi- vidual's level of satisfaction with family functioning. The instrument may prove particularly useful to family physicians as a quick method of assessing family functioning as a social support resource in relation to the health status of the patient.

Research utility: Validity studies of the Family APGAR are promising. The instrument has potential for use in research situations calling for a subject's global assessment of family functioning.

SUMMARY EVALUATION

The Family APGAR will probably be most useful as a screening instrument for physicians or for others who need to make quick assessments of family func- tioning. Similarly, the instrument may be useful as a rough and global assess- ment of an individual's perception of family functioning for research that re- lates social support to behavioral and physical health outcomes. Limitations of this global screening device include the inability to differentiate variability of functioning within the family (e.g., subsystems) and the deceptiveness of measuring complex variables with a single item. One advantage of the instrument is that it was designed for use with single persons and nontraditional families as well as with traditional nuclear families. Validity studies to date appear promising.

REFERENCES

Good, M. D., Smilkstein, G., Good, B. J., Shaffer, T., & Arons, T. (1979). The Family APGAR INDEX: A study of construct validity. *Journal of Family Practice, 8,* 577–582.

McNabb, T. R. (1982). Family function and depression. *Journal of Family Practice, 16,* 169–171.

Smilkstein, G. (undated). *Instructions for use of the Family APGAR, a family function screening questionnaire.* (Available from G. Smilkstein, School of Medicine, University of Washington, Seattle, WA)

Smilkstein, G. (1978). The Family APGAR: A proposal for a family function test and its use by physicians. *Journal of Family Practice, 6,* 1231–1239.

Smilkstein, G. (1980). Assessment of family function. In G. M. Rosen, J. P. Geyman, & R. H. Layton (Eds.), *Behavioral science in family practice.* New York: Appleton-Century-Crofts.

Smilkstein, G., Ashworth,C., & Montano, D. (1982). Validity and reliability of the Family APGAR as a test of family function. *Journal of Family Practice, 15,* 303–311.

Smilkstein, G., Helsper-Lucas, A., Ashworth, C., Montano, D., & Pagel, M. (1984). Prediction of pregnancy complications: An application of the biopsychosocial model. *Social Science and Medicine, 18,* 315–321.

AUTHOR'S RESPONSE

No additional comments.

W-6
Family Assessment Measure (FAM-III)

GENERAL INFORMATION

Date of publication: 1984.

Authors: Harvey A. Skinner, Paul D. Steinhauer, and Jack Santa-Barbara.

Source/publisher: Addiction Research Foundation, Toronto.

Availability: Available from Dr. Harvey Skinner, Addiction Research Foundation, 33 Russell St., Toronto, Ontario, Canada M5S 2S1. Plans are in progress for the formal publication of this assessment measure and a manual.

Brief description: The FAM is a self-report measure of family strengths and weaknesses from three perspectives: the family as a system, dyadic relationships, and individual family members.

Purpose: The FAM is designed for use as a diagnostic tool, as a measure of therapy process and outcome, and as a measure of family process in research.

Theoretical base: The Process Model of Family Functioning. This model, an elaboration of two earlier models, the Family Categories Schema and the McMaster Model of Family Functioning, emphasizes family dynamics and the interaction between individual and family process.

PHYSICAL DESCRIPTION OF QUESTIONNAIRE

Physical features: The FAM is composed of three scales: a 50-item, nine subscale General scale; a 42-item, seven-subscale Dyadic-Relationships scale; and a 42-item, seven-subscale Self-Rating scale. All items have the same four possible responses. "strongly agree," "agree," "disagree," and "strongly disagree." The FAM is considered appropriate for family members over 10 to 12 years of age (Skinner, Steinhauer, & Santa-Barbara, 1984).

Unit of study: Whole family; dyadic relationships, individual within the family.

Respondent: Individual family members, independently.

Scales and dimensions: The FAM consists of three scales: (1) a 50-item General scale, which measures the overall level of family health–pathology; (2) a 42-item Dyadic-Relationships scale, which examines how each member views each of his or her dyadic relationships; (3) a 42-item Self-Rating scale, which allows each member to rate his or her functioning within the family. Family functioning, from these three perspectives, is evaluated across seven dimensions: Task Accomplishment, Role Performance, Communication, Affective Expression, Affective Involvement, Control, Values and Norms. Thus, items reflecting each dimension appear within each of the three scales. An overall rating for each scale is simply the average of the seven clinical scales. In addition to the clinical scales, a Social Desirability scale and a Denial-Defensiveness scale are built into the General scale.

Manual: An administration and interpretation guide is currently available for the FAM, and development of a formal manual is in progress (Skinner et al., 1984). The guide includes information on administration, scoring, and interpretation of measurement results.

Standardization and norms: The FAM was standardized on a group of 475 families (933 adults, 502 children). The sample appeared representative across socioeconomic groups. No information regarding ethnicity is provided. Of the standardization sample, 28% were designated problem families, defined on the basis of one or more family members having received professional help for psychiatric, school-related, or legal problems. Differentiating demographic characteristics of the problem families are not provided (Skinner, Steinhauer, & Santa-Barbara, 1983).

Evaluation of physical description of questionnaire: *Strengths:* (1) Multilevel assessment perspective across consistent dimensions; (2) standardization and normative data; (3) response format that permits range of response. *Limitations:* (1) The standardization sample may be biased, as recruitment occurred via health and social service organizations. (2) Information regarding the problem families sample is limited.

ADMINISTRATIVE PROCEDURES

Directions: Respondents are instructed to read the directions appearing on the front of the test booklet (one provided for each scale) to decide how well the statement describes their family, then to circle the corresponding letter on the answer sheet. Distribution of only one questionnaire and corresponding answer sheet at a time is recommended. Questionnaires and answer sheets are color-coded. Completion of the measure will take from 20 to 60 minutes, depending on the number of questionnaires administered and the number of people (dyadic relationships) in the family. Family members complete the measures individually.

Ease of use: The FAM instructions are self-explanatory. Administrative procedures are simple, and, when they are followed, this measure would appear easy to use. No information is provided regarding individual versus group administration.

Training for administration and scoring: Guidelines regarding administration and scoring are clearly explicated (Skinner et al., 1984).

Scoring procedures: Answer sheets are composed of two parts: a top sheet upon which the respondent marks and a bottom scorer's sheet upon which the numerical value of the response is transferred automatically. First, raw scores for each subscale of each questionnaire are derived by summing the value of the responses per subscale. Raw scale scores are then converted to standard scores, based on conversion tables provided for adults and for adolescents. Finally, standard scores are plotted onto a separate profile for each scale.

Evaluation of administrative procedures: *Strengths:* The FAM is relatively easy to administer and to score. The use of answer sheets permits recycling of test booklets. Profile forms enhance the clinical interpretation of the data. *Limitations:* Depending on the size of the family, administration of the FAM may become quite lengthy, which may result in less valid responses. Additionally, sequential administration of individual questionnaires appears of considerable importance for the respondent to be able to maintain the perspective requested. A concern deserving empirical investigation is the extent to which children who have not attained a formal operations cognitive developmental level are able to respond reliably to the FAM, particularly to the multiple Dyadic-Relationships scale.

EVALUATION OF CONSTRUCTS MEASURED

Reliability: Reliability data were obtained from statistical analyses of the standardization sample (Skinner et al., 1983). Internal consistency reliability estimates (coefficient alpha) for the overall ratings were substantial: General scale (adults, .93; children, .94); Dyadic-Relationships scale (adults, .95; children, .94); Self-Rating scale (adults, .89; children, .86). The median reliability for the briefer individual scale reliabilities was lower. For adult respondents, General scale subscale reliability ranged from .67 to .87 (median, .73); Dyadic-Relationships scale subscale reliability ranged from .64 to .82 (median, .72); and Self-Rating scale subscale reliability ranged from .39 to .67 (median, .53).

Intercorrelations among the subscales were moderate to high in a sample of clinical families: General scale, .39 to .70; Dyadic-Relationships scale, .63 to .82; Self-Rating scale, .25 to .63. The median correlation of subscales with social desirability was $-.53$ (General scale), $-.35$ (Dyadic-Relationships), and $-.35$ (Self-Rating). The median correlation with defensiveness was $-.48$ (General scale), $-.28$ (Dyadic-Relationships), and $-.28$ (Self-Rating). Significance data regarding the correlations is not provided (Skinner, 1987).

No test–retest reliability for the FAM has yet been published.

Validity: *Criterion:* The discriminating power of FAM-III in differentiating problem from nonproblem families was examined by Skinner et al. (1983). A multiple discriminant analysis found that four discriminant functions were statistically significant $(p < .001)$; however, two functions were the major discriminators, accounting for 84% of group differences. One dimension (Control, Values/Norms, and Affective Expression) differentiated adults from children; the second dimension (Role Performance and Involvement) significantly discriminated between problem and nonproblem families.

In a study of anorexia nervosa, several FAM subscales were found to discriminate between groups. Mothers were differentiated significantly on the subscales of Task Accomplishment, Role Performance, Communication and Affective Expression, and Social Desirability. Adolescents were significantly differentiated on Task Accomplishment, Role Performance, and Social Desirability (Garfinkel et al., 1983).

A number of research studies are currently being conducted that are expected to provide additional external validation information.

Clinical utility: The FAM has demonstrated clinical utility in corroborating and expanding upon clinical impressions (Skinner et al., 1983; Steinhauer, 1984).

Research utility: Preliminary evidence suggests that the FAM has research utility (e.g., Garfinkel et al., 1983); however, as FAM authors acknowledge, this measure continues to be in the development phase, with research utility yet to be determined and significantly dependent, at present, on psychometric considerations.

SUMMARY EVALUATION

The FAM-III provides a unique contribution to the existing self-report measures of family process with its three-level analysis of family functioning. In addition to this structural strength, the FAM is easily administered and scored, with normative data and interpretative guidelines available. Limitations of the FAM-III center on limited reliability and validity studies completed to date. Of particular psychometric concern are the high subscale intercorrelations obtained, suggesting that constructs within scales are not distinct; the lack of test–retest reliability data; and the low internal consistency evident for the Self-Rating scale subscales.

REFERENCES

Garfinkel, P. E., Garner, D. M., Rose, J., Darby, P. L., Brandes, J. S., O'Hanlon, J., & Walsh, N. (1983). A comparison of characteristics in the families of patients with anorexia nervosa and normal controls. *Psychological Medicine, 13,* 821–828.

Skinner, H. A. (1987). Self-report instrument for family assessment. In T. Jacob (Ed.), *Family interaction and psychopathology: Theories, methods and findings.* New York: Plenum.

Skinner, H. A., Steinhauer, P. D., & Santa-Barbara, J. (1983). The Family Assessment Measure. *Canadian Journal of Community Mental Health, 2*(2), 91–105.

Skinner, H. A., Steinhauer, P. D., & Santa-Barbara, J. (1984). *The Family Assessment Measure: Administration and interpretation guide.* Toronto: Addiction Research Foundation.

Steinhauer, P. D. (1984). Clinical applications of the Process Model of Family Functioning. *Canadian Journal of Psychiatry, 29,* 98–111.

Steinhauer, P. D., Santa-Barbara, J., & Skinner, H. (1984). The Process Model of Family Functioning. *Canadian Journal of Psychiatry, 29,* 77–87.

AUTHOR'S RESPONSE

Additional references are available from the author. See the FAM Clinical Rating Scale abstract (in Section V) for author comments.

W-7
Family Environment Scale (FES)

GENERAL INFORMATION

Date of publication: 1974.

Authors: R. Moos and B. Moos.

Source/publisher: Consulting Psychologists Press, 577 College Ave., Palo Alto, CA 94306.

Availability: Manual (2nd ed., 1986) and specimen set available from source (above).

Brief description: The FES is 90-item, true–false, self-report questionnaire that assesses the social environment characteristics of all types of families. It is composed of 10 subscales that assess three underlying dimensions: interpersonal relationships, personal growth emphases, and basic organizational structure. The FES has three forms: the Real Form (Form R), which measures members' perceptions of their conjugal or nuclear family environment; the Ideal Form (Form I), which measures conceptions of ideal family environments; and the Expectations Form (Form E), which measures people's expectations of a new family environment (e.g., foster family) following a major family life cycle event.

Purpose: The FES is designed to assess systematically the social or interpersonal climate of families so that a taxonomy and clinically useful typology of family environments can be constructed and a family change can be assessed.

Theoretical base: Social-ecological-psychological theory, family systems theory.

PHYSICAL DESCRIPTION OF QUESTIONNAIRE

Physical features: The FES is composed of 90 true–false items. The reading level is appropriate for adults and for children 11 years of age and over (Moos & Moos, 1981).

Unit of study: Whole family.

Respondent: Individual family members over age 11.

Scales and dimensions: The FES contains 10 subscales (nine items each) within three family social climate dimensions:

1. Relationship dimension
   Cohesion
   Expressiveness
   Conflict
2. Personal Growth dimension
   Independence
   Achievement Orientation
   Intellectual-Cultural Orientation
   Active-Recreational Orientation
   Moral-Religious Emphasis
3. System Maintenance dimension
   Organization
   Control

Manual: An FES manual is available from Consulting Psychologists Press (see "Source/publisher"). The manual includes a description of the measure, its rationale and development, administration and scoring directions, interpretation guidelines for research and clinical applications, and reliability and validity data.

Standardization and norms: The FES has been standardized and normed on a sample of 1,125 normal and 500 distressed families. The normal sample included both single-parent and multigenerational families from several ethnic minorities in various stages of the family life cycle and from several geographic sections of the United States. There is some question regarding the social class representativeness of the normal sample, which was predominantly high socioeconomic status. The distressed sample consisted of families in which a member exhibited a diagnosed psychiatric disorder, including substance abuse, delinquent or criminal behavior, and other family crises. Means and standard deviation scores are published for the clinical and normal families (Moos & Moos, 1981). Clinic families do not appear to have been matched on critical variables (e.g., socioeconomic status) with normal families.

Evaluation of physical description of questionnaire: *Strengths:* (1) Theoretically based; (2) standardized and normed; (3) comprehensive manual available; (4) items easily understood by respondents. *Limitations:* (1) Inadequate information is presented in the manual regarding variations in socioeconomic status, education, and ethnicity among the standardization samples. The FES may have differential predictive validity and discriminatory power with low-income and less-educated families. (2) Item content generally reflects whole-family functioning, whereas responses might differ for certain individuals or dyads within the family.

ADMINISTRATIVE PROCEDURES

Directions: Respondents are instructed to read the item in the test booklet and to mark an X in the appropriate box (true–false) on the answer sheet. Family members complete the measure independently. There is no time limit.

Ease of use: No special administrative procedures are required. Directions and items are self-explanatory. The FES can be administered to individuals or groups. The answer sheet format may pose some initial difficulty for respondents and should be supervised for the first few items.

Training for administration and scoring: No training is required beyond reading the directions provided in the manual.

Scoring procedures: The answer sheet is arranged so that each column represents one of the 10 subscales. An answer sheet key (template) can be superimposed on the answer sheet and the ''true'' responses for each subscale summed, giving a score for the subscale. Subscale scores are converted to standard scores and placed on a profile form, which permits a visual depiction of family environment factors that exceed the normal range.

Evaluation of administrative procedures: *Strengths:* The FES is easy to administer and to score. The use of answer sheets permits recycling of test booklets. The profile form enhances clinical interpretation of the data. *Limitations:* The true–false response format may not provide an adequate range of response.

EVALUATION OF CONSTRUCTS MEASURED

Reliability: The 10 FES subscales demonstrate adequate internal consistency, ranging from .61 to .78. Test–retest reliabilites range from .68 to .86 for a 2-month interval and .52 to .89 for a 12 month interval (Moos & Moos, 1981), indicating considerable stability. Average subscale intercorrelations vary considerably, with a range of .01 to .45 (absolute mean intercorrelation, .25). Subscale intercorrelations within dimensions are not consistently greater than between dimensions. Thus, the FES subscales, to a varying degree, measure distinct though somewhat related aspects of family social environments.

Validity: *Construct:* Although the FES was constructed with factor analysis procedures, several investigations have challenged its dimensional structure. Fowler (1981, 1982a), using a varimax-rotation factor analysis with the original FES normative sample, found a two-factor solution to be most appropriate. The two factors were a bipolar interpersonal dimension and a unipolar control dimension. The two dimensions were replicated in a subsequent research with a college sample (Fowler, 1982b). Robertson and Hyde (1982), using a principal-components factor analysis procedure with high school–aged sample, similarly found that the FES does not contain 10 dimensions. Rather, seven dimensions were identified, four of which replicated. Nelson (1984), using a principal-components factor analysis of the FES with a sample of middle school–aged children, identified three factors: a bipolar support-structure versus conflict factor; a bipolar cohesion versus control factor; and a unipolar independence-achievement orientation. *Criterion:* The validity of the FES has been established in more than 200 studies in which it has been found to discriminate normal from disturbed families, to differentiate family types, and to relate to treatment outcomes in predictable ways (Moos, Clayton, & Max, 1979; Moos & Spinrad, 1984). Recent studies corroborate these research findings, with the FES differentiating the families of social maladjusted adolescents (Fox, Rotatori, Macklin, Green, & Fox, 1983) and the families of former psychiatric inpatients (Spiegel & Wissler, 1983). The FES Relationship dimension has been found to vary with changes in the level of family social support (Mitchell & Moos, 1984), and the Conflict scale has been found to differentiate children's functioning in postdivorce family situations (Dancy & Handel, 1984). FES variables differentially predicted treatment gains and relapse in an alcoholic sample (Moos & Moos, 1984).

Clinical utility: Numerous published articles (Moos et al., 1979; Moos & Spinrad, 1984) attest to the clinical utility of the FES, both as a diagnostic device and as a measure of treatment effectiveness.

Research utility: The FES has demonstrated research utility, as evidenced by the numerous studies supporting the criterion-related validity of the measure. Less clearly evaluated is the differential predictive utility of the FES across socioeconomic groups. Additionally, the factor structure of the FES remains controversial. Therefore, researchers are advised to replicate the FES subscale intercorrelations and factor analyses with adequate sample sizes to determine fit with their particular samples.

SUMMARY EVALUATION

The FES is a 90-item, true–false questionnaire that assesses family members' perceptions of their family social climate along three dimensions: Interpersonal Relationships, Personal Growth, and System Maintenance. Strengths of the FES include adequate standardization and normative data; a clear and comprehensive manual; ease of administration, scoring, and data reduction; and extensive validation research. Caution remains appropriate regarding interpretation of this measure with lower socioeconomic groups. Additionally, the most parsimonious factor structure of the FES may vary across samples.

REFERENCES

Dancy, B. L., & Handal, P. J. (1984). Perceived family climate, psychological adjustment, and peer relationships of black adolescents: A function of parental marital status or perceived family conflict? *Journal of Community Psychology, 12,* 222–229.

Fox, R., Rotatori, A. F., Macklin, F., Green, H., & Fox, T. (1983). Socially maladjusted adolescents perceptions of their families. *Psychological Reports, 52,* 831–834.

Fowler, P. C. (1981). Maximum likelihood factor structure of the Family Environment Scale. *Journal of Clinical Psychology, 37* (1), 160–164.

Fowler, P. C. (1982a). Factor structure of the Family Environment Scale: Effects of social desirability. *Journal of Clinical Psychology, 38* (2), 285–292.

Fowler, P. (1982b). Relationship of family environment and personality characteristics: Canonical analyses of self-attributions. *Journal of Clinical Psychology, 38* (4), 804–810.

Mitchell, R. E., & Moos, R. H (1984). Deficiencies in social support among depressed patients: Antecedents or consequences of stress? *Journal of Health and Social Behavior, 25,* 438–452.

Moos, R. H., Clayton, J., & Max, W. (1979). *The social climate scales: An annotated bibliography.* Palo Alto, CA: Consulting Psychologists Press.

Moos, R. H., & Moos, B. S. (1981). *Family Environment Scale manual.* Palo Alto, CA: Consulting Psychologists Press.

Moos, R. H., & Moos, B. S. (1984). The process of recovery from alcoholism: III. Comparing functioning in families of alcoholics and matched control families. *Journal of Studies on Alcohol, 45* (2), 111–118.

Moos, R. H., & Spinrad, S. (1984). *The social climate scales: An annotated bibliography.* Palo Alto, CA: Consulting Psychologists Press.

Nelson, G. (1984). The relationship between dimensions of classroom and family environments and the self-concept, satisfaction, and achievement of grade 7 and 8 students. *Journal of Community Psychology, 12,* 276–287.

Robertson, D. U., & Hyde, J. S. (1982). The factorial validity of the Family Environment Scale. *Educational and Psychological Measurement, 42,* 1233–1241.

Spiegel, D., & Wissler, T. (1983). Perceptions of family environment among psychiatric patients and their wives. *Family Process, 22,* 537–547.

AUTHOR'S RESPONSE

No additional comments.

W-8
Family Evaluation Form (FEF)

GENERAL INFORMATION

Date of publication: 1980; revised version, 1984.

Authors: Robert S. Emery, Sheldon Weintraub, and John M. Neale.

Source/publisher: Sheldon A. Weintraub, Department of Psychology, SUNY, Stony Brook, NY 11794.

Availability: Available from author (see "Source/publisher," above).

Brief description: The original Family Evaluation Form is a 136-item self-report instrument. The finished version includes 17 scales. A 7-point rating scale is the response format for the first 125 items. The response format for the remaining 8 items is forced-choice. The revised form of the instrument has 128 items, which make up 18 scales.

Purpose: The Family Evaluation Form was developed as an easy-to-use yet comprehensive measure of family functioning for researchers.

Theoretical base: The theoretical base of the Family Evaluation Form is best described as eclectic. Items were derived empirically and from relevant theoretical constructs in the literature in order to provide an "omnibus" measure of family functioning (Emery, Weintraub, & Neale, 1980).

PHYSICAL DESCRIPTION OF QUESTIONNAIRE

Physical features The original version of the Family Evaluation Form consists of 136 items (revised version, 125 items). Most of the items are statements about family members, which are rated on a 7-point scale according to how well they describe the family ("not at all," "a little," "somewhat," "moderately," "quite a lot," "very much," and "extremely"). Some of the items are rated twice, once for the husband once for the wife. Several additional questions are asked, which are answered using a forced-choice format, with specific alternatives (four to seven choices) provided.

Unit of study: Whole family.

Respondent: Husband and wife in the family.

Scales and dimensions: Scales included in the 1984 (revised) version are Family Centeredness, Conflict and Tension, Open Communication, Emotional Closeness, Community Involvement, Children's Relations, Children's Adjustment, Parenting—Nurturance, Parenting—Independence Training, Parenting—Effective Discipline, Parenting—Strict/Punitive Discipline, Parenting—Negative Style, Husband/Wife Dominance, Marital Satisfaction, Homemaker Role, Worker Role, Financial Problems, and Extrafamilial Support.

Manual: None available.

Standardization and norms: Copies of the Family Evaluation Form were mailed to a stratified (by social class) random sample in a suburban New York county, and normative data were compiled on 132 forms returned from 88 families, including 44 families with responses from both husband and wife, 34 families with responses from only one parent and 10 single-parent families. Means and standard deviations are given separately for mothers and fathers of the total sample and for high-, middle-, and low-income census tracts (mothers and fathers combined). Correlations between mothers' and fathers' ratings on each scale are also given (Emery et al., 1980).

Evaluation of physical description of questionnaire: *Strengths:* Reading level and response format seem appropriate; local norms are available. *Limitations:* So far, norms are limited, and the length of the FEF could be a liability. Item content reflects whole-family functioning, whereas responses could differ when referring to specific individuals or dyads within the family.

ADMINISTRATIVE PROCEDURES

Directions: Simple directions for the respondent are provided with the instrument.

Ease of use: The instrument is easy to administer, requiring only the items and a pencil. It could be computer-scored

Training for administration and scoring: The FEF could be administered by nonprofessionals. Scoring for the instrument will probably be simple to learn once written instructions are provided.

Scoring procedures, including calculation of summary scores: Written scoring procedures are not given with the instrument. It seems that the score for each scale is composed of the mean of ratings of items making that scale. Since the number of responses varies among items, clear scoring instructions are essential. The instrument does come with a list of items that belong to each scale, and items with reversed scoring are marked with an asterisk.

Evaluation of administrative procedures: *Strengths:* ease of administration. *Limitations:* Lack of clearly written scoring procedures.

EVALUATION OF CONSTRUCTS MEASURED

Reliability: Alpha coefficients are given for mothers' and fathers' separate and combined scores. Alphas for the combined scores ranged from .41 to .89, with only four of the scales included in the original instrument falling below .62. Two-week test–retest reliabilities for a small sample ($n = 15$) for the various scales ranged from .94 to .40 (Emery et al., 1980). The only psychometric data available on the 1984 (revised) version of the FEF are alpha coefficients, which range from .88 to .61 for the 18 scales that make up the new version.

Validity: Significant correlations between mothers' and fathers' scores were found for all but one of the scales (Marital Satisfaction) in the original finished version. Significant differences among census tract groups (with higher-income families scoring in a more desirable direction) on four scales and significant differences between spouses on three scales were offered by the authors as evidence of validity (Emery et al., 1980).

Clinical utility: Demonstration of the clinical utility of the Family Evaluation Form awaits its use with a wider variety of families and a broader standardization sample.

Research utility: Although the instrument has potential, further validation studies are essential to demonstrate its usefulness for research.

SUMMARY EVALUATION

Work in progress (including more normative work and work on test–retest reliability and construct validation) with the revised version of the Family Evaluation Form should add to our knowledge of the instrument's usefulness. At present, the instrument lacks clear scoring instructions, a broadly based normative sample, and adequate evidence of validity. The instrument is long and is composed of many (possibly redundant) scales, which have not been factor analyzed. The FEF is designed for use with single-parent as well as two-parent families.

REFERENCES

Emery, R. E., Weintraub, S., & Neale, J. M. (1980, August). *The Family Evaluation Form: Construction and Normative data.* Paper presented at the annual meeting of the American Psychological Association, Montreal.

Forman, B. D., & Hagan, B. J. (1983). A comparative review of total family functioning measures. *American Journal of Family Therapy, 11,* 25–40.

AUTHOR'S RESPONSE

No additional comments.

W-9
Family Functioning in Adolescence Questionnaire (FFAQ)

GENERAL INFORMATION

Date of publication: 1985.

Authors: Ronelle Roelofse and Margaret Middleton.

Source/publisher: Roelofse, R., & Middleton, M. R. (1985). The Family Functioning in Adolescence Questionnaire: A measure of psychosocial family health during adolescence. *Journal of Adolescence, 8,* 33–45.

Availability: Available from Dr. Margaret R. Middleton, Dept. of Psychology, The Australian National University, GPO Box 4, A.C.T. 2601, Australia.

Brief description: The FFAQ is a 42-item self-report measure with a four-choice response format that was developed to assess family functioning as perceived by adolescents.

Purpose: The purpose of the FFAQ is to assess the adolescent's perception of the psychosocial health of the family during the stage in which it had adolescent children, focusing on six dimensions of the family system as they bear on the developmental tasks and identity formation of the adolescent.

Theoretical base: Family systems theory, family development theory, Erikson's identity formation theory.

PHYSICAL DESCRIPTION OF QUESTIONNAIRE

Physical features: The FFAQ includes 42 items, each responded to on a 4-point scale: "almost always true," "often true," "sometimes true," and "hardly ever true."

Unit of study: Whole family.

Respondent: The individual adolescent in the family.

Scales and dimensions: The six dimensions (subscales) are Structure, Affect, Communication, Behavior Control, Value Transmission, and External System.

Manual: A manual is available from the authors. It includes instructions for administration, the items, and a scoring key.

Standardization and norms: Formal norms are unavailable. Roelofse and Middleton (1985) report means, standard deviations, and ranges for the six scale scores on a sample of 413 Australian adolescents

Evaluation of physical description of questionnaire: *Strengths:* Response format, length, and reading level seem appropriate and comprehensible. *Limitations:* There is a lack of normative data. Questions refer to whole-family functioning, whereas perceptions might vary as a function of the individual family member or subsystem being referred to. Item format assesses two distinct constructs on several items. Minor revisions in phrasing may be necessary for cross-cultural use.

ADMINISTRATIVE PROCEDURES

Directions: Directions to the respondent are clear and explicit regarding the appropriate frame of reference to be adopted.

Ease of use: The FFAQ is easy to administer, requiring only the items, an answer sheet, and a pencil. It can easily be computer-scored.

Training for administration and scoring: The FFAQ could be administered and scored by nonprofessionals.

Scoring procedures, including calculation of summary scores: Scoring procedures are provided in the manual. Responses are assigned a score of 1, 2, 3, or 4, and then summed. For most items, number scores correspond directly to the degree of frequency indicated. Notably, however, some items (on the Structure, Cohesion, and External Systems scales) are scored to allow for the curvilinear relation between the item and family health.

Evaluation of administrative procedures: *Strengths:* Easy to administer and score; curvilinear relation to family health explicitly recognized. *Limitations:* None noted.

EVALUATION OF CONSTRUCTS MEASURED

Reliability: The alpha coefficient for the entire instrument is .90. Alphas for subscales are as follows: Structure, .57; Affect, .77; Communication, .79; Behavior Control, .49; Value Transmission, .51; and External System, .40. All subscale intercorrelations are very high (r ranges from .76 to .89). No test–retest results are reported.

Validity: *Construct:* Factor analysis yielded a single factor with eigenvalue greater than 1.0, accounting for 54% of the variance. *Criterion-related:* Adolescents who were able to use a wider variety of appropriate means in solving problems perceived their families as functioning better; inappropriate problem solving (e.g., cheating, aggression) was negatively related to reported family functioning. The correlation between the FFAQ and the Erikson Psychosocial Stage Inventory was .46.

Clinical utility: The FFAQ has questionable clinical utility until more complete normative data are available. It does have the potential to be clinically useful for those working with adolescents. Item responses could be springboards for discussion in therapy.

Research utility: The instrument is potentially useful in research, but it needs further validity study.

SUMMARY EVALUATION

This instrument shows promise but is still largely untested. Further research will be necessary to establish its usefulness. Because of the high internal consistency of the full scale and the single factor that emerged in the factor analysis, the instrument may be measuring one overall dimension rather than six distinguishable constructs.

REFERENCES

Roelofse, R., & Middleton, M. R. (1985). The Family Functioning in Adolescence Questionnaire: A measure of psychosocial family health during adolescence. *Journal of Adolescence, 8,* 33–45.

AUTHOR'S RESPONSE

No additional comments.

W-10
Family Process Scales (FPS), Form E

GENERAL INFORMATION

Date of publication: 1985.

Authors: Oscar A. Barbarin and Renee Gilbert.

Source/publisher: Family Development Project, Ann Arbor, MI

Availability: Available from Oscar A. Barbarin, Family Development Project Lab, Dept. of Psychology, University of Michigan, 580 Union Dr., Ann Arbor, MI 48109.

Brief description: The Family Process Scales include 50 items, each of which is responded to on a 5-point Likert-type scale, from "strongly agree" to "strongly disagree."

Purpose: The purpose of the Family Process Scales is to assess interdependence of family members, dynamic homeostasis in the family, and the family's ability to provide an environment that fosters healthy psychological development and promotes a sense of well-being in its members.

Theoretical base: Family systems theory.

PHYSICAL DESCRIPTION OF QUESTIONNAIRE

Physical features: The FPS includes 50 items, which are responded to on a 5-point Likert-type scale ranging from "strongly agree" to "strongly disagree." Although not specified, the reading level would probably be suitable for early adolescents through adults.

Unit of study: Whole family.

Respondent: Individual family member.

Scales and dimensions: Five factor-analytically derived scales, each including 10 items, are measured: Enmeshment, Mutuality, Flexibility, Support, and Satisfaction.

Manual: No manual is provided; information concerning the measure was obtained from published articles and preprints.

Standardization and norms: According to a profile provided in Barbarin (undated): "high" scores on each scale range from 40 to 50, "medium" scores range from 26–39, and "low" scores range from 10 to 25. The derivation of these norms is unknown.

Evaluation of physical description of questionnaire: *Strengths:* The FPS is empirically derived and grounded in family theory. It has a clear response format with adequate range; items are of comprehensible length; and reading level is appropriate for adolescents and adults. *Limitations:* Further information concerning norms, standardization procedures, and so forth, is needed. The content of some items reflects whole-family functioning, whereas perceptions might vary for different individuals or subsystems within the family.

ADMINISTRATIVE PROCEDURES

Directions: Respondents are asked to indicate the extent to which each of 50 items describes how they see their family.

Ease of use: The FPS is very easy to use.

Training for administration and scoring: Very little training is required. The instrument may be hand-scored or computed-scored.

Scoring procedures: The five summary scores are computed by summing the respondent's answers to the 10 items on each scale.

Evaluation of administrative procedures: *Strengths:* The FPS is very easy to administer, use, and score. *Weaknesses:* Ease of use and scoring may mask the complexity of the constructs being assessed.

EVALUATION OF CONSTRUCTS MEASURED

Reliability: Cronbach's alphas in two studies: Support = .91, .96; Matuality = .86, .86; Satisfaction = .86, .87; Flexibility = .74, .87; Differentiation-Enmeshment = .75, .87 (Barbarin, undated; Barbarin & Tirado, 1985).

Validity: *Criterion-related:* The FPS Enmeshment scale correlated significantly with the Cohesion scale on the FACES ($r = -.25$) and the Cohesion scale on the Family Environment Scale ($r = -.29$); the Flexibility subscale correlated .52 with the FACES Adaptability scale; the Support scale correlated .55 with

FES Expressiveness and .75 with FACES Cohesion; Satisfaction correlated .80 with FACES Cohesion (Barbarin & Tirado, 1985). The FPS Support scale correlated .55 with the Deger-McCullough Cohesion scale.The Satisfaction scale correlated .76 with the Deger-McCullough Happiness-Contentment scale. Mutuality correlated significantly with FACES Cohesion, and Differentiation-Enmeshment correlated negatively with Cohesion ($r = -.48$) (Barbarin, undated). The Enmeshment scale successfully discriminated between families whose interactions seem to influence successful maintenance of weight loss from families whose interactions do not (Barbarin & Tirado, 1985). *Construct-related:* Correlation of FPS scales with conceptually similar scales (see above) and higher monotrait, heteromethod than heterotrait, monomethod correlations for each of the FPS scales are presented as evidence of convergent and discriminant validity (Barbarin, undated).

Clinical utility: The FPS can be used prior to an initial therapy session as an intake instrument and can be used in controlled studies of the effects of particular types of interventions on families. Illustrations of clinical use of the FPS may be found in Barbarin (undated).

Research utility: Researchers may use the FPS as dependent variables in studies or to classify families in research projects.

SUMMARY EVALUATION

The FPS was derived from family systems theory rather than empirically. It has undergone several revisions and a fair amount of testing, and it is easy to administer, take, and score. It has demonstrated adequate internal consistency and has accrued some evidence in support of cirterion-related and construct validity. On the other hand, the FPS is not a comprehensive measure of family process.

REFERENCES

Barbarin, O. A. (undated). *Measuring basic family processes: Development and use of the FPS.* Manuscript submitted for publication.

Barbarin, O. A., & Gilbert, R. (1979). *Family Process Scales.* Ann Arbor, MI: Family Development Project.

Barbarin, O. A., & Tirado, M. (1985) Enmeshment, family processes, and successful treatment of obesity. *Family Relations, 34,* 115–121.

AUTHOR'S RESPONSE

No additional comments.

W-11
Family Relationship Questionnaire (FRQ)

GENERAL INFORMATION

Date of publication: 1980.

Authors: Scott W. Henggeler and Joseph B. Tavormina.

Source/publisher: Scott W. Henggeler, Department of Psychology, Memphis State University Memphis, TN 38152.

Availability: Available from Scott Henggeler at the above address.

Brief description: The FRQ consists of 11 Likert-type items with 5-point response formats for rating family functioning along the dimensions of affect, conflict, and dominance.

Purpose: The FRQ was designed to measure each family member's perception of the affect, conflict, and dominance within family dyads. The FRQ was developed for use with families that vary in cultural composition and socioeconomic status, including families with low literacy rates.

Theoretical base: The three dimensions measured by the FRQ—family affect, conflict, and dominance—are based on scales developed by Hetherington and Frankie (1965, cited in Henggeler, Borduin, & Mann, 1987) and are derived from research in the child development and psychiatric literature relating those dimensions of family functioning to various child clinical problems.

PHYSICAL DESCRIPTION OF QUESTIONNAIRE

Physical features: Eleven items are included in the FRQ. Each is rated according to a 5-point response format (e.g., "never" to "always" and "mother always get her own way" to "father always get his own way"). Although designed for low-literacy respondents, the response format varies somewhat across domains, thus increasing response difficulty. Dyadic and whole-family relationship queries are merged within domains. The reading level is simple.

Unit of study: Dyadic relationships: mother–father, mother–adolescent, father–adolescent.

Respondent: Adult or adolescent family member.

Scales and dimensions: Three dimensions are measured by the FRQ: Affect, Conflict, and Dominance.

Manual: None available.

Standardization and norms: None available.

Evaluation of physical description of questionnaire: *Strengths:* The simplicity and easy reading level of the FRQ recommend it for use with families with low educational levels. Items are of comprehensible length, and the response format range is adequate. *Limitations:* Norms are not available for the FRQ, and, although it is purportedly a measure of dyadic relationshps, several items reflect whole-family functioning.

ADMINISTRATIVE PROCEDURES

Directions: Simple directions are provided with the questionnaire. However, they are limited in specificity.

Ease of use: The FRQ is easy to administer, requiring only the items and a pencil.

Training for administration and scoring: The FRQ could be administered by nonprofessionals although scoring procedures are not explicit.

Scoring procedures, including calculation of summary scores: Although explicit scoring procedures are not given, the assumption is that scores for each of the three scales are summed.

Evaluation of administrative procedures: *Strengths:* Ease of administration and scoring. *Limitations:* Directions that discourage socially desirable responses are not provided. Items are possibly too simple to tap complex family variables adequately.

EVALUATION OF CONSTRUCTS MEASURED

Reliability: Mean test–retest reliabilities of .67 and .70 (Henggeler et al., 1987; Henggeler & Tavormina, 1980) are given for a period of 1 to 2 weeks. Although the instrument uses a numbering format that shows only one item per scale, each of the items has several parts that appear to be separate items. No evidence has been presented for internal consistency within each of the three scales.

Validity: Several studies support the criterion-related validity of the Affect and Conflict dimensions of the FRQ. The affective relationship between father and child predicted membership in delinquent versus nondelinquent groups for black, lower-class boys (Borduin, Pruitt, & Henggeler, 1986). In another study (Hanson, Henggeler, Haefele, & Rodick, 1984), the parent–child affective relationship predicted several types of adolescent offender status. Mother–son conflict differentiated delinquent from nondelinquent adolescent boys (Borduin et al., 1986) and violent adolescent felons from nonviolent and control groups (Henggeler, Hanson, Borduin, Watson, & Brunk, 1985). No studies to date have provided validity support for the Dominance dimension or for the FRQ as a whole.

Clinical utility: The FRQ was developed for use in research. No norms are available, and the instrument is probably not suitable for use in a clinical setting.

Research utility: Several demensions of the FRQ show promise for use in family research. However, the instrument's current usefulness is limited until adequate evidence of the reliability and validity of all dimensions of the FRQ has been established.

SUMMARY EVALUATION

The FRQ has potential for use in family research because of its simplicity, which lends itself to use with diverse types of families. However, the usefulness of the measure is limited by a lack of normative data and a lack of psychometric support, particularly evidence of validity.

REFERENCES

Borduin, C. M., Pruitt, J.A., & Henggeler, S. W. (1986). Family interactions in black, lower-class families with delinquent and nondelinquent adolescent boys. *Journal of Genetic Psychology, 147,* 333–342.

Hanson, C. L., Henggeler, S. W., Haefele, W. F., & Rodick, J. D. (1984). Demographic, individual, and family relationship correlates of serious and repeated crime among adolescents and their siblings. *Journal of Consulting and Clinical Psychology, 52,* 528–538.

Henggeler, S. W., Borduin, C. M. & Mann, B. J. (1987). Intrafamily agreement: Association with clinical status, social desirability, and observational ratings. *Journal of Applied Developmental Psychology, 8,* 97–111.

Henggeler, S. W., Hanson, C. L. Borduin, C. M., Watson, S. M., & Brunk, M. A. (1985). Mother–son relationships of juvenile felons. *Journal of Consulting and Clinical Psychology, 53,* 942–943.

Henggeler, S. W., Rodick, J. D., Borduin, C. M., Hanson, C. L., Watson, S. M., & Urey, J. R. (1986). Multisystemic treatment of juvenile offenders: Effects on adolescent behavior and family interactions. *Developmental Psychology, 22,* 132–141.

Henggeler, S. W., & Tavormina, J. B. (1980). Social class and race differences in family interaction: Pathological, normative, or confounding methodological factors? *Journal of Genetic Psychology, 137,* 211–222.

AUTHOR'S RESPONSE

No additional comments.

W-12
Index of Family Relations (IFR)

GENERAL INFORMATION

Date of publication: 1977.

Author: Walter W. Hudson.

Source/publisher: The Dorsey Press, 1818 Ridge Rd., Homewood, IL 60430.

Availability: Available as part of the Clinical Measurement Package.

Brief description: The Index of Family Relations (IFR) is a 25-item questionnaire in which a family member responds with perceptions of his or her family as a whole on a 5-point scale ranging from "rarely or none of the time" to "most or all of the time."

Purpose: The IFR, part of the Clinical Measurement Package (CMP), was developed for repeated use with a client to monitor and evaluate progress in therapy. The instrument was designed to measure the magnitude of a problem in family members' relationships as seen by the respondent and can be viewed as a measure of intrafamilial stress. Although the scale can be used in a variety of settings, the initial use was in single-subject, repeated-measures designs to monitor and guide treatment.

Theoretical base: Not explicitly stated; consistent with an interactionist perspective.

PHYSICAL DESCRIPTION OF QUESTIONNAIRE

Physical features: The IFR includes 25 items, each of which is responded to on a 5-point scale ranging from "rarely or none of the time" to "most or all of the time." Approximately half of the items are worded in a positive direction and half in a negative direction in order to control response set. The author suggests that the IFR not be administered to children under age 12.

Unit of study: whole family.

Respondent: Individual family member.

Scales and dimensions: The IFR was designed to be a unidimensional scale.

Manual: The CMP manual includes descriptions and sample copies of the nine scales (of which the IFR is one), instructions for scoring and administration of the scales, reliability and validity information, suggestions for using the scales, answers to pertinent questions, and references. The reading level is simple and is appropriate for adults and children over age 12.

Standardization and norms: A clinical cutting score of 30 or above indicates that the client has significant problems in the area of family relationships. The appropriateness of this score has been demonstrated in several validity studies (see below.)

Evaluation of physical description of questionnaire: *Strengths:* The IFR is a straightforward measure that is easy to understand. A comprehensive manual is available. The clinical cutting score of 30 seems appropriate for the instrument's clinical uses. The response format is clear and has an adequate range. *Limitations:* Since the nine Clinical Measurement Package scales are sold as a set, the IFR cannot be purchased separately. Anchor points are vague, and responses to some items that reflect whole-family functioning may vary among individual family members.

ADMINISTRATIVE PROCEDURES

Directions: Respondents are asked to respond to each item on a 5-point scale. To minimize the possibility that the subject might give socially desirable answers, the clinican should emphasize that the results will be used for the client's benefit and therefore need to be as accurate as possible.

Ease of use: The IFR is easy to use, as the questions are simple, and the instrument is easy to administer and score.

Training for administration and scoring: Little specialized training is needed for administration or scoring. Instructions concerning interpretation of the results are provided in the CMP manual.

Scoring procedures: Items written in a positive direction must first be reversed-scored. (The numbers of those items that require reverse-scoring are listed below the copyright notation at the bottom of the scale. (After reverse-scoring, the total score is computed by summing item scores and subtracting 25. If items have been omitted, the score is calculated as $S = (Y-N)(100)/[(N)(4)]$, where N is the number of items properly completed by the respondent.

Any item left blank or scored outside the 1–5 range is given a score of 0. This method of scoring yields a score ranging from 0 to 100, with higher scores indicating more problematic relationships. A score above 30 indicates that the person has a clinically significant problem in the area being measured.

Evaluation of administrative procedures: *Strengths:* The IFR is easy to administer, complete, and score. *Limitations:* Because of the nature of the questions, the administrator must take steps to minimize social desirability responses. In the clinical setting, Hudson recommends that the therapist tell the client that the measure must be completed honestly in order to benefit him or her. In a research setting, subjects might not so readily feel motivated to respond honestly.

EVALUATION OF CONSTRUCTS MEASURED

Reliability: In three studies cited in the manual, coefficient alphas were .91, .98, and .97 in samples of 198, 120, and 200, respectively. Hudson feels that test–retest reliability is "of dubious value" because of the instrument's use in clinical settings, in which change is expected.

Validity: *Criterion-related:* Discriminant validity has been well established for the IFR. Therapy clients who were determined independently to have or not have family relationship problems completed the IFR. The point-biserial correlation between group membership and IFR score was .92 (Hudson, Acklin, & Bartosh, 1980). The IFR was also significantly related ($r = .56$) to college students' answers to a question about family problems. *Construct-related:* In another study cited in the manual, correlations were computed between IFR items and scores on several other measures. As predicted, the items correlated better with scales they were theoretically related to than with those they were not related to.

Clinical utility: The primary purpose of the IFR is for use in a clinical setting. The CMP scales have been widely used and do appear to help clinicians monitor and guide their treatment and obtain improved estimates of the severity of client problems.

Research utility: The scale's high reliability and validity coefficients and its ease of administration, completion, and scoring would make it highly desirable in many research settings. Drawbacks, however, include the scale's atheoretical background and the possibility of social desirability response set.

SUMMARY EVALUATION

The IFR is a short-form, easily administered self-report measure of the severity of family relationship problems as seen by one or more family members. It has been shown to have acceptable reliability and validity. Because it is a self-report measure, it suffers from all the weaknesses and threats to validity that are common to this type of instrument: the intent of the items is quite transparent, and subjects could easily make themselves appear trouble-free; and there may be subjective variation in the vague anchor points on the scale. In addition, the questions on the IFR refer to the family as a whole, whereas a subject may note within-family variations in the accuracy of a particular statement. As was intended by the author, the measure would appear to be more useful and valid in a clinical setting than a research setting, since clients may be more willing to respond honestly.

REFERENCES

Hudson, W. W. (1982). *The Clinical Measurement Package.* Homewood, IL: Dorsey Press.

Hudson, W. W., Acklin, J. D., & Bartosh, J. C. (1980). Assessing discord in family relationships. *Social Work Research and Abstracts, 16*(3), 21–29.

Kurlychek, R. T. (1984). Review of *The Clinical Measurement Package. Journal of Personality Assessment, 48,* 107–108.

AUTHOR'S RESPONSE

No additional comments.

W-13
Inventory of Family Feelings (IFF)

GENERAL INFORMATION

Date of publication: 1973.

Author: Joseph C. Lowman.

Source/publisher: Joseph C. Lowman, PhD. Dept. of Psychology. The University of North Carolina, Chapel Hill, NC 27514.

Availability: Available from the author (see above).

Brief description: The IFF is a 38-item scale in which each family member indicates agreement with items in terms of his or her feelings at that moment toward every other family member.

Purpose: The IFF is designed to determine the affective structure of the family, particularly the strength of positive affect.

Theoretical base: Lowman proposes the Multilevel Model of Family Functioning (Lowman, 1981)—including the behavioral, cognitive and affective levels—which is compatible with family systems theory.

PHYSICAL DESCRIPTION OF QUESTIONNAIRE

Physical features: The IFF contains 38 items regarding feelings toward another family member, to which each member responds "agree," "disagree," or "neutral." The IFF takes approximately 20 minutes to complete, is written at a fifth-grade reading level, and can be completed by most children at least 12 years of age.

Unit of study: Whole family, dyadic relationships, individual member.

Respondent: Individual family member.

Scales and dimensions: Two scales were derived from factor analysis: Subjective Feelings and Perceived Feelings. These are positively and highly correlated; therefore, they are combined to produce a single affect score or dimension.

Manual: None available.

Standardization and norms: None available. Means and standard deviations on a small sample are provided in Lowman (1980).

Evaluation of physical description of questionnaire: *Strengths:* (1) Simplicity and clarity of the construct measured. (2) Opportunity for assessment of multiple family levels. *Limitations:* (1) Use of 3-point response format. (2) Although items are written at a fifth-grade reading level, the use of double negatives may increase the difficulty of comprehension. (3) Lack of norms.

ADMINISTRATIVE PROCEDURES

Directions: Self-explanatory directions are provided with the measure. Directions are somewhat lengthy and are likely to require some initial monitoring by a test administrator.

Ease of use: Directions are self-explanatory, but as the format is somewhat unique, assistance is likely to be necessary.

Training for administration and scoring: No training is required.

Scoring procedures: Each item indicated as the correct response on the scoring key is scored + 1. Several kinds of scores are provided with the IFF:

Individual scores: one member's affective rating of a given other member
Dyad score: an average of two members' individual scores toward each other
Response score: an average of individual scores a member produces toward the members of his or her family as a group
Reception score: the average individual scores given to one member by the others
Family unit score: the average individual scores produced by an entire family

Evaluation of administrative procedures: *Strengths:* (1) Scoring is simple. (2) Multiple relationship scores can be derived, producing, in effect, an emotional family sociogram. *Limitations:* (1) Scoring procedures are not clearly delineated in the directions. (2) Normative data and a manual are not available for interpretation of scores.

EVALUATION OF CONSTRUCTS MEASURED

Reliability: A split-half internal consistency coefficient of .98 was obtained. Test–retest reliability of response scores, over a 2-week period with a sample of college students, was .96 (Lowman, 1980).

Validity: *Criterion-related:* IFF scores were significantly correlated with Marital Adjustment Test scores in couples (Lowman, 1980). Clinical ratings of affect, using a system based on Leary's interpersonal model, were correlated .49 with the IFF self-report scores (Fineberg & Lowman. 1975). IFF scores significantly differentiated families with a pathological family member from nonclinical families, with pathological families demonstrating greater negative affect; negative IFF scores significantly related to degree of individual psychopathology. IFF scores significantly differentiated maritally distressed from maritally satisfied couples (Lowman, 1980).

Clinical utility: The IFF demonstrates clinical promise as a pre–post treatment measure and as a diagnostic assessment device for determining covert affective patterns (e.g., alliances, scapegoating). Clinical utility is currently limited by the absence of stable normative data and a manual to guide scoring and interpretation.

Research utility: The IFF demonstrates research utility as a method of comparing affective structures across family types as well as for process and outcome treatment evaluation. Evidence of good reliability and validity support the use of this measure for the dimension of family affect. However, additional concurrent validity studies with the affective dimensions of other family measures appear warranted.

SUMMARY EVALUATION

The IFF is a 38-item questionnaire that evaluates the affective structure of the family—specifically, the degree to which family relationships are laden with positive affect. Strengths of the measure include single dimensionality, ease of scoring, potential multiple relationship perspectives or scores, and good psychometric evaluation to date. Limitations include the lack of normative data, a relatively more difficult item format and language than is customary in self-report measures, and inadequate published information regarding scoring and interpretation.

REFERENCES

Fineberg, B. L., Lowman, J. (1975). Affect and status dimensions of marital adjustment. *Journal of Marriage and the Family, 37,* 155–160.

Lowman, J. (1980). Measurement of family affective structure. *Journal of Personality Assessment, 44*(2). 130–141.

Lowman, J. (1981). Love, hate, and the family: Measures of emotion. In E. E. Filsinger & R. A. Lewis (Eds.). *Assessing marriage: New behavioral approaches* (pp. 55–73). Beverly Hills, CA: Sage.

AUTHOR'S RESPONSE

No additional comments.

W-14
McMaster Family Assessment Device (FAD), Version 3

GENERAL INFORMATION

Date of publication: 1982.

Authors: Nathan B. Epstein, Lawrence M. Baldwin, and Duane S. Bishop.

Source/publisher: The Brown University/Butler Hospital Family Research Program, Butler Hospital, 345 Blackstone Blvd., Providence, RI 02906.

Availability: Available from above source.

Brief description: The FAD is a self-report screening instrument that assesses family functioning on seven dimensions and distinguishes between healthy and unhealthy families.

Purpose: The FAD is designed to permit clinicians and researchers to screen for health and pathology of family functioning on a variety of clinically relevant dimensions.

Theoretical base: The McMaster Model of Family Functioning (Epstein, Bishop, & Levin, 1978), a clinical model based on the assumption that family functioning is related to the accomplishment of essential functions and tasks. The model, which is compatible with systems theory, describes the structural and organizational properties of the family unit and the patterns of transactions among family members that have been found to distinguish healthy and unhealthy families.

PHYSICAL DESCRIPTION OF QUESTIONNAIRE

Physical features: The FAD consists of 60 items (with 7 items added to three of the scales to increase reliability of the original 53-item version) about the family. Degree of agreement or disagreement with each statement is rated on a 4-point likert scale, with responses ranging from ''strongly agree'' to ''strongly disagree.'' The reading level is approximately sixth grade.

Unit of study: Whole family.

Respondent: Individual family members age 12 and older.

Scales and dimensions: The FAD scales are as follows:

Problem Solving (6 items)
Communication (9 items)
Roles (11 items)
Affective Responsiveness (6 items)
Affective Involvement (7 items)
Behavior Control (9 items)
General Functioning (12 items)

Manual: None.

Standardization and Norms: A sample of 503 individuals (294 clinical members of 112 families and 209 nonclinical introductory psychology students) completed the FAD. Means and standard deviations for the clinical and nonclinical groups ($N = 218$ and $N = 98$, respectively) are provided (Epstein, Baldwin, & Bishop, 1983). Recommended health–pathology cutoff scores are reported in Miller, Epstein, Bishop, and Keitner (1985).

Evaluation of physical description of questionnaire: *Strengths:* Items are clearly written, comprehensible, and single in focus. Response directions are clear, and the response format easy to complete. The FAD dimensions address a broad range of family functioning areas. The measure is theoretically based. *Limitations:* Normative data are limited and the sample is inadequate. No manual is provided. Item content reflects whole-family functioning, whereas the accuracy of a statement might vary across persons or subsystems within the family.

ADMINISTRATIVE PROCEDURES

Directions: Clearly written directions to the respondent are provided with a sample of stimulus items and response format.

Ease of use: The FAD directions are self-explanatory, and the response format is easy to complete and interpret. Questionnaire completion reportedly takes 15 to 20 minutes.

Training for administration and scoring: Minimal training is needed for either administration or scoring, as directions are clear and self-explanatory.

Scoring procedures: To score the FAD, all responses are coded from 1 (''strongly agree'') to 4 (''strongly disagree''). Then the scores for items describing unhealthy functioning are transformed by subtracting 5. Scored responses to the items of each scale are averaged to provide seven scale scores with a range from 1.00 (healthy) to 4.00 (unhealthy). If more than 40% of the items on a scale are incomplete, the scale score is not calculated. A scoring sheet is provided, or computer scoring is available, for a fee, from the Brown/Butler Family Research Program.

Evaluation of administrative procedures: *Strengths:* The FAD is optimal to administer. Directions for completion and scoring are clear and self-explanatory. Scoring involves simple addition and subtraction. Time to complete the questionnaire is reasonable. *Limitations:* Normative data are limited.

EVALUATION OF CONSTRUCTS MEASURED

Reliability: *Internal consistency:* Item selection for a scale stopped when the scale reliability was over a minimum alpha level of .70. Internal consistency ranges across scales from .72 to .92. Scale intercorrelations range from .37 to .76. Partial correlations, however, approach zero when the General Functioning scale is held constant (Epstein et al., 1983). *Test–Retest:* Estimates over a 1-week period ($N=45$) yielded the following: Problem-Solving, .66; Communication, .72; Roles, .75; Affective Responsiveness, .76; Affective Involvement, .67; Behavior Control, .73; General Functioning, .71 (Miller et al., 1985).

Validity: *Criterion (concurrent):* A discriminant analysis of individual FAD scores ($N=218$ nonclinical, $N=98$ clinical) predicted 67% of the nonclinical group and 64% of the clinical group ($p<.001$) (Epstein et al., 1983). A regression analysis found the FAD to predict 28% (R = .53) of the variance on the Locke Wallace Marital Satisfaction Scale (Epstein et al., 1983).*Criterion (predictive):* In a comparison of the FAD and Locke Wallace, the FAD was found to be a more powerful predictor (i.e., contributed more of the variance in a regression analysis) of morale scores in a geriatric population ($N=178$ couples) (Epstein et al., 1983). *Construct:* Correlations of scales theoretically expected to be related were examined for three family self-report measures: the FAD, the Family Adaptability and Cohesion Scale (FACES-II) and the Family Unit Inventory (FUI). Obtained correlations between the FAD scales and the FUI were very close to a priori predictions. Using analysis of variance procedures, comparison of the FACES-II and FAD did not find extreme groups on the FACES-II to score more pathological on the FAD. Only disengaged and rigid subjects on the FACES-II scored more pathologically, whereas enmeshed and chaotic subjects scored healthier (Miller et al., 1985). Correlations between the FAD and the Marlowe-Crowne Social Desirability Scale were uniformly low, ranging from − .06 to − .19. FAD scores compared with clinical ratings of healthy and unhealthy families ($N=36$), using the same theoretical model, found six of seven dimensions to correspond significantly. Behavior Control did not correspond across methods (Miller et al., 1985).

Clinical utility: The psychometric evaluation data to date suggest that the FAD has considerable clinical utility as a screening measure. It taps areas of family functioning not easily or immediately observed. Although not empirically investigated, the FAD profile can be expected to be useful to the clinician for identifying family strengths and weaknesses and for guiding intervention (with the exception of the Behavior Control scale, which may not yield insider–outsider congruence of perspective). Currently limiting the clinical utility of this measure is the lack of a manual, adequate standardization, and clarification of interpretation of multiple family member perspectives.

Research utility: Additional reliability and validity studies are essential for determining the utility of FAD for research purposes. Currently, test–retest reliability had been assessed only for a 1-week period. Although good discriminant validity is demonstrated regarding clinical–nonclinical groups, studies examining the diffential predictive validity of the FAD are warranted.

SUMMARY EVALUATION

The FAD has the potential of being a useful instrument for clinicians and researchers. It is an economical screening device that provides information regarding family functioning across multiple relevant dimensions. The FAD is theoretically based. Psychometric evaluation to date is promising and suggests that the FAD is internally consistent, reliable over short periods, unrelated to measures of social desirability, and successful in discriminating clinical from nonclinical groups. The differential clinical and predictive utility of the FAD, as well as its research utility, remains to be demonstrated.

REFERENCES

Epstein, N. B., Baldwin, L. M., & Bishop, D. (1983). The McMaster Family Assessment Device. *Journal of Marital and Family Therapy, 9*(2), 171–180.

Epstein, N. A., Bishop, D. S., & Levin, S. (1978). The McMaster Model of Family Functioning. *Journal of Marital and Family Counseling, 4,* 19–31.

Miller, I. V., Epstein, N. B., Bishop, D. S., & Keitner, G. I. (1985). The McMaster Family Assessment Device: Reliability and validity. *Journal of Marital and Family Therapy, 11*(4), 345–356.

AUTHOR'S RESPONSE

No additional comments.

W-15
Personal Authority in the Family System
Questionnaire (PAFS-Q)

GENERAL INFORMATION

Date of publication: 1984.

Authors: J. H. Bray, D. S. Williamson, and P. E. Malone.

Source/publisher: James H. Bray, Texas Women's University, 1130 M. D. Anderson Blvd., Houston, TX 77030.

Availability: Available from James H. Bray at the above address.

Brief description: The PAFS-Q is a self-report instrument with 132, 122, or 84 items (depending on the version used), which are rated on a 5-point Likert scale.Questions relate to an individual's perception of trigenerational family relationships.

Purpose: The PAFS-Q is designed to assess an individual's perception of important relationships in the three-generation family system.

Theoretical base: Intergenerational family theory (Bowen, 1978; Williamson, 1981, 1982a, 1982b; Williamson & Bray, in press).

PHYSICAL DESCRIPTION OF QUESTIONNAIRE

Physical features: The PAFS-Q uses 5-point Likert scales with varying formats (e.g., quality of relationships rated "excellent" to "very poor," degree of agreement with a statement rated "strongly agree" to "strongly disagree"). There are three versions of the instrument: Version A, for adults with children (132 items); Version B, for adults without children (122 items); and Version C, for college students without children (84 items). The reading level appears appropriate for adults with high school reading ability. Unmarried individuals may respond to "spousal" items by referring to their "significant other" or to their "most likely or most recent significant other."

Unit of study: Relationships within the three-generation family system.

Respondent: Adult family member.

Scales and dimensions: The PAFS-Q has eight scales: Spousal Intimacy, Spousal Fusion/Individuation, Nuclear Family Triangulation, Intergenerational Intimacy, Intergenerational Fusion/Individuation, Intergenerational Triangulation, Intergenerational Intimidation, and Personal Authority. Nuclear Family Triangulation is not included in versions for persons without children (Versions B and C).

Manual: A 23-page manual is available; it includes theoretical information, information on questionnaire development, reliability and validity data, an interpretation guide, scoring directions, and references.

Standardization and norms: The PAFS-Q has been standardized on nonclinical ($N = 312$ to 525, depending on the scale) and clinical ($N = 83$) samples (Bray, Williamson, & Malone, 1984a, undated). Means and standard deviations for these groups are given in the manual. Persons in the clinic group were asked to fill out two PAFS-Qs after completing intergenerational family therapy, one in reference to their present functioning and another in reference to functioning before therapy. Means and standard deviations are given for the clinic groups' PAFS-Q scores for both of these times (i.e., perceptions of family relationships after therapy and retrospective reports of those relationships before therapy). Norms for the college student version (Version C) appear in Bray and Harvey (undated). Means, standard deviations, and interscale correlations are given separately for men ($N = 345$) and women ($N = 367$) undergraduates. In addition, Bray and Williamson (1986) give typical profiles for individuals experiencing cutoff or fused intergenerational relationships.

Evaluation of physical description of questionnaire: *Strengths:* Versions available for single or married adults, with or without children, and for college students; availability of norms for nonclinical populations (adult and college students) and of norms using a smaller sample for clinical populations; availability of a manual containing psychometric data and clear scoring instructions. *Limitations:* Need for norming with larger clinical samples; length.

ADMINISTRATIVE PROCEDURES

Directions: Clear directions are given with the instrument.

Ease of use: The PAFS-Q is easy to administer, requiring only the items, and answer sheet, and a pencil. It can easily be computer-scored or administered to groups.

Training for administration and scoring: Administration is simple. Scoring, though not difficult, is likely to be time-consuming and requires careful attention to instructions, which are provided in the manual.

Scoring procedures, including calculation of summary scores: A different procedure is used (e.g., subtracting sums from a certain number) to derive a scaled score for each of the eight scales.

Evaluation of administrative procedures: *Strength:* Easy to administer; clear scoring instructions provided in manual. *Limitations:* Scoring possibly time-consuming.

EVALUATION OF CONSTRUCTS MEASURED

Reliability: Alpha coefficients for a sample of nonclinical adults ($N = 90$) ranged from .82 to .95 at time 1 and from .80 to .95 at time 2, with means of .90 and .89. Alpha coefficients were computed for scales derived from a factor analysis of the scores of another sample of nonclinical adults ($N = 400$). Alpha coefficients for the empirically derived factors ranged from .74 to .96 (Bray, Williamson, & Malone, 1984b). Alphas ranged from .75 to .96 in one clinical sample ($N = 83$) (Bray et al., 1984a, 1984b, undated) and from .77 to .96 in another another clinical sample ($N = 80$) (Bray, Harvey, & Williamson, undated). Alpha coefficients for Version C of the PAFS-Q ranged from .97 to .85 and from .73 to .92 in two samples of undergraduate college students ($N = 321$ and 712). Alphas of .75 to .92 were found for a clinical sample of 62 undergraduates (Bray & Harvey, undated; Bray et al., undated). All scales except Intergenerational Fusion demonstrated acceptable 2-week test–retest reliability with the sample of 90 nonclinical adults. Estimates ranged from .55 to .95, with a mean of .75 (Bray et al., 1984a). Scores from Version C used with the college student sample ($N = 321$) resulted in 2-month test–retest reliabilities ranging from .56 to .80. Estimates for all scales were above .66, except for the Intergenerational Intimidation scale, which had a reliability of .56.

Validity: *Criterion-related:* Relationships found between the PAFS-Q and other measures of family functioning suggest that the PAFS-Q overlaps with these measures to some degree but also taps different aspects of family functioning. In the nonclinical sample of 90 adults, correlations between PAFS-Q scales and the Adaptability scale of the Family Adaptability and Cohesion Evaluation Scales (FACES) were low (from $-.15$ to $-.03$). Two PAFS-Q scales, Spousal Intimacy and Intergenerational Intimacy, correlated significantly with the FACES Cohesion scale, and several PAFS-Q scales correlated significantly with the Dyadic Adjustment Scale (DAS) (Bray et al., 1984a).

For a clinical sample of 80, Bray, et al. (undated) found significant zero-order correlations between all but one (Intergenerational Intimacy) of the PAFS-

Q scales and the Symptom Index (a measure of physical and psychosomatic symptoms and stress). Zero-order correlations were also found between various scales of the PAFS-Q and portions of the Family Adaptability and Cohesion Evaluation Scales II (FACES II, rated twice for nuclear family and family of origin relationships) and the DAS. In a multiple-regression analysis using the family process measures (PAFS-Q, FACES II, DAS) to predict health distress (Symptom Index scores), PAFS-Q scores added to the predictive power of the other two measures further indicating that the PAFS-Q, although related to the other measures, assesses aspects of family process not assessed by FACES II or the DAS. The analysis also indicates that individuals who are more individuated from parents and spouse (PAFS-Q Intergenerational Individuation/Fusion and Spousal Individuation/Fusion scales) tend to experience fewer health problems (Bray et al, undated).

In another study, the PAFS-Q scores of college students were negatively correlated with measures of life stress and health distress. Multiple-regression analysis indicated that less life stress plus less Intergenerational Intimidation, *less* Personal Authority, and more individuation with parents and the significant other predict better health. According to the authors, the fact that lower scores on the Personal Authority scale predict better health supports Williamson's (1981, 1982a, 1982b) developmental theory that lack of personal authority in the family system is age-appropriate prior to approximately the fourth decade of life (Bray et al., undated).

In a sample of 712 college students, PAFS-Q scores correlated in the expected direction with measures of psychological well-being and subscales of the Structural Family Interaction Scale. When multiple analysis of variance was used to compare the PAFS-Q scores of this group of college students with the scores of a clinical college group ($N = 62$), significant differences in the expected direction were found on all PAFS-Q scales except Intergenerational Intimidation (Bray & Harvey, undated).

Construct-related: Factor analysis of the PAFS-Q scores of 400 nonclinical adults resulted in 23 factors. A scree test of these factors led to a seven-factor solution (an eighth factor, representative of Nuclear Family Triangulation, was found for scores of persons with children). Overall, the conceptual scales were confirmed by the factor structure, with the exception of an overlap of items from the Spousal Fusion/Individuation scale with items from the Spousal Intimacy scale. Correlations among the eight factors were moderate to low (range, .59 to −.05), indicating that the scales measure different aspects of personal authority in the family system relatively independently.

An exploratory factor analysis of the PAFS-Q, Version C, used with 321 college students, resulted in seven factors roughly replicating the factors found previously with Versions A and B. In another sample of 712 college students, PAFS-Q scores were analyzed using the LISREL VI computer program to compare the previous seven-factor model with three other possible models. The seven-factor structure found with the previous sample was the best fitting model for the data (Bray & Harvey, undated).

In a comparison of a group of individuals completing intergenerational family therapy for marital or relational problems with a group of individuals with similar problems completing system-oriented therapy (control group), the intergenerational family therapy group's PAFS-Q scores improved significantly more than those of the control group on the Intergenerational Triangulation and Personal Authority scales. These individuals had significantly more positive posttest scores on these two scales and on the Intergaenerational Intimidation scale. However, persons in the control group showed significantly more improvement on the Spousal Intimacy scale. Retrospective PAFS-Q ratings of relationships before intergenerational family therapy were significantly lower than those of a normative sample, and PAFS-Q scores following intergenerational family therapy were significantly higher than those of the normative sample on most of the scales. (Bray et al., undated).

The PAFS-Q has been used in other studies investigating intergenerational family processes (Curry, 1986, de la Sota, 1985; Harvey & Bray, undated; Harvey, Curry, & Bray, 1986).

Clinical utility: Norms are available based on clinical and nonclinical adult and college student samples. Norms using larger clinical samples and further work with PAFS-Q profiles would further enhance the clinical utility of the instrument. According to Bray and Williamson (1986), the instrument has multiple clinical applications. It can be used as an assessment device to measure current family functioning. Comparisons of family members' scores can be used to enhance mutual understanding, and the PAFS-Q, given at different points in therapy, can help to measure change and enhance self-evaluation. Finally, the PAFS-Q is useful as an intervention tool to help clients examine their intergenerational family relationships.

Research utility: The PAFS-Q is the only measure of intergenerational family relationships available to researchers of intergenerational family functioning. Validity studies, although showing relationships between the PAFS-Q and other family process measures, show that the PAFS-Q taps unique aspects of family functioning. Internal consistency of the scales has been excellent, and test–retest reliability has usually been adequate. Promising evidence has been presented for the validity of this instrument for investigating the complexities of intergenerational family theory.

SUMMARY EVALUATION

The PAFS-Q has the advantages of a sound theoretical base, norms calculated from several samples, good internal consistency and adequate test–retest reliability, dimensions generally supported by factor analysis, and promising evidence of validity. This instrument, which seems to be the only measure of intergenerational family functioning available, should be especially useful to practitioners and researchers who are interested in intergenerational family functioning.

REFERENCES

Bowen, (1978). *Family in clinical practice.* New York: Aronson.

Bray, J. H., & Harvey, D. M. (undated). *A measure of family and peer relationships for college students.* Unpublished manuscript.

Bray, J. H., Harvey, D. M., & Williamson, D. S. (undated). *Intergenerational family relationships: An evaluation of theory and measurement.* Unpublished manuscript.

Bray, J. H., & Williamson, D. S. (1986). Assessment of intergenerational family relationships. In A. J. Hovestadt & M. Fine (Eds.), *Family of origin therapy: Applications in clinical practice. Family therapy collections.* Rockville, MD: Aspen Press.

Bray, J. H., Williamson, D. S., & Malone, P. E. (1984a). Personal authority in the family system: Development of a questionnaire to measure personal authority in intergenerational family processes. *Journal of Marital and Family Therapy, 10,* 167–178.

Bray, J. H., Williamson, D. S., & Malone, P. E. (1984b) *Personal Authority in the Family System Questionnaire manual.* Houston, TX: Houston Family Institute.

Bray, J. H., Williamson, D. S., & Malone, P. E. (undated). *An evaluation of an intergenerational consultation process to increase personal authority in the family system.* Unpublished manuscript.

Curry, C. J. (1986). *Intergenerational family processes of college students and their parents: Determinants of physical and psychological well-being.* Unpublished doctoral dissertation, University of Texas, Austin.

de la Sota, E. M. (1985). *Perceived family relationships of college males and females and their effect on psychological adjustment and capacity for intimacy and achievement.* Unpublished doctoral dissertation, University of Texas, Austin.

Harvey, D. M., & Bray, J. H. (undated). *Evaluation of an intergenerational theory of personal development: Family process determinants of psychological health and distress.* Unpublished manuscript.

Harvey, D. M., Curry, C. J., & Bray, J. H. (1986, August). *Individuation/ Intimacy in intergenerational relationships and health: Patterns across two generations.* Paper presented at the annual convention of the American Psychological Association, Washington, DC.

Williamson, D. S. (1981). Personal authority via termination of the intergenerational hierarchical boundary: A "new" stage in the family life cycle. *Journal of Martial and Family Therapy, 7,* 441–452.

Williamson, D. S. (1982a). Personal authority in family experience via termination of the intergenerational hierachical boundary: Part III. Personal authority defined, and the power of play in the change process. *Journal of Marital and Family Therapy 8,* 309–323.

Williamson, D. S. (1982b). Personal authority via termination of the intergenerational hierachical boundary: Part II. The consultation process and the therapeutic method. *Journal of Marital and Family Therapy 8,* 23–37.

Williamson, D. S., & Bray, J. H. (in press). Family development and change across the generations: An intergenerational perspective. In C. J. Falicov (Ed.), *Family transitions: Continuity and change over the life cycle.* New York: Guilford Press.

AUTHOR'S RESPONSE

No additional comments.

W-16
Self-Report Family Inventory (SFI)

GENERAL INFORMATION

Date of publication: 1985.

Authors: W. R. Beavers, Robert Hampson, and Yosaf Hulgus.

Source/publisher: Beavers, W. R., Hampson, R. B., & Hulgus, Y. F. (1985). Commentary: The Beavers Systems approach to family assessment. *Family Process, 24,* 398–405.

Availability: The scale is printed in the published source listed above. The complete assessment system, including descriptive manual and additional psychometric information, is available from the Southwest Family Institute, 12532 Nuestra, Dallas, TX 75230.

Brief description: The SFI is a 36-item self-report instrument that uses a 5-point response scale.

Purpose: The SFI assesses the constructs of Family Health, Conflict, Family Communication, Family Cohesion, Directive Leadership, and Expressiveness. It was designed to translate observational constructs from the Beavers Systems Model into a self-report format. The SFI is designed to be combined with observational ratings in order to provide "insider" and "outsider" perspectives of family functioning.

Theoretical base: Beavers Systems Model.

PHYSICAL DESCRIPTION OF QUESTIONNAIRE

Physical features: The SFI includes 36 items, each of which is responded to on a 5-point scale from "Yes: Fits our family very well" to "No: does not fit our family."

Unit of study: Whole family.

Respondent: Individual family member.

Scales and dimensions: Family Health (19 items); Conflict (12 items); Family communication (4 items); Family Cohesion (5 items); Directive Leadership (3 items); Expressiveness (5 items). Second-order factors: Health/Competence, Style, and Expressiveness. When combined with the Beavers-Timberlawn Family Evaluation Scale and the Centripetal/Centrifugal Family Style Scale, a multimethod, multilevel family systems evaluation is provided.

Manual: Scoring instructions, test items, normative data, and psychometric information are available from the authors (see ''Availability,'' above).

Standardization and norms: Means and standard deviations from a sample of 186 families are given for mothers, fathers, 9- to 16-year-old children, and children over 16 (Hulgus, personal communication, November 14, 1986).

Evaluation of physical description of questionnaire: *Strengths:* Items easy to understand and respond to; clear response format with adequate range; norms and manual available. *Limitations:* None noted.

ADMINISTRATIVE PROCEDURES

Directions: ''For each question, mark the answer that best fits how you see your family now. If you feel that your answer is between two of the labeled numbers (the odd numbers), then choose the even number that is between them.''

Ease of use: The SFI is easy to administer and score; it could easily be computer-scored.

Training for administration and scoring: Little experience or training is necessary. The authors believe that familiarity with family systems theory—specifically with the Beavers Systems Model of Family Functioning—would be helpful for interpretation of scores.

Scoring procedures, including calculation of summary scores: Reverse necessary items within each factor; then add all items associated with a given factor and divide by the number of items included for that factor. This average reflects the average SFI factor score.

Evaluation of administrative procedures: *Strengths:* Easy to administer. *Limitations:* Item overlap across some scales.

EVALUATION OF CONSTRUCTS MEASURED

Reliability: Internal consistency reliability coefficients (Cronbach's alpha) were computed for two samples. Reliabilities for the full 44-item set were .88 and

.84; alphas for a reduced item set in which factor loadings exceeded .40 were .84 and .78. No reliability coefficients for the individual scales were reported. Test–retest reliabilities for factor scores over 30- and 90-day periods ranged from .30 to .87. All were statistically significant at $p < .01$ (Hulgus, personal communication, November 14, 1986).

Validity: *Criterion-related:* The SFI Health/Competence And Expressiveness factors have been used to distinguish previously rated high- and low-functioning families. Concurrent validity was assessed by comparing SFI scale scores to scores on the Bloom Family Evaluation Scale, FACES II, FACES III, the Family Environment Scale, and the Family Assessment Device. in general, convergence of the SFI with scales from these measures is good (tables available from the authors). SFI scores are uncorrelated with the Marlowe-Crowne Social Desirability Scale across three time periods. A canonical correlation of .62 was obtained between Beavers System observational ratings of Health/ Competence and Style and SFI scores. Discriminant validity was assessed by correlating the SFI with the State-Trait Anxiety Inventory. Eight of 12 correlations were statistically significant, ranging from .03 to .49. Thus, the discriminant validity of the instrument is questionable. Because of differential patterns of correlations, depending on the scales, the authors concluded that there were some areas of family functioning that were observable with high agreement by insiders and outsiders, but that other domains were observed differently by the two parties. (It is unclear whether the validity studies cited above used the original 44-item version or the revised 36-item version of the SFI).

Clinical utility: The availability of norms enhances the clinical utility of the SFI. Further work with a diversity of families would enhance the usefulness of the instrument. The authors recommend that the SFI be used in combination with observational measures of family functioning.

Research utility: The instrument has potential research utility, but further reliability and validity work will be essential. Assessment of the internal consistency of the individual scales is necessary.

SUMMARY EVALUATION

The SFI is easy to administer and score, is written in simple language, and appears to capture some important dimensions of family functioning. Instructions for scoring and administration and norms are available. The instrument has a sound basis in theory and was designed for use with observational measures that have the same theoretical basis. The process of validation is still in the early stages, and the instrument may require further refinement before a final version is ready for use. Internal consistency and independence or distinctiveness of scales has not yet been established.

REFERENCES

Beavers, W. R., Hampson, R. B., & Hulgus, Y. F. (1985). Commentary: The Beavers Systems approach to family assessment. *Family Process, 24,* 398–405.

Beavers, W. R., & Voeller, M. N. (1983). Family models: Comparing and contrasting the Olson Circumplex Model with the Beavers Systems Model. *Family Process, 22,* 85–98.

Green, R. G., Kolevzon, M. S., & Vosler, N. R. (1985). The Beavers-Timberlawn Model of Family Competence and the Circumplex Model of Family Adaptability and Cohesion: Separate but equal? *Family Process, 24,* 385–398.

Hulgus, Y. (undated). *Results of the psychometric evaluation of the SFI.* Unpublished manuscript. (Available from the Southwest Family Institute, Dallas, TX).

Hulgus, Y. F. (1985). *Evaluation of the Self-Report Family Instrument.* Unpublished master's thesis, Texas Woman's University, Denton.

AUTHOR'S RESPONSE

No additional comments.

W-17
Structural Family Interaction Scale
(SFIS)

GENERAL INFORMATION

Date of publication: 1981 (original); third revision unpublished.

Author: Linda M. Perosa.

Source/publisher: Linda M. Perosa, PhD, 206 E. Willard Hall, Education Bldg., University of Delaware, Newark, DE 19716.

Availability: Measure available from the author at the address above.

Brief description: The SFIS is a 185-item, 4-point Likert-type self-report questionnaire composed of 21 scales that assess variables of family functioning as posited by Minuchin's structural family therapy model. The SFIS-R Form A (Perosa, 1986) consists of 76 items combined into eight scales.

Purpose: The SFIS is designed to provide an objective self-report measure of family interaction patterns as conceptualized by Minuchin's model of structural family therapy.

Theoretical base: Structural family therapy model.

PHYSICAL DESCRIPTION OF QUESTIONNAIRE

Physical features: Three revisions of the SFIS have been completed. The initial SFIS contained 85 items and 23 subscales (Perosa, Hansen, & Perosa, 1981). The second revision, done in 1981, consists of 105 items and 21 scales (Prather, 1981). The most recent revision (SFIS-R Form A) consists of 76 items and 8 scales (Perosa, 1986). Respondents indicate the extent to which each item is true on a 4-point scale ("very true," "more true than false," "more false than true," very false"). The SFIS is designed for children aged 12 years and older. Currently, an ideal version of the SFIS-R Form A, a clinical rating scale based on it, and a form allowing repondents to compare each child in the family on items referring to "this child in the family" are being developed and used in research.

Unit of Study: Subscales apply either to the whole family or to specific dyadic relationships.

Respondent: Individual family members over age 12.

Scales and dimensions: The SFIS-R Form A contains eight subscales:

> Spouse Conflict—with Resolution/without Resolution
> Parent Coalition/Cross-Generational Triads
> Father–Child Cohesion/Estrangement
> Mother–Child Cohesion/Estrangement
> Flexibility/Rigidity
> Enmeshment/Disengagement
> Family Conflict Avoidance/Expression
> Overprotection/Autonomy

Manual: None

Standardization and norms: None available.

Evaluation of physical description of questionnaire: *Strengths:* It is theory-based. *Limitations:* The most recent revision, the SFIS-R Form A, was unavailable for examination; therefore, limitations noted may be inappropriate. (1) Item content suggests that a particular child is being referenced. Although the author suggests that the respondent be directed to insert a particular child's name in place of "child" (personal communication), this appears to limit the validity of the measure for examining the whole family unit. (2) The sibling subsystem and socioenvironmental components of the theoretical model are not measure. (3) There is no manual or normative data. (4) The content of some items may be reactive.

ADMINISTRATIVE PROCEDURES

Directions: The essential directions to the respondent contain jargon (e.g., "family interaction patterns"), which may not be understood.

Ease of use: With the exception of lack of clarity in specific item content, the measure is straightforward to administer.

Training for administration and scoring: No information provided.

Scoring procedures: Items receive weighted scores ($4 = A$ to $1 = D$) according to a scoring key. Summary scores per scale are derived. To get a measure for a family, if more than one member takes the questionnaire, each member's score per scale is summed and divided by the number of family members. A Family Incongruency score for each scale is obtained by subtracting all possible dyad scores and dividing the sum by the number of subtractions. According to the author, various scoring systems can be devised, depending on the purpose of the research (Perosa, 1986).

Evaluation of administrative procedures: *Strengths:* Scoring is simple. *Limitations:* Lack of documentation; no control in the directions for social desirability.

EVALUATION OF CONSTRUCTS MEASURED

Reliability: *SFIS (85-item version):* Reliability estimates are based upon a sample of 50 families (25 with a learning disabled child) (Perosa 1981). Internal consistencies of the 13 primary subscales found 9 subscales to meet the acceptable alpha level of .5. Several subscales approached the criterion (Overprotection, .49; Parent-Management, .47; Flexibility, .44). Neglect (.25) demonstrated inadequate internal consistency. Secondary subscales yielded, in general, inadequate internal consistency, with the exception of the Father Neglect (.56) and Parent Conflict Resolution (.54) subscales. Item subscale correlations were more stable, with a range of .50 to .70 for the primary subscales and a range of .70 to .83 for the secondary subscales. Average interitem correlations, describing homogeneity of variables, were mixed. Using an alpha criterion of .25, 6 of the 13 primary subscales reached criterion. Combining subscales theoretically lowered the correlation coefficient, indicating that subscales stand better alone than on a continuum, as predicted theoretically. No test–retest reliability is reported.

SFIS-R Form A: Test–retest reliability falls within the .80 to .90 range for every scale (personal communication, August 19, 1987).

Validity: *SFIS (85-item version): Content*—Interjudge reliability for the content of items by six expert judges (family therapists) yielded a correlation coefficient of .950. *Construct*—Subscale intercorrelations are congruent with hypothesized theoretical relationships. *Criterion*—Significant differences on numerous SFIS variables were obtained between nonclinical families and families with a learning-disabled child (Perosa & Perosa, 1982). Corsica (1981) found differences in the family dynamics that correlated with school adjustment in intact, reconstituted, and father-absent families.

SFIS (105-item version): Construct—Subscale intercorrelations are congruent with hypothesized theoretical relationships (Walrath, 1984). *Criterion:* The in-

strument differentiated families of unwed pregnant adolescents from other families (Prather, 1981); families of anorectic and bulemic adolescents from control
families (Kramer, 1983); families of women with severe premenstral syndrome
from families of a control group; families of emotionally disturbed adolescents
from other families (Walrath, 1984); and families of runaway youth from other
families (Krawitz, 1985). In addition, the SFIS has been used successfully to
identify family variables related to the psychological well-being of the adolescent family member (Walsh, 1985). Harding (1986) found no differences between families of female anorectics and families of a female college student
control group.

SFIS-R Form A: Content:—A factor analysis of the SFIS-R Form A yielded
eight scales with the following alpha loadings: Spouse Conflict, .90; Parent
Coalition, .81; Father–Child Cohesion, .91; Mother–Child Cohesion, .85;
Flexibility/Rigidity, .81; Enmeshment/Disengagement, .93; Family Conflict
Avoidance/Expression, .82; and Overprotection/Autonomy, .76. *Criterion:*—
The instrument distinguished family factors related to the identity status and
coping styles of young adults (Perosa & Perosa, 1987). Additional validation
studies of the SFIS Form A are under way, as are plans to develop a young
child's version (Perosa, 1986).

Clinical utility: The SFIS represents the only effort to date to capture the
structural family therapy theory of Minuchin in a self-report questionnaire. As
such, the SFIS potentially has considerable clinical utility, particularly for
structural family therapists, in differentiating healthy from pathological families
and in identifying specific types of dysfunctional relationships. Currently, however, the clinical utility of the SFIS is limited by a lack of empirical data on
the psychometric properties of the measure, continuous revision, and a lack of
normative data.

Research utility: Several studies have provided promising evidence of the research utility of the SFIS (Perosa, 1986; Perosa & Perosa, 1982); One limitation of the SFIS—the numerous subscales or variables included in the measure—appears to be resolved in the SFIS-R Form A. The research utility of the
SFIS-R Form A, however, remains to be determined.

SUMMARY EVALUATION

The most recent revision of this measure, the SFIS-R Form A, is a 76-item
questionnaire, with 8 scales, that identifies family interaction patterns according
to Minuchin's structural family therapy theory. As the only self-report measure
based on structural theory, the SFIS represents a significant contribution to the
family assessment field. Current utilization of the measure is limited (1) by its
continuous revision, which renders investigation of the measure's psychometric

properties obsolete, and (2) by lack of adequate psychometric investigation on the updated version.

REFERENCES

Corsica, J. (1981). *The relationship of changes in family structure to the academic performance and school behavior of adolescents from a middle class, suburban high school.* Unpublished doctoral dissertation, State University of New York at Buffalo.

Harding, T. (1985). *Family interaction patterns and locus of control as predictors of the presence and severity of anorexia nervosa.* Unpublished doctoral dissertation, Fairleigh-Dickinson University, Rutherford, NJ.

Kramer, S. (1983). Bulimia and related eating disorders: A family systems perspective. Unpublished doctoral dissertation, California School of Professional Psychology, San Diego.

Krawitz, G. (1985). *The relationship of family structures to runaway behavior.* Unpublished doctoral dissertation, State University of New York at Buffalo.

Perosa, L. M. (1986). *The revision of the Structural Family Interaction Scale.* Unpublished manuscript.

Perosa, L., Hansen, J., & Perosa, S. (1981). Development of the Structural Family Interaction Scale. *Family Therapy, 8*(2), 77–90.

Perosa, L. M., & Perosa, S. L. (1982). Structural interaction patterns in families with a learning disabled child. *Family Therapy, 9*(2), 175–187.

Perosa, S., & Perosa, L. (1987, August). *The relationship between family structure, identity status, and coping style.* Paper presented at the annual meeting of the American Psychological Association, New York.

Prather, F. (1982). *Family environment, self-esteem and the pregnancy states of adolescent females.* Unpublished doctoral dissertation, State University of New York at Buffalo.

Walrath, R. (1984). *Measures of enmeshment and disengagement in normal and disturbed families.* Unpublished doctoral dissertation, Nova University, Fort Lauderdale, FL.

Walsh, T. (1985). *The perception of family environment and its relationship to the psychological well-being of the adolescent.* Unpublished doctoral dissertation, Syracuse University.

AUTHOR'S RESPONSE

Several validity studies are under way. Currently, an ideal version of the SFIS-R Form A, a clinical rating scale based on it, and a form allowing respondents to compare each child in the family on items referring to "this child in the family" are being developed and used in research.

Regarding the limitations of designating one child, it should be noted that although a version of the SFIS-R Form A has been used in research in which the respondent is directed to refer only to a particular child in the family, another version of the SFIS-R Form A, currently being used in research, compares each child in the family on items referring to "this child in the family." This format was developed so the instrument could tap into the whole family unit. However, there are no items referring specifically to siblings relating to each other. Therefore, while each child's relationship with the parent is examined separately, children's relationships with each other are not.

Section VII
Abstracts of Self-Report Questionnaires: Family Stress and Coping

FC-1
Family Crisis Oriented Personal Scales
(F-COPES)

GENERAL INFORMATION

Date of publication: 1982.

Authors: Hamilton McCubbin, Andrea S. Larsen, and David H. Olson.

Source/publisher: Family Social Science Department, University of Minnesota.

Availability: Available through Dr. Hamilton McCubbin, Dept. of Child and Family Studies, University of Wisconsin, 1300 Linden Drive, Madison, WI 53706; also available from Dr. David Olson, Dept. of Family Social Science, University of Minnesota, St. Paul, MN 55108, in *Family Inventories* (see "References," below.)

Brief Description: The F-COPES contains 29 statements regarding families' possible responses to family problems or difficulties. The respondent is asked to determine to what degree, based on a 5-point scale, he or she agrees or disagrees with each statement.

Purpose: The F-COPES was developed to record problem-solving attitudes and behavior with which families respond to problems or difficulties.

Theoretical base: The F-COPES was drawn from a sociological research tradition based on the family stress literature (Hill, 1958; McCubbin, 1979). The measure attempts to integrate both the research regarding coping strategies as an intrafamily process and the research concerning the value of the community in the management of family stress.

PHYSICAL DESCRIPTION OF QUESTIONNAIRE

Physical features: The F-COPES consists of 29 statements, each of which describes an attitude and behavior in response to family problems or difficulties. The measure begins with the opening stem, "When we face problems or difficulties in our family, we respond by:" The opening comment is then followed by the 29 descriptive statements. Each statement is followed by a 5-point Likert scale on which the respondent may indicate the degree to which he or she agress or disagrees with each statement. The scale ranges from "strongly disagree" (1) to "strongly agree" (5).

Unit of study: Whole family.

Respondent: Parent or adolescent.

Scales and dimensions: Using factor-analytic methods, five conceptual scales have been derived from the item pool:

1. Acquiring Social Support (9 items)
2. Reframing (8 items)
3. Seeking Spiritual Support (4 items)
4. Mobilizing Family to Acquire and Accept Help (4 items)
5. Passive Appraisal (4 items)

Each factor had an eigenvalue greater than 1.0, and each item had a factor loading greater than .35.

Manual: A manual is available from the Family Social Science Department (University of Minnesota) in D. H. Olson et al. *Family Inventories,* or from Dr. McCubbin at his address listed above. (University of Wisconsin).

Standardization and norms: Separate norms are available for adults and adolescents by sex for each subscale and the total scale score.

Evaluation of physical description of questionnaire: *Strengths:* The F-COPES is a very brief and relatively clearly written self-report measure. The reading level is simple, the response format is clear, and the measure would not appear to be difficult to complete for adolescent or adult respondents. A manual and norms are available. *Weaknesses:* Because all items are keyed in a positive direction, the instrument is vulnerable to a response bias. Social desirability response bias is likely. Because each family member may view the problem differently, variation in the interpretation of anchor points may occur across family members.

ADMINISTRATIVE PROCEDURES

Directions: The respondent is asked to indicate how well each statement discribes his or her family's attitudes or behaviors in response to problems or difficulties. Responses are given on a Likert-type scale of 1 ("strongly disagree") through 5 ("strongly agree.") Prior to completing the measure, the respondent is asked to refer to his or her family of origin or procreation when responding to the questions.

Ease of use: The F-COPES is easy to administer and score and requires very little time to complete.

Training for administration and scoring: The instrument requires little training for administration; scoring could be done by computer.

Scoring procedures: The numbers 1 through 5 are assigned to the 5-point response options. Summary scores can be obtained for each subscale and the total scale by summing the appropriate items.

Evaluation of administrative procedures: *Strengths:* The F-COPES is concise and easy to complete, administer, and score; it could be administered to large groups. *Weaknesses:* Such a simple measure may not adequately capture the complexity of family coping strategies. The meaning of the Passive Appraisal scale needs clarification. In one study (Barnes & Olson, 1985), families rated high in communication had low scores on this scale.

EVALUATION OF CONSTRUCTS MEASURED

Reliability: Cronbach's alpha was computed for each factor separately and for the scale as a whole for two random samples. The overall alpha for Sample 1 was .86; that for Sample 2 was .87. The alpha reliability of the five individual subscales ranged from .62 (Passive Appraisal) to .84 (Acquiring Social Support). Test–retest reliability for the five factors over a 4-week interval ranged from .61 (Reframing) to .95 (Seeking Spiritual Support). Text–retest reliability for the total scale was .81.

Validity: Construct validity was assessed through factor analysis. Eight initial factors were collapsed into five factors, each having an eigenvalue greater than 1.0.

Clinical utility: The F-COPES recognized that family management of stress requires the integration of intrafamilial resources with community resources. From a clinical perspective, by using the F-COPES to assess the family's means of coping with stress, the clinician may become aware of the active strategies that are involved in the family coping process. Diagnostically, the clinician can then suggest changes, if needed, in the family's coping mechanisms. However, the instrument is relatively new, and whether such a self-report measure is sensitive enough to capture the complexities of family coping strategies is as yet unknown.

Research utility: The concept of family stress has been used in both clinical and research literatures, though it is often elusive and unclear in definition. Measures like the F-COPES continue to examine questions regarding whether coping behaviors are definable, measurable, and unique dimensions of family resources in the management of stress (McCubbin, 1979). Through further research, the F-COPES may clarify which coping behaviors may or may not be functional. Further validity studies would be desirable.

SUMMARY EVALUATION

The instrument may prove to be an important tool in trying to discover how families manage stress. It is straightforward and easy to administer, take, and score. A manual and norms are available. However, the measure may be inadequately sensitive to family processes. The meaning of the total score is unclear, in that all strategies from "Watching TV" to "Seeking assistance from community agencies and programs" are given equal weight. The meaning of items comprising the Passive Appraisal scale is especially problematic. The scale has demonstrated adequate internal consistency, but factor analysis has been the only validity work done to date.

REFERENCES

Barnes, H. L., & Olson, D. H. (1985). Parent–adolescent communication and the circumplex model. *Child Development, 56,* 438–447.

Hill, R. (1958). Generic features of families under stress. *Social Casework, 39,* 130–150.

McCubbin, H. I. (1979). Integrating coping behavior in family stress theory. *Journal of Marriage and the Family, 41,* 237–244.

Olson, D. H., McCubbin, H. I., Barnes, H., Larsen, A., Muxen, M., & Wilson, M. (1982). *Family inventories: Inventories used in a national survey of families across the family life cycle.* (Available from Family Social Science, 290 McNeal Hall, University of Minnesota, St. Paul, MN 55108).

AUTHOR'S RESPONSE

At the time of this writing, the Family Social Science Department has records of approximately 100 studies that have used or are using the F-COPES scale. Abstracts of these studies are available from the department.

FC-2
Family Function Questionnaire (FFQ)

GENERAL INFORMATION

Date of publication: Not known (approximately 1984–1985).

Author: R. J. Sawa.

Source/publisher: R. J. Sawa, University of Calgary, Calgary General Hospital, 841 Centre Avenue E, Calgary, Alberta, Canada T2E OA1.

Availability: Available from the author (see "Source/publisher," above)

Brief description: The Family Function Questionnaire is composed of 49 items in two sections plus a table for listing information about family members. Various response formats are used. The questionnaire is designed to be completed by each family member independently.

Purpose: The FFQ is part of a method for assessing families (Primary Care Family Assessment) formulated by the author for use by physicians and other health care workers. Within this assessment system, family members' answers to the questionnaire are used to formulate hypotheses about a family's coping difficulties.

Theoretical base: The Primary Care Family Assessment method was derived from family systems theory—specifically, from the McMaster Model of Family Functioning.

PHYSICAL DESCRIPTION OF QUESTIONNAIRE

Physical features: Part 1 consists of 26 questions responded to on the basis of a forced-choice (yes or no) format, followed by space for comments and a grid on which the name of each family member, along with information about that person, is listed. The 23 questions in Part II feature a variety of response formats, including listing, a 5-point rating scale, and specified choices.

Unit of study: Whole family.

Respondent: The questionnaire is designed to be completed by each family member independently. Although age of children is not specified, the length and reading level required would probably exclude children younger than 12.

Scales and dimensions: The dimensions measured by the FFQ are Connectedness, Life Cycles, Internal Family Function, and Health and Coping.

Manual: None available

Standardization and norms: No formal norms are available. Two hundred seventy-four forms filled out by 113 families requiring counseling were used to generate percentages descriptive of these families (e.g., percentage expressing the need for more time together, percentage reporting unclear communication). Major presenting problems for this sample, as well as profiles for families with problems in the four dimensions measured, are also presented.

Evaluation of physical description of questionnaire: *Strengths:* Percentages of major presenting problems and profiles of families with problems in the four dimensions could possibly prove interesting to clinicians. *Weaknesses:* Lack of norms; length of the questionnaire.

ADMINISTRATIVE PROCEDURES

Directions: Directions are provided with the questionnaire.

Ease of use: The FFQ should be easy to administer, requiring only the questionnaire and a pencil. Some family members might show resistance to filling out an instrument of this length, particularly during an evaluation for medical problems.

Training for administration and scoring: The FFQ could be administered by nonprofessionals; a scoring system is not yet available.

Scoring procedures, including calculations of summary scores: Scoring procedures are not yet available. According to the author, further studies will be needed to quantify the four dimensions.

Evaluation of administrative procedures: *Strengths:* Ease of administration. *Weaknesses:* Lack of quantifiable scoring procedures.

EVALUATION OF CONSTRUCTS MEASURED

Reliability: No reliability data are given. According to the author, studies of reliability are now in progress.

Validity: A sample of families having problems coping were given the Family APGAR as well as the FFQ. Forty-four percent of the families scored in the "disturbed" range on the Family APGAR. Since no FFQ scores are available for this sample, the meaning of this information is not clear. Studies of the instrument's validity are in progress.

Clinical utility: Use with a variety of families and normative data are necessary before the clinical utility of this instrument will be demonstrated. The Family Function Questionnaire may be too long to be used as a screening instrument by practicing physicians.

Research utility: A quantifiable scoring system is a must before the Family Function Questionnaire becomes useful for research. Data on the reliability and validity of the instrument are also necessary.

SUMMARY EVALUATION

The Family Function Questionnaire is still in a stage of development. An objective scoring system and psychometric data are needed before the instrument can be judged useful for more than getting a qualitative feel for the functioning of a family. It seems doubtful that most physicians will have the time to use such a lengthy instrument for screening purposes, and family professionals are likely to prefer instruments with normative data, quantifiable scoring, and demonstrated psychometric properties.

REFERENCES

Sawa, R. J., Falk, W. A., & Pablo, R. Y. (1986). *Assessing the family in primary care*. Unpublished manuscript.
Sawa, R. J., Falk, W. A., & Pablo, R. Y. (1986). *Family Function Questionnaire*. Unpublished manuscript.

AUTHOR'S RESPONSE

No additional comments.

FC-3
Family Functioning Index (FFI)

GENERAL INFORMATION

Date of publication: 1973.

Authors: I. B. Pless and Betty Satterwhite Stevenson.

Source/publisher: Pless, I. B., & Satterwhite, B. (1973). A measure of family functioning and its application. *Social Science and Medicine, 7,* 613–621 (copy of measure not included).

Availability: The instrument and scoring instructions are available from Betty Satterwhite Stevenson, Assistant to the Chairman of the Department of Pediatrics, University of Rochester Medical Center, 601 Elmwood Ave., Rochester, N.Y. 14642.

Brief description: The Family Functioning Index is a brief, easily administered 15-question self-report questionnaire or interview for assessing the dynamics of family interaction. The response format varies from two to five choices.

Purpose: The FFI was developed for clinical and research use to examine the relationship between family functioning and the psychological adjustment of children with chronic illness. The authors emphasize that the clinical purpose of the index is screening of families that require further attention.

Theoretical base: The authors describe their choice of questions as eclectic, but they seem to be derived from sociological family role theory.

PHYSICAL DESCRIPTION OF QUESTIONNAIRE

Physical features: The Family Functioning Index includes 15 questions. The response format is item-specific, varying from two choices (yes or no) to a 5-point rating scale. Some of the questions concern dyadic relationships within the family (e.g., sibling, martial relationships): others concern the family as a whole (e.g., is the family happier than other families?). Parallel forms for husband and wife are available. The FFI has been modified to a 5-point Likert-type scale by Seeman, Tittler, and Friedman (1985).

Unit of study: Whole family.

Respondent: Husband or wife in the family.

Scales and dimensions: The principal components to emerge from a factor analysis were marital satisfaction, frequency of disagreements, happiness, communications, weekends together, and problem solving.

Manual: None available.

Standardization and norms: Although no formal norms are available, the means and standard deviations for components of the scale are given for the families of 399 school children (209 chronically ill, 190 healthy) who were part of a 1% random sample of the children of Monroe County, New York (Pless & Satterwhite, 1973).

Evaluation of physical description of questionnaire: *Strengths:* Length and reading level seem appropriate. *Limitations:* No manual is available, and the instrument lacks normative data. The response format is not uniform.

ADMINISTRATIVE PROCEDURES

Directions: Brief directions are provided with the instrument.

Ease of use: The respondent might need guidance in filling out the instrument because of the confusing response format. Scoring instructions are confusing.

Training for administration and scoring: Although the instrument requires care in administration and scoring, it could be administered and scored by non-professionals.

Scoring procedures, including calculation of summary scores: Responses are assigned scores of 0 to 4 (with the exception of two items rating marital satisfaction, which have a possible combined score of 11) and summed. Score range is 0 to 35, with higher scores indicating more desirable functioning. Scoring directions must be followed carefully because of varying response formats and score assignments for the different items.

Evaluation of administrative procedures: *Strengths:* None noted. *Weaknesses:* Although not difficult, scoring is confusing because of lack of uniformity in response format and in assigning scores to responses. Items are assigned different weights with no apparent rationale for doing so.

EVALUATION OF CONSTRUCTS MEASURED

Reliability: Correlations between the dimensions derived from factor analysis and total scores ranged from .07 to .96 for fathers and from .21 to .95 for mothers. Husband/wife agreement was .72, with greater agreement shown in low-scoring families ($r = .41$ for families with high scores $r = .60$ for families with intermediate scores, and $r = .74$ for families with low scores) (Pless & Satterwhite, 1973). Using a portion ($n = 30$) of the original group of families with chronically ill children, Satterwhite, Zweig, Iker, and Pless (1976) found a 5-year test–retest reliability of .83 for the total scores. Test–retest correlations for the 15 individual items were all positive (range $= .04$ to .71), with correlations for 8 of the items showing statistical significance ($p < .05$). An alpha coefficient of .69 and a 6-week test–retest reliability of .79 ($p < .01$) was obtained for a modification of the index into a 5-point Likert-type scale (Seeman, et al., 1985).

Validity: *Construct-related:* Correlations between FFI scores for new registrants at family counseling agencies and caseworker ratings of family functioning were .48 ($p < .01$) for mothers and .35 ($p < .01$) for fathers. The correlation between ratings of paraprofessional counselors and parents' FFI scores for families of children with chronic physical disorders with .39 ($p < .01$) (Pless & Satterwhite, 1973). The FFI was correlated .80 with scores on the Family APGAR (Good, Smilkstein, Good, Shaffer, & Arons, 1979).

   Criterion-related: Families with low FFI scores were more likely to have children with low psychosocial adjustment scores as measured by various tests and ratings, and significant mean difference ($t = 7.7, p < .001$) were shown on the FFI between families from a random sample and from a group seeking the services of a family counseling agency (Pless & Satterwhite, 1975a). However, in a study by Heller, Rafman, Zvagulis, and Pless (1985), no relationship was found between scores on the FFI and "progressive or persistent maladjustment" as measured by the Achenbach Child Behavior Check List.

Clinical utility: The FFI has potential for use as a screening instrument by physicans. However, its utility is limited by weak psychometric construction and the need for more complete normative data. Clarification of the relationship between scores on FFI and psychological maladjustment in children would add to its clinical utility.

Research utility: Reliability and validity data appear mixed. The instrument shows potential for use in research, but further validity studies need to be done, especially in relation to the criterion of psychological maladjustment in children.

SUMMARY EVALUATION

The Family Functioning Index has potential as a screening device for physicians and as a research instrument for measuring general family functioning. The instrument as a whole has shown impressive temporal stability, but mixed results cast doubts on the coherence of the dimensions and the validity of the instrument as a predictor of psychological maladjustment in children. One source of difficulty may be the atheoretical nature of the measure. Furthermore, the response format of the FFI is inconsistent and confusing to score. The Family Functioning Index is unsuitable for use with single-parent families because of the number of items concerned with marital adjustment. A modification of this measure (Seeman et al., 1985) may prove more useful.

REFERENCES

Good, M. D., Smilkstein, G., Good, B. J., Shaffer, T., & Arons, T. (1979). The Family APGAR Index: A study of construct validity. *Journal of Family Practice, 8,* 557–582.

Heller, A., Rafman, S., Zvagulis, I., & Pless, I. B. (1985). Birth defects and psychosocial adjustment. *American Journal of Diseases of Children, 139,* 257–263.

Pless, I. B., Roghmann, K., & Haggerty, R. J. (1972). Chronic illness, family functioning, and psychological adjustment: A model for the allocation of preventive mental health services. *International Journal of Epidemiology, 1,* 217–277.

Pless, I. B., & Satterwhite, B. B. (1972). Chronic illness in childhood: Selection, activities, and evaluation of non-professional counselors. *Clinical Pediatrics, 11,* 403–410.

Pless, I. B., & Satterwhite, B. B. (1973). A measure of family functioning and its application. *Social Science and Medicine, 7,* 613–621.

Pless, I. B., & Satterwhite, B. B. (1975a). Chronic illness. In R. J. Haggerty, K. J. Roghmann, & I. B. Pless (Eds.), *Child health and the community* (pp. 78–94). New York: Wiley.

Pless, I. B., & Satterwhite, B. B. (1975b). Family functioning and family problems. In R. J. Haggerty, K. J. Roghmann, & I. B. Pless (Eds.), *Child health and the community* (pp. 41–54). New York: Wiley.

Satterwhite, B. B., Zweig, S. R., Iker, H. P., & Pless, B. (1976). The Family Functioning Index: Five-year test–retest reliability and implications for use. *Journal of Comparative Family Studies, 7,* 111–116.

Seeman, L., Tittler, B. I., & Friedman, S. (1985). Early interactional change and its relationship to family therapy outcome. *Family Process, 24,* 59–68.

AUTHOR'S RESPONSE

No additional comments.

FC-4
Family Inventory of Life Events and Changes (FILE)

GENERAL INFORMATION

Date of publication: 1982.

Authors: Hamilton McCubbin, Joan M. Patterson, and Lance R. Wilson.

Source/publisher: Published in *Family Inventories* (Olson et al., 1982).

Availability: Available from David H. Olson, Dept. of Family Social Science, 290 McNeal Hall, University of Minnesota, St. Paul, MN 55108.

Brief description: The FILE is a 71-item self-report instrument designed to record the normative and nonnormative life events and changes experienced by a family unit in the past year.

Purpose: The FILE assesses the ''pile-up'' or sum of normative and nonnormative stressors and intrafamilial strains experienced by members of the family.

Theoretical base: Family systems theory and family stress theory, based on the assumption that the accumulation of life events plays a role in the etiology of various psychiatric disorders.

PHYSICAL DESCRIPTION OF QUESTIONNAIRE

Physical features: The FILE is a 71-item self-report instrument. Family members are asked to respond by checking whether or not each event occured within the past year.

Unit of study: Whole family.

Respondent: Individual adult family member. (Another measure, the A-FILE, was developed for use with adolescents, who respond about changes in their families.)

Scales and dimensions: The FILE consists of the following 9 scales:

1. Intrafamily Strains
   a. Conflict
   b. Parenting Strains
2. Marital Strains
3. Pregnancy and Childbearing Strains
4. Finance and Business Strains
   a. Family Finances
   b. Family Business
5. Work–Family Transitions and Strains
   a. Work Transitions
   b. Family Transitions and Work Strains
6. Illness and Family "Care" Strains
   a. Illness Onset and Child Care
   b. Chronic Illness Strains
   c. Dependency Strains
7. Losses
8. Transitions "In" and "Out"
9. Legal

Manual: The manual is well organized and easy to use and includes information on test development and validation. However, it is not comprehensive; the user is referred to other works for more complete explanations.

Standardization and norms: National norms were based on approximately 980 couples (1,960 individuals). This sample included couples across the family life cycle, from young married couples to retired couples. The subjects were primarily Lutheran and Caucasian.

Evaluation of physical description of questionnaire: The inventory is easy to use, with a clear response format, norms available, and a simple reading level.

ADMINISTRATIVE PROCEDURES

Directions: The directions for using the FILE are on the inventory itself. They are clear and straight forward.

Ease of use: The FILE is very easy to use.

Training for administration and scoring: Minimal training is required to use the FILE. The directions are self-explanatory and are printed on the measure. Scoring consists of simply summing yes and no responses.

Scoring procedures: A total sum score of the no responses is used for scoring. A higher score implies lower stress. The authors state that the unweighted sum is as useful as any weighting procedure.Scores of 55 and below are considered to depict "high" stress; however, the basis for this judgment is unclear.

Evaluation of administrative procedures: *Strengths:* The FILE is easy to administer and score. *Weaknesses:* Equal weighting of stressful events assumes that each one has equal import to the respondent, or at least that statistical weighting does not add much information.

EVALUATION OF CONSTRUCTS MEASURED:

Reliability: The overall scale reliability (Cronbach's alpha) was .81, varying from .30 to .73 on the subscales. Because the subscales are less reliable, the authors recommend that only the total scale score be used. Pearson r for test–retest reliability over a 4- to 5-week period ranged from .64 to .84 (total scale = .80). Use of test–retest reliability for an instrument that purports to be sensitive to change over time seems questionable.

Validity: Factor analysis was used to examine the construct validity of the instrument. This was problematic because of the wide variance in the frequency of occurrence of items and affected the factor structure. Therefore, decisions about final item selection were based on conceptual groupings rather than purely empirical groupings. Correlations between the FILE and the Moos Family Environment Scale (FES) ranged from $-.41$ to $+.42$ for subscales and from $-.24$ to $+.23$ on the total scale score. FES Conflict was correlated $+.23$ with total life changes ($p < .05$); Cohesion was correlated $-.24$ ($p < .05$) with total life changes.

Clinical utility: The FILE appears to be a useful clinical instrument. It can give the person working with a family some idea of the accumulation of stressors in the family that have influenced their present situation.

Research utility: The FILE appears to be a promising research instrument. It operationalizes the concept of accumulated life stress in a manner that allows the study of family behavior in response to stress. Since it has been used in few empirical studies to date, research utility awaits further evaluation.

SUMMARY EVALUATION

The FILE is a 71-item self-report measure developed to assess the accumulation of normative and nonnormative life events and changes experienced by a family. Conceptually, the FILE is appealing. It is too early to assess its clinical or research utility, but there appears to be potential for both. The most significant weaknesses seem to be in the unreliability of the subscales, the lack of interpretive guidelines for scores, the lack of weights for items, and the lack of attention to chronic stressors. (Although the manual states that the FILE also records events experienced prior to the past year, no provision for this is made on the instrument itself.) The FILE, like any self-report instrument, is susceptible to social desirability in responding. A respondent who wished to portray the family in an inaccurate way could easily do so.

REFERENCES

Olson, D. H., McCubbin, H. I., Barnes, H., Larsen, A., Muxen, M., & Wilson, M. (1982). *Family inventories: Inventories used in a national survey of families across the family life cycle.* (Available from Family Social Science, 290 McNeal Hall, University of Minnesota, St. Paul, MN 55108).

AUTHOR'S RESPONSE

Although the lack of weights for items could possibly be a weakness for clinical use, it should not be so for research use.

FC-5
Family Relationships Index (FRI)

GENERAL INFORMATION

Date of publication: 1981 (Family Environment Scale published in 1974).

Authors: C. J. Holahan and Rudolf H. Moos.

Source/publisher: Consulting Psychologists Press, 577 College Avenue, Palo Alto, CA 94306.

Availability: The manual for the Family Environment Scale (2nd ed.) is available from consulting Psychologists Press; a specimen set is also available.

Brief description: The Family Relationships Index (FRI) consists of the items from three subscales of the Family Environment Scale (FES): Cohesion, Expressiveness, and Conflict (reversed in scoring). These scales include 27 true–false items.

Purpose: The purpose of this special scale is to assess the quality of support found in social relationships within the family environment.

Theoretical base: Ecological psychology theory

PHYSICAL DESCRIPTION OF QUESTIONNAIRE

Physical features: The FRI includes 27 true–false items.

Unit of study: Whole family climate.

Respondent: Individual family member above age 11.

Scales and dimensions: Since the FRI is an index derived from a larger instrument (the FES), the FRI is viewed as a unitary dimension of family support in research studies using it (e.g., Holahan & Moos, 1985).

Manual: A comprehensive manual is available for the FES (Moos, 1986). Since the FRI items are a direct subset of the FES, much of the information in the larger manual applies to the FRI as well.

Standardization and norms: See FES abstract.

Evaluation of physical description of questionnaire: *Strengths:* The index is simple and straightforward and shares many of the strengths of the well-validated FES. *Weaknesses:* None

ADMINISTRATIVE PROCEDURES

Directions: The respondent replies "true" or "false" to each of 27 items.

Ease of use: The FRI is very easy to use.

Training for administration and scoring: Very little is required.

Scoring procedures: The three FES subscales of Cohesion, Expressiveness, and Conflict are scored according to the key in the manual. Scores on the Conflict scale are reversed before they are summed so that all of the scales are scored in the same direction. Raw scores are converted to standard scores and may be plotted on profiles.

Evaluation of administrative procedures: *Strengths:* The instrument is easy to administer and score and has an adequate response range. *Limitations:* none.

EVALUATION OF CONSTRUCTS MEASURED

Reliability: Internal consistency (Cronbach's alpha) for the FRI is .89.

Validity: The FRI has been used in several studies of the role of family support in resistance to stress (Holahan & Moos, 1981, 1982, 1983, 1985, 1986). For example, in one study, results supported the prediction that decreases in support in the family and work environments were related to increases in psychological maladjustment over a 1-year period (Holahan & Moos, 1981).

Clinical utility: Although the FRI has primarily been used in research, it is expected to be clinically useful, as the FES has demonstrated clinical utility.

Research utility: The research utility of the instrument has been amply demonstrated in several studies (see "References," below). The psychometric qualities of the index are strong, and the theoretical basis of the instrument is clear.

SUMMARY EVALUATION

The Family Relationships Index, a measure composed of a subset of 27 items from the Family Environment Scale, is a useful, theoretically grounded instrument for assessing support in family relationships. The instrument is easy to administer, complete, and score. Results of studies using the instrument have demonstrated its usefulness in the research setting.

REFERENCES

Holahan, C. J., & Moos, R. H. (1981). Social support and psychological distress: A longitudinal analysis. *Journal of Abnormal Psychology, 90,* 365–370.

Holahan, C. J., & Moos, R. H. (1982). Social support and adjustment: Predictive benefits of social climate indices. *American Journal of Community Psychology, 10,* 403–415.

Holahan, C. J., & Moos, R. H. (1983). The quality of social support: Measures of family and work relationships. *British Journal of Clinical Psychology, 22,* 157–162.

Holahan, C. J., & Moos, R. H. (1985). Life stress and health: Personality, coping, and family support in stress resistance. *Journal of Personality and Social Psychology, 49,* 739–747.

Holahan, C. J., & Moos, R. H. (1986). Personality, coping, and family resources in stress resistance: A longitudinal analysis. *Journal of Personality and Social Psychology, 51,* 389–395.

Moos, R. H. (1986). *Manual for the Family Environment Scales* (2nd ed.). Palo Alto, CA: Consulting Psychologists Press.

AUTHOR'S RESPONSE

No additional comments.

FC-6
Family Routines Inventory

GENERAL INFORMATION

Date of publication: 1983.

Authors: Eric W. Jensen and W. Thomas Boyce.

Source/publisher: Jensen, E. W., James, S. A., Boyce, W. T. & Hartnett, B. A. (1983). The Family Routines Inventory: Development and validation. *Social Science and Medicine, 17,* 201–211.

Availability: Available from Eric W. Jensen, School of Medicine, 207H, Wing B, Box 5, Chapel Hill, NC 27514.

Brief description: The Family Routines Inventory is a 2B-item self-report inventory using a four-choice format to rate the frequency of occurrence of a routine in the family and a three-choice format to rate the importance of a routine to the family.

Purpose: The purpose of the Family Routines Inventory is to measure an individual family's endorsement of and adherence to positive routines that are thought to protect family members against ill health.

Theoretical base: The inventory is based on the social-epidemiological model that postulates stressful life change as a contributor to disease susceptibility and social support as a buffer against disease susceptibility. Family routines are seen as contributing to family health by promoting consistency and serving as symbols of permanence during times of major life change.

PHYSICAL DESCRIPTION OF QUESTIONNAIRE

Physical features: The inventory presents 28 family routines. A four-choice format is used to rate the routines' frequency of use (always-everyday, 3–5 times a week, 1–2 times a week, or almost never). The importance of each routine is also rated (very important, somewhat important, or not at all important). Reading level is appropriate for literate adult respondents.

Unit of study: Whole family.

Respondent: Parent in the family.

Scales and dimensions: The 28 family routines were designed to tap 10 domains of family life: Workday Routines, Weekend and Leisure Time, Children's Routines, Parent(s) Routines, Bedtime, Meals, Extended Family, Leaving and Homecoming, Disciplinary Routines, and Chores.

Manual: None available.

Standardization and norms: None available.

Evaluation of physical description of questionnaire: *Strengths:* The response format, length, and reading level seem appropriate. One of the criteria for choosing items was that the item not discriminate among families on the basis of race (black or white) or social class. The inventory, therefore, is likely to be appropriate for heterogeneous families as well as for families of different social classes. *Limitations:* The inventory lacks normative data. Items were chosen on the basis of interviews and mothers' judgments of the items' importance. Further research is needed to ascertain if the routines chosen for the inventory are important as buffers against stress for the family. The keying of all items in a positive direction may increase the possibility of socially desirable responses.

ADMINISTRATIVE PROCEDURES

Directions: No directions are available.

Ease of use: The instrument is easy to administer, requiring only the items, an answer sheet, and a pencil. It can easily be computer-scored.

Training for administration and scoring: The measure could be administered and scored by nonprofessionals.

Scoring procedures, including calculation of summary scores Responses to items are weighted (daily performance = 3; 3–5 times a week = 2; 1–2 times a week = 1; and almost never = 0) and the weights are summed to yield a frequency score ranging from 0 to 84. Although the authors discussed assigning weights to the ratings of family routines' importance and deriving an "importance score," this score was dropped prior to studies of reliability and validity because it was thought to reflect attributes similar to those of the frequency score.

Evaluation of administrative procedures: *Strengths:* The instrument is easy to administer and score. *Limitations:* The portion of the instrument in which the importance of family routines is rated seems to have little utility, since responses to this portion of the instrument are not scored. Depletion of ratings of importance would result in a shorter instrument and little information would be lost. Instructions to discourage socially desirable responding are not included with the instrument.

EVALUATION OF CONSTRUCTS MEASURED

Reliability: Thirty-day test–retest reliability ($n = 271$) was .79 for the frequency score (Jensen, James, Boyce, & Hartnett, 1983). No internal consistency reliabilities are available.

Validity: *Construct-related:* Family Routines Inventory scores correlated positively and significantly with a question about general family satisfaction ($r = .33$, $p < .001$) and with Family Environment Scale subscales Cohesion, Organization, and Control ($r = .35$, .36, and .20, $p < .001$ for all). The correlation with Family Environment Scale subscale Conflict was negative ($r = .10$, $p < .001$). Multiple-regression analyses supported the role of the Family Routines Inventory score as a predictor variable in relation to the five validity indices discussed, even after controlling for 15 other relevant variables (Jensen et al., 1983).

Criterion-related: Family rhythmicity as measured by the Family Routines Inventory predicted mothers' sense of competence as parents in a study of 285 families with infants between 2 and 13 months of age (Sprunger, Boyce, & Gaines, 1985).

Clinical utility: Without normative data, the clinical utility of this instrument is limited. However, the instrument could be used as an informal means of assessing extent of routinization in families and, as such, could be useful in focusing intervention.

Research utility: Research to date suggests that the instrument is useful, especially in studies investigating the role of family routines as a buffer against stress.

SUMMARY EVALUATION

The Family Routines Inventory is an instrument with demonstrated research potential for assessing the degree of predictability and routinization in family life. Strengths of the inventory include use with heterogeneous populations, since the authors attempted to minimize the effects of race and social class on the instrument, and ease of administration and scoring. Social desirability may be a problem with the Family Routines Inventory because of the keying of all items in a positive direction and the lack of instructions to discourage socially desirable responses. Further studies, especially normative studies and studies of reliability and validity, would be useful in further evaluating the utility of the instrument.

REFERENCES

Boyce, W. T., Jensen, E. W. Cassel, J. C., Collier, A. M., Smith A. H. & Ramsey, C. T. (1977). Influence of life events and family routines on childhood respiratory tract illness. *Pediatrics, 60,* 609–615.

Boyce, W. T., Jensen, E. W. James, S. A., & Peacock, J. L. (1983). The Family Routines Inventory: Theoretical origins. *Social Science and Medicine, 17* 193–200.

Jensen, E. W., James, S. A., Boyce, W. T. & Hartnett, S. A. (1983). The Family Routines Inventory: Development and validation. *Social Science and Medicine, 17,* 201–211.

Sprunger, L. W., Boyce, W. T., & Gaines, J. A. (1985). Family-Infant congruence: Routines and rhythmicity in family adaptations to a young infant. *Child Development, 56,* 564–572.

AUTHOR'S RESPONSE

No additional comments.

FC-7
Family Strengths

GENERAL INFORMATION

Date of publication: 1982.

Authors: David H. Olson, Andrea S. Larsen, and Hamilton I. McCubbin.

Source/publisher: Published in *Family Inventories* (Olson et al., 1982).

Availability: Available from David H. Olson, Dept. of Family Social Science, 290 McNeal Hall, University of Minnesota, St. Paul, MN 55108.

Brief description: Family Strengths is a 12-item self-report measure designed to measure several aspects of resources available to families.

Purpose: Family Strengths assesses family pride (including loyalty, trust and respect) and accord, or a family's sense of competency.

Theoretical base: Derived from sociological family theories concerning family resources; consistent with family systems theory.

PHYSICAL DESCRIPTION OF QUESTIONNAIRE

Physical features: Family Strengths includes 12 items, each of which is responded to on a scale of 1 ("strongly disagree") to 5 ("strongly agree"). The reading level is simple, appropriate for children 10 and above and adults.

Unit of study: Whole family.

Respondent: Individual family member.

Scales and dimensions: The final instrument includes two dimensions: Pride (including pride, loyalty, trust, and respect) and Accord (tapping a family's sense of competency).

Manual: The manual, which is part of a larger collection of descriptions of family inventories (Olson et al., 1982), includes information on theoretical formulation, empirical validation, and psychometric data.

Standardization and norms: National norms, developed on the Lutheran sample of 1,140 couples and 412 adolescents reported in the manual, are reported.

Evaluation of physical description of questionnaire: *Strengths:* The inventory is easy to use and has a clear response format and length, an adequate response range, and normative data. *Weaknesses:* The normative sample is limited in terms of generalizability. Item content reflects whole-family functioning, whereas perceptions might vary for different individuals or subsystems in the family.

ADMINISTRATIVE PROCEDURES

Directions: Respondents are asked to rate each of 12 items on a Likert-type scale of 1 ("strongly disagree") to 5 ("strongly agree").

Ease of use: The instrument is very easy to use.

Training for administration and scoring: Very little training is required.

Scoring Procedures: The instrument can easily be scored by hand. Scores on negatively worded items are reversed before scores are summed.

Evaluation of administrative procedures: *Strengths:* Easy to administer and score. *Weaknesses:* Vulnerable to social desirability response bias.

EVALUATION OF CONSTRUCTS MEASURED

Reliability: Cronbach's alphas for Pride were .87–.88; for Accord, .72–.73; for the total score, .83. Test–retest reliability (Pearson correlation) over a 4-week interval was .73 for Pride, .79 for Accord, and .58 for the total score.

Validity: Factor analysis performed on the 12 items replicated across two samples, yielding two factors. In the manual, however, factor loadings are reported only for the primary factor on which each item loaded.

Clinical utility: At this point, the clinical utility of the instrument is unknown. Presumably, responses on this scale would give a clinician a general index of family members' optimism and positive outlook about their family.

Research utility: At this point, the research utility is unknown. The instrument's rather transparent purpose and items make it very susceptible to socially desirable responding.

SUMMARY EVALUATION

Family Strengths is a short self-report measure designed to assess family members' views concerning their strengths and, hence, their family resources. Simple test construction and ease of use are strengths of this measure. Limitations center on the content and construct validity of the measure and its susceptibility to socially desirable responding. These limitations await further research in order to assess the clinical and research utility of the measure. The usefulness of "family strengths" as a theoretical construct also awaits further work.

REFERENCES

Olson, D. H., McCubbin, H. I., Barnes, H., Larsen, A., Muxen, M., & Wilson, M. (1982). *Family inventories: Inventories used in a national survey of families across the family life cycle*. (Available from Family Social Science, 290 McNeal Hall, University of Minnesota, St. Paul, MN 55108)

AUTHOR'S RESPONSE

No additional comments.

FC-8
Feetham Family Functioning Survey
(FFFS)

GENERAL INFORMATION

Date of publication: 1983.

Authors: Suzanne L. Feetham and Carolyn S. Roberts.

Source/publisher: Roberts, C. S., & Feetham, S. L. (1982). Assessing family functioning across three areas of relationships, *Nursing Research, 31,* 231–235.

Availability: Available from Suzanne L. Feetham, Director of Nursing for Education and Research, Children's Hospital National Medical Center, 111 Michigan Ave. NW, Washington, DC 20012.

Brief description: The Feetham Family Functioning Survey is a 27-item self-report inventory designed to evaluate relationships within the family as well as relationships between the family and the social environment. Each item is rated in relation to its present existence in the family, its desired existence, and its importance.

Purpose: The FFFS was first developed to measure the effect on families of having a child with myelodysplasia (spina bifida) for the purpose of planning nursing interventions. The instrument is also considered useful for measuring family functioning under many other conditions, including the birth of a child, and may be repeated to determine a pattern of changes in family functioning over time.

Theoretical base: Family ecological theory, family systems theory.

PHYSICAL DESCRIPTION OF QUESTIONNAIRE

Physical features: The 1983 revision of the FFFS consists of 27 items. The format consists of a stem that provides a referent for three questions: (1) How much is there now? (2) How much should there be? and (3) How important is this to me? The respondent is required to rate each question on a 7-point scale (from 1 = "little" to 7 = "much"). Persons with less than high school education may have difficulty with this format, as anchor points are defined only for the extremities. The measure may be completed by either parent and takes approximately 10 minutes to complete.

Unit of study: Whole family.

Respondent: Adult/parent (The FFFS is not suitable for single-parent families.)

Scales and dimensions: The FFFS measures three major areas of family functioning as relationships: (1) relationships between the family and broader social units, (2) relationships between the family and subsystems, and (3) relationships between the family and each individual within the family. The existing degree of need fulfillment, the discrepancy between achieved and expected levels, and the importance of the content of each stem are scored. More recently, the instrument has been interpreted as a measure of social support in addition to the foregoing three dimensions.

Manual: None available.

Standardization and norms: Item-by-item means and standard deviations are given for all four scores (how much exists, how much there should be, discrepancy score, and importance score) for a sample of 103 mothers of children with myelodysplasia (Roberts & Feetham, 1982), and mean discrepancy scores are given for 45 parents of children with myelodysplasia for the periods just prior to birth and 3 months, 6 months, 12 months and 18 months after birth. Although the FFFS was used with parents of normal children in two studies, statistics for these studies are not available in published articles (Feetham & Humenick, 1982). Work in progress includes testing the instrument with larger samples of families of healthy children, families with infants at risk for apnea, and families of children receiving new health care procedures.

Evaluation of physical description of questionnaire: *Strengths:* Several scores can be derived, and both intra- and extra-familial environments are assessed with the FFFS. Some normative data are available, and the measure is short. *Limitations:* Although the purpose of the instrument is the measurement of whole-family functioning, items refer to one person's perception of family life. The format is not suitable for parents with less than a high school education, requiring individual administration in an interview format. Norms are not yet available; therefore, the instrument may not be suitable for use in a nonmedical setting with families of normal children. (*Note:* Psychometric data for normal children should soon be available from work now in progress: S. L. Feetham, personal communication, September, 12, 1986.)

ADMINISTRATIVE PROCEDURES

Directions: Clear directions are provided with the instrument. Directions do not discourage socially desirable responding or inform the respondent of the purpose of the measure, which may lower the respondent's motivation.

Ease of use: The FFFS is moderately easy to use. The measure can be self-administered or administered as an interview for respondents with a low educational level. No significant differences in distribution of responses were found attributable to method of administration (Roberts & Feetham, 1982).

Training for administration and scoring: The instrument could be administered by nonprofessionals with little training. Scoring would require some training.

Scoring procedures, including calculation of summary scores: The discrepancy score is obtained by summing the differences between ratings of the first and second question for each item. The discrepancy score can then be converted to an absolute score in order to eliminate negative score values. The importance score is obtained by summing the ratings of the importance of each item.

Evaluation of administrative procedures: *Strengths:* Moderately easy to use; different administration methods can be used; scoring requires some training but is not extremely difficult. *Limitations:* Persons with less than a high school education may need help filling out the measure because of the complicated format. Socially desirable responding is not discouraged in the directions of the measure.

EVALUATION OF CONSTRUCTS MEASURED

Reliability: Alpha coefficients were .66 for "How much is there?" items, .75 for "How much should there be?" items, .81 for the discrepancy score, and .84 for the importance score. Two-week test–retest reliability was .85 (Roberts, 1979, cited in Roberts & Feetham, 1982).

Validity: *Construct-related:* The correlation between the FFFS and Pless and Satterwhite's Family Functioning Index was $-.54$ ($p < .001$). The authors expected a moderate correlation, since the FFFS measures relationships between the family and the environment in addition to the intrafamily functioning measured by the Family Functioning Index. Factor analysis of the FFFS responses of 103 mothers supported the three areas of relationships that the instrument was constructed to measure. All but three of the items of the FFFS loaded with eigenvalues of at least .43 on one of three factors representing relationships between the family and individual family members, between the family and other subsystems, and between the family and broader social systems. The three items were retained in the FFFS for further testing (Roberts & Feetham, 1982).

Clinical utility: Although the authors recommend that the FFFS be used as a research instrument rather than a clinical instrument until its clinical utility is confirmed by further testing, the instrument may prove to be useful for planning and assessing care of families of children with birth defects. Normative data are needed to demonstrate the usefulness of this instrument with other types of families.

Research utility: The instrument may be useful for nursing research, especially in relation to families that have children with birth defects. Repeated use of the instrument over time to measure changes in family functioning seems especially promising.

SUMMARY EVALUATION

The FFFS is unique in that it recognizes the importance of the relationship of the family to the environment. The discrepancy score, together with the importance score, can help to identify areas of dissatisfaction and their importance for family members. Repeated use of the instrument to measure changes in family functioning may prove useful for assessment and research. Limitations include a moderately difficult response format, lack of a manual, and currently inadequate normative data. Further research needs to be done to demonstrate the usefulness of the measure with different types of families. The FFFS is now being tested with samples of families with healthy children, families with infants at risk for apnea, and families of children on new health care procedures.

REFERENCES

Feetham, S. L., & Humenick, S. S. (1982). Feetham Family Functioning Survey. In S. Humenick (Ed.), *Analysis of current assessment strategies in the health care of young children and childbearing families* (pp. 259–268). Norwalk, CT: Appleton-Century-Crofts.

Roberts, C. S., & Feetham, S. L. (1982). Assessing family functioning across three areas of relationships. *Nursing Research, 31,* 231–235.

Speer, J. J., & Sachs, B. (1985). Selecting the appropriate family assessment tool. *Pediatric Nursing, 11,* 349–355.

Thomas, R. B., & Barnard, K. E. (1986). Understanding families: A look at measures and methodologies. *From Zero to Three, 6*(5), 11–14.

AUTHOR'S RESPONSE

No additional comments.

FC-9
Procidano Perceived Social Support Questionnaire—Family (PSS-Fa)

GENERAL INFORMATION

Date of publication: 1983.

Authors: M. E. Procidano and K. Heller.

Source/publisher: Procidano, M. E., & Heller, K. (1983). Measures of perceived social support from friends and family. Three validation studies. *American Journal of Community Psychology, 11*(1), 1–24.

Availability: Scale is printed in cited source.

Brief description: The Perceived Social Support Questionnaire—Family is a 20-item measure of perceived family support.

Purpose: The PSS-Fa is designed to measure the extent to which an individual perceives that his or her needs for support, information, and feedback are fulfilled by the family.

Theoretical base: Prevention/community psychology.

PHYSICAL DESCRIPTION OF QUESTIONNAIRE

Physical features: The PSS-Fa consists of 20 declarative statements to which the individual answers "Yes," "No," or "Don't know."

Unit of study: Individual.

Respondent: Individual.

Scales and dimensions: The PSS-Fa consists of a single scale. A second scale, the Perceived Social Support—Friends (PSS-FR) is also available.

Manual: None available.

Standardization and norms: None available.

Evaluation of physical description of questionnaire: *Strengths:* Items and response format are straightforward and easily completed in a brief administration. *Limitations:* Questionnaire construction appears to have been determined solely on a college-age sample, which may have resulted in the retention of items primarily characteristic of this developmental stage and may have limited generalizability of this measure to other populations.

ADMINISTRATIVE PROCEDURES

Directions: Respondents are clearly directed to circle one of three possible answers provided next to each question.

Ease of use: Maximum ease.

Training for administration and scoring: None needed.

Scoring procedures: For each item, the response indicative of social support is scored + 1, so that scores range from 0, indicating no support, to 20, indicating maximum support.

Evaluation of administration procedures: *Strengths:* Administrative procedures are very simple. *Limitations:* None noted.

EVALUATION OF CONSTRUCTS MEASURED

Reliability: The PSS-Fa was found to be internally consistent, with a Cronbach's alpha of .90. The PSS-Fa was found to be unaffected by manipulation of respondent mood. No test–retest data were reported for the final version of the measure.

Validity: *Construct-related:* The PSS-Fa was significantly and negatively related to the MMPI subscales of D, Pt, and Sc ($p < .001$) and positively related to K. ($r = .20$; $p < .05$). Although positively related to social desirability ($p < .001$), partial correlations, with social desirability controlled, remained significant.

Clinical utility: Based on preliminary construct validation, the PSS-Fa may have clinical utility with a college-age population; however, additional psychometric evaluation is essential to confirm as well as to determine the utility of this measure for additional populations.

Research utility: The internal consistency and ease of administration and scoring suggest that the PSS-Fa may be useful in research, at present, with college samples only.

SUMMARY EVALUATION

The strengths of the PSS-Fa lie in its simplicity of administration and scoring. Therefore, it represents a potentially useful measure of perceived social support in the family. Psychometric investigation of the measure is preliminary and is limited to college samples, thereby limiting the current clinical and research utility of the measure.

REFERENCES

Procidano, M. E., & Heller, K. (1983). Measures of perceived social support from friends and family: Three validation studies. *American Journal of Community Psychology, 11*(1), 1–24.

AUTHOR'S RESPONSE

Studies, as yet unpublished, subsequent to the initial validation of the PSS instruments also have demonstrated their reliability and validity. For instance, internal consistency estimates (Cronbach's alphas) for PSS-Fa were .89 (90 female high school students) and .91 (60 male adult multiple sclerosis patients). Test–retest reliability estimates over a 1-month period were .80 (female high school students) and .91 (115 college dormitory residents). The PSS-Fa was related positively to adjustment and/or negatively to symptomatology in studies of female high school students, 110 adult college students, male adult multiple sclerosis patients, and 90 Vietnam veterans. Some evidence for the stress-buffering hypothesis was also obtained. Perceived social support appears to be a better predictor of adjustment than structural social network characteristics. Normative and construct validation data are available from the author, and a user's manual is in preparation.

Section VIII
Abstracts of
Self-Report Questionnaires:
Parent–Child Relationships

PC-1
Adult–Adolescent Parenting Inventory (AAPI)

GENERAL INFORMATION

Date of publication: 1984.

Author: Stephen J. Bavolek, PhD.

Source/publisher: Family Development Resources, Inc.

Availability: Available from Family Development Resources, Inc., 767 2nd Ave., Eau Claire, WI, 54703.

Brief description: The AAPI consists of 32 items assessing the attitudes of adults and adolescents in each of four parenting patterns: inappropriate developmental expectations of children; lack of an empathetic awareness of children's needs; strong parental belief in the use of corporal punishment; reversing parent–child family roles. Specific information regarding current or potential parenting strengths and weaknesses is gathered from an individual's response to the inventory.

Purpose: The purpose of the AAPI is to assess high-risk parenting attitudes and child-rearing practices of adolescents and adults. Data from the AAPI provide an index of risk (high, medium, low) for practicing abusive and neglecting parenting and child-rearing behaviors.

Theoretical base: Socialization theory.

PHYSICAL DESCRIPTION OF QUESTIONNAIRE

Physical Features: The AAPI is a 32-item self-report attitudinal inventory. Individuals respond to the 32 items by circling a response reflecting their degree of support for each statement. The responses appear in a 5-point Likert format ("strongly agree," "agree," "uncertain," "disagree," "strongly disagree") beneath each item.

Unit of Study: Adolescents aged 12 to 19 and adults aged 20+.

Respondent: Individual adolescents aged 12 to 19 and adults aged 20+.

Scales and dimensions: Four parenting scales derive from the 32-item inventory: Inappropriate Expectations (6 items), Empathy (8 items), Corporal Punishment (10 items), and Role Reversal (8 items).

Manual: The manual includes an introduction to the AAPI, an explanation of its design and construction, information about the diagnostic and discriminatory validity of the AAPI, and data collection and scoring procedures. It also includes the development of the standardization and norms of the AAPI and the norm tables used for interpreting responses to the inventory.

Standardization and Norms: More than 8,800 adults and adolescents from around the country have participated in the standardization of the AAPI. Twenty norm tables are available for converting raw scores into standard scores for the purpose of understanding a respondent's scores on the AAPI. Norm tables are presented by age (adult and adolescent), sex (male, female, and combined), race (white, black, and combined), and status (abused/nonabused and abusive/nonabusive). To determine degree of risk for abuse, individual responses can be compared to the responses of abusive parents or abused adolescents.

Evaluation of physical description of questionnaire: *Strengths:* Based on existing research, the four parenting scales of the AAPI provide adequate distinction among abusive/abused versus nonabusive/nonabused populations. The manual is clear and useful and provides direct information regarding the standardization and norms of the AAPI. *Limitations:* As with any self-report assessment, the possibility of social desirability response bias is always present.

ADMINISTRATIVE PROCEDURES

Directions: Respondents are asked to read the 32 statements in the test booklet and decide the degree to which they agree or disagree with each statement by circling one of the responses located under each statement.

Ease of use: The AAPI appears to be quite easy to use. The measure can be administered either individually or in small groups.

Training for administration and scoring: No special training is required for administration of the measure. Scoring instructions are included in the manual.

Scoring procedures: Using scoring stencils, total raw scores for each parenting scale are calculated for each respondent. Raw scores in each parenting scale are then converted into standard scores by selecting the correct norms tables found in the manual. The standard scores are then plotted on two parenting profiles (either nonabusive and abusive adult population profile or nonabused and abused adolescent population profile). The profiles can then be used to determine parenting strengths and weaknesses.

Evaluation of administrative procedures: *Strengths:* The AAPI is easy to administer and score. Standardized scores and the availability of normative data permit the assessment of a respondent's degree of risk for abuse. *Limitations:* The AAPI requires a sixth-grade reading level to complete the inventory's items; however, the test can be administered orally to nonreaders.

EVALUATION OF CONSTRUCTS MEASURED:

Reliability: Internal reliability alpha coefficients for both adults and adolescents ranged from .70 to .86, indicating a fairly high internal reliability within the four AAPI constructs (Bavolek, 1984). The alpha coefficients were generally higher for adults than for adolescents. The test–retest reliability of the items ranges from $-.10$ to .91; among the four constructs, the coefficients ranged from .39 to .89. Overall, adolescent responses to the items in the construct Empathic Awareness have the highest test-retest reliability (.89), while the construct Parental Expectations had the lowest (.39). The average test–retest reliability over all 32 items is .76.

Validity: *Criterion:* In general, the AAPI found significant mean differences between abused and nonabused adolescents and adults, male and female adolescents and adults, and older and younger mothers (Bavolek, 1984). *Construct:* Parent AAPI scores predicted males' exposure to but not preference for violent, fantasy, superhero, and loner TV programs. Results for females were nonsignificant (Price, 1985). Further predictive and construct validity studies are currently in progress (Gordon & Gordon, undated).

Clinical Utility: Data obtained from the AAPI can be used to provide treatment and remediation to parents and adolescents whose attitudes indicate a high risk for child abuse. The AAPI can also be used to screen foster parent applicants, child care staff, and volunteers for education and training purposes.

Research utility: As a research assessment tool, the AAPI can be used to assess the parenting and child-rearing attitudes of adults and adolescents prior to parenthood and the role that these attitudes may play in the parent–child relationship. The AAPI can also be useful in providing pre- and posttest data to assess treatment and parent education effectiveness.

SUMMARY EVALUATION

The AAPI is an effective assessment tool for identifying high-risk parenting attitudes and child-rearing practices of adolescents and adults. The strengths of this measure include its ease of administration and scoring and its potentially *proactive*, rather than reactive, approach to child abuse. Although the measure can not "predict" potential child abusers, the AAPI can identify those individuals who are at higher risk for abusive behavior, based on the normative data.

REFERENCES

Bavolek, S. J. (1984). *Adult–Adolescent Parenting Inventory*. Eau Claire, WI: Family Development Resources.

Bavolek, S. J. (1980a). *Primary prevention of child abuse: Assessing the parenting and child rearing attitudes of adolescents in inner city Baltimore.* Technical report, University of Wisconsin—Eau Claire.

Bavolek, S. J. (1980b). *Primary prevention of child abuse: Identification of high risk parents.* Educational Resources Information Center (ERIC).

Gordon, R. H., & Gordon, P. E. (undated). *The Adult–Adolescent Parenting Inventory and the MMPI "AT RISK" Scale: A clinical validity study.* Unpublished manuscript. (Available from Applied Mental Health Consultants, 1341 N. Wright Rd., Janesville, WI 53545)

Price, J. (1985, August). *Aspects of the family and children's television viewing content preferences.* Paper presented at the annual meeting of the American Psychological Foundation, Toronto.

AUTHOR'S RESPONSE

No additional comments.

PC-2
Child Abuse Potential (CAP) Inventory

GENERAL INFORMATION

Date of publication: 1986.

Author: Joel S. Milner.

Source/publisher: Psytec, Inc., P.O. Box 564, DeKalb, IL 60115.

Availability: Available from the publisher (above).

Brief description: The CAP Inventory includes 160 items answered in a simple agree/disagree format. The scales that tap physical abuse are Distress, Rigidity, Unhappiness, Problems with Child and Self, Problems with Family, and Problems from Others.

Purpose: The CAP Inventory was designed as a screening tool for the detection of physical child abuse.

Theoretical base: Empirically constructed to detect abuse; grounded in psychiatric and interpersonal theories concerning family stress and mental health.

PHYSICAL DESCRIPTION OF QUESTIONNAIRE

Physical features: The CAP Inventory includes 160 items, each of which is responded to as "agree" or "disagree." The Inventory is self-administered. It has a third-grade readability level and requires from 12 to 20 minutes to complete.

Unit of study: Individual parent, parent–child dyad.

Respondent: Parent.

Scales and dimensions: The CAP Inventory includes a 77-item scale that taps six abuse factors: Distress, Rigidity, Unhappiness, Problems with Child and Self, Problems with Family, and Problems from Others. It also includes three validity scales—a lie scale, a random-response scale, and an inconsistency scale—

that form faking good, faking bad, and random-response indices. Filler and experimental items are included to bring the total to 160 items.

Manual: A comprehensive, well-written manual is available from the publisher. It contains detailed information on administration, scoring, interpretation, test construction, reliability, validity, and research issues.

Standardization and norms: Clinical cutoff scores were derived from a sample of 110 physical child abusers and a control group of 836 parents. The manual also presenting mean abuse scores from more than than 5,000 individuals in more than 60 studies representing maltreating parents, the general population, and nurturing groups.

Evaluation of physical description of questionnaire: *Strengths:* The CAP Inventory has a clear (agree/disagree) response format, a simple reading level, and a comprehensive manual with normative data from multiple samples. *Limitations:* The agree/disagree response format may force the subject into constrained choices.

ADMINISTRATIVE PROCEDURES

Directions: The CAP Inventory is easily self-administered.

Ease of use: The CAP Inventory is easy to administer and complete.

Training for administration and scoring: Administration is quite straightforward. Scoring is quite complex and requires the use of multiple templates (with complex item weights) or a computer scoring program, both available from the publisher. The manual notes the ease with which errors in scoring and calculation can be made with the template scoring method.

Scoring procedures: The instrument may be scored by template or with computer software. Although scoring is mechanical (although hand-scoring is vulnerable to errors in computation), interpretation of the profile requires considerable judgment because of the issues involved with labeling suspected abuse.

Evaluation of administrative procedures: *Strengths:* The CAP Inventory is easy to administer. Computer scoring is available for investigators with personal computers. *Limitations:* Hand-scoring is vulnerable to errors in computation; interpretation requires care and skill.

EVALUATION OF CONSTRUCTS MEASURED

Reliability: Internal consistency reliabilities for the abuse scales range in the .90's. Subscale reliabilities are generally lower but still acceptable. Test–retest reliabilities range from the low .90's across a 1-day to 1-week interval to .83 and .75 for 1- and 3-months intervals, respectively. Detailed reliability data from multiple studies are presented in the manual.

Validity: The manual provides detailed information about content, construct, and criterion-related validity from multiple studies. Extensive data using CAP Inventory scores to discriminate abusing from nonabusing parents are reported. In addition, data reporting changes in CAP Inventory abuse scores as a function of an intervention program are reported.

Clinical utility: The CAP Inventory has demonstrated considerable utility as a screening device for identifying physically abusive or potentially abusive parents. Its ease of administration makes it very accessible for clinic use.

Research utility: The CAP Inventory has considerable research utility. Although most of the studies cited in the manual have addressed issues of discriminant validity, the research potential of the measure is significant but as yet untapped. A bibliography of more than 90 research publications is available from the author.

SUMMER EVALUATION

The Child Abuse Potential Inventory is a significant addition to the group of measures used to assess parenting behavior. The measure has been carefully validated, and the manual contains excellent documentation of the measure's development and use. The CAP Inventory is easy to administer and complete and requires a minimal reading level. The scoring of the measure is straightforward, but hand-scoring is vulnerable to errors. Clinical interpretation of individual profiles concerning abuse requires considerable care.

REFERENCES

Milner, J. S. (1986). *The Child Abuse Potential Inventory Manual* (2nd ed.). Webster, NC: Psytech.
Milner, J. S. (in press). An ego-strength scale for the Child Abuse Potential Inventory. *Journal of Family Violence.*
Milner, J. S., Gold, R. G., Ayoub, C., & Jacewitz, M. M. (1984). Predictive validity of the Child Abuse Potential Inventory. *Journal of Consulting and Clinical Psychology, 52,* 879–884.
Milner, J. S., Gold, R. G., & Wimberley, R. C. (1986). Prediction and explanation of child abuse: Cross-validation of the Child Abuse Potential Inventory. *Journal of Consulting and Clinical Psychology, 54,* 865–866.
In addition, a bibliography of more than 90 related publications is available from the author.

AUTHOR'S RESPONSE

In addition to the existing CAP Inventory technical manual (Milner, 1986), an applied user's manual and a related self-instructional text are under development (estimated publication date, early 1989). The applied manual is intended to supplement, not replace, the existing manual. It is designed for professionals, such as protective services workers, who have only limited training in the use of psychological tests but are required to evaluate caretakers reported for child maltreatment. The self-instructional text is designed to provide an overview of basic psychometric principles. Beyond general test reliability and validity, users of any psychological test must be aware of a variety of related psychometric issues, such as the probabilistic nature of test scores, the attenuation in prediction due to changes in sample base rates and differences between test samples and normative population characteristics, and other limitations of self-report questionnaire data. A new ego-strength scale has recently been developed (Milner, in press).

PC-3
Child Behavior Toward Parent Inventory
(CBTPI)

GENERAL INFORMATION

Date of publication: 1975 (revised); short form, 1977.

Authors: E. S. Schaefer and N. W. Finkelstein.

Source/publisher: E. S. Schaefer, Department of Maternal and Child Health, School of Public Health, University of North Carolina, Chapel Hill, NC 27514.

Availability: Available from the author (see "Source/publisher," above).

Brief description: The CBTPI is a 155-item parent self-report questionnaire that assesses 6- to 16-year-old children's behaviors toward the parent on the dimensions of control, acceptance/rejection, and independence/dependence.

Purpose: The CBTPI is designed to assess the child's behavior toward the parent from the perspective of the parent and to complement the Child's Report of Parental Behavior Inventory (CRPBI) (Schaefer, 1965), so that reciprocity in parent–child interaction can be measured.

Theoretical base: Phenomenology, cognitive-developmental psychology. It is assumed that parental perceptions of their child's behavior exert a stronger influence on parents' actions than the child's actual behavior does.

PHYSICAL DESCRIPTION OF QUESTIONNAIRE

Physical features: The CTBPI is a parent self-report questionnaire that consists of 31 five-item subscales (155 items). Parents describe their children's behavior toward them by circling one of four possible responses: "very much like," "somewhat like," "a little like," or "not at all alike." Schaefer and Edgerton (1977) report a version of the CTBPI that consists of five five-item scales.

Unit of study: Parent (mother's or father's perception of the child's behavior).

Respondent: Individual parent.

Scales and dimensions: Through factor analyses (Schaefer and Finkelstein, 1975), five major dimensions were identified from the 31 subscales. The dimensions and number of associated subscales (in parentheses) were Control (12), Acceptance versus Rejection (10), Independence versus Dependence (4), Considerateness (5), and Helpfulness (4). The three factors of Control, Acceptance versus Rejection, and Independence versus Dependence were replicated and considered stable (Schaefer & Finkelstein, 1975). The short form assesses five dimensions: Positive Relationship, Control, Independence, Obedience, and Detachment.

Manual: None available.

Standardization and norms: None available.

Evaluation of physical description of questionnaire: *Strengths:* Items are easy to read and understand. *Limitations:* The 155-item questionnaire is lengthy, which may affect parents' responses. The 25-item short form provides much of the information of the longer form.

ADMINISTRATIVE PROCEDURES

Directions: Parents are asked to read the items describing different behaviors that children do and indicate the extent to which the behavior is similar to what their child does with them. Completion time is about 30 to 40 minutes.

Ease of use: The CBTPI instructions are very clear and simple. Parents should have no trouble responding to questionnaire items.

Training for administration and scoring: No guidelines are provided other than the instructions on the test form.

Scoring procedures: None available. Scoring appears to be done manually, with scores derived by summing responses to individual items for each subscale. Items associated with each dimension and subscale are identified by a scoring form available from the author.

Evaluation of administrative procedures: *Strengths:* The CBTPI instructions are clear, and completion should present no problems for parents. *Limitations:* The 155-item version of the CBTPI is long, especially if parental perceptions of more than one child are being assessed. Manual scoring is time-intensive.

EVALUATION OF CONSTRUCTS MEASURED

Reliability: Reliability data were obtained from the sample of 34 parents used in the factor analysis of the 31 scales. Internal consistency (KR-20) coefficients for the 31 scales ranged from .69 to .95 (mean = .87; Schaefer & Finkelstein, 1975). Internal consistency (alpha) coefficients from a sample of 332 mothers for the short form ranged from .60 to .81 (Schaefer & Edgerton, 1977).

Validity: *Construct.* The factor analysis of the long form shows that the 31 scales load separately on the three major dimensions of child behavior (control, acceptance/rejection, and independence/dependence). The authors have reported significant correlations between CBTPI scales and other parent and teacher ratings of children's behavior, but indicate that further validity studies are needed (Schaefer, Sayers, & St. Clair, 1987).

Clinical utility: None demonstrated.

Research utility: None demonstrated. The possible role of the CBTPI in the investigation of the influence of parental perceptions of their child's behavior on their interactions with their child and on their child's later adjustment remains to be shown.

SUMMARY EVALUATION

The CBTPI focuses on the influence of parental perceptions of children's behavior on the children's social and personality development. In conjunction with the CRPBI—a measure of children's perceptions of the parents' behavior (Schaefer, 1965)—researchers may investigate how children's and parents' perceptions of each other's behavior influence the course and outcomes of their interactions. However, the factors identified on the long form may be unstable because of the low subject–scale ratio. Further reliability and validity studies are needed for both the short and long forms.

REFERENCES

Schaefer, E. S. (1965). Children's reports of parental behavior: An inventory. *Child Development, 36,* 413–424.

Schaefer, E. S., & Edgerton, M. (1977). *Parent Report of Child Behavior to the Parent: Short form.* (Available from Department of Maternal and Child Health, School of Public Health, University of North Carolina, Chapel Hill, NC 27514)

Schaefer, E. S., & Finkelstein, N. W. (1975, August). *Child Behavior Toward Parent: An inventory and factor analysis.* Paper presented at the annual meeting of the American Psychological Association, Chicago.

Schaefer, E. S., Sayers, S. L., & St. Clair, K. L. (1987, August). *Mother-child relationship correlations of mothers' reports of child behavior.* Paper presented at the 95th Annual Meeting of the American Psychological Association, Baltimore.

PC-4
Child-Rearing Practices Report (CRPR)

GENERAL INFORMATION

Date of Publication: 1965.

Author: Jeanne H. Block.

Source/publisher: Department of Psychology, University of California at Berkeley.

Availability: Available from NAPS-2 or Jack Block, Department of Psychology, Tolman Hall, University of California, Berkely, CA 94720.

Brief description: The CRPR is a 91-item Q-sort that contains socialization-relevant behaviorally anchored statements. The statements are appropriate for the description of maternal and paternal child-rearing orientations and values.

Purpose: The purpose of the CRPR is to assess child-rearing attitudes, values, and goals through a method that minimizes the occurrence of possible response sets.

Theoretical base: The CRPR was derived from an eclectic theoretical base employing recognitions from the developmental and clinical literature.

PHYSICAL DESCRIPTION OF QUESTIONNAIRE

Physical features: The CRPR is a self-report attitudinal measure. The measure consists of a deck of 91 cards containing child-rearing statements and seven corresponding sorting envelopes. Both a first-person form and a third-person form of the Q-sort are available. The third-person form is completed by adolescents or young adults to describe the child-rearing orientations of their parents. The respondent arranges the 91 statements on a 7-point scale ranging from "most descriptive" to "least descriptive," using a forced-choice Q-sort format with 13 items at each scale point. The seven envelopes correspond to the seven categories and are ordered on a 7-point scale ranging from "most descriptive statements" (7) to "least descriptive statements" (1). Following the respondent's formulation of the 7-point rectangular distribution of statements, the card stacks are put into their corresponding envelopes.

Unit of study: The parent.

Respondent: The parent (first-person form) or the child (third-person form).

Scales and dimensions: Using factor-analytic methods, 28 + scales have been developed out the 91-item CRPR pool. The number of CRPR items varies within each scale. The scales include Encouraging Openness to Experience, Emphasis on Achievement, Authoritarian Control, and Affective Quality of Parent–Child Interaction. (For a complete listing of the scales, see Roberts, Block, & Block, 1984.) The scales are an alternative form of analyzing the CRPR responses and are not always employed as an analytic technique.

Manual: A manual is available from the author. It includes information regarding the development of the Q-sort, scoring procedures, and psychometric data.

Standardization and Norms: The CRPR has been administered to more than 6,000 persons from diverse age groups, socioeconomic levels, educational levels, and national origins. The Q-sort has been translated into several languages and is suitable for cross-cultural studies.

Evaluation of physical description of questionnaire: *Strengths:* A primary strength of this measure is the Q-sort format, which minimizes the possibility of response sets and the respondent's differential perceptions of category definitions. The individual Q-sort cards provide the respondent with the advantage of moving a response before making a final response commitment to any one category. The Q-sort statements are comprehensive and clear. *Limitations:* The measure is rather time-consuming to complete. A sixth-grade reading level is required for completion of the measure.

ADMINISTRATIVE PROCEDURES

Directions: The directions are very clearly and precisely indicated in the CRPR manual. Mothers and fathers complete the Q-sort *independently.*

Ease of use: The CRPR Q-sort is straightforward, although a number of sorting steps are required for completion, and the actual sorting process can be time-consuming.

Training for administration and scoring: No special training is required for administration or sorting of the CRPR. The CRPR can be administered individually or in groups.

Scoring procedures: Four methods have been designed for scoring the CRPR. Depending on the nature of the questions being asked, different approaches can be taken to analyze the data received from the CRPR: (1) item analysis—comparisons of the means of each of the 91 items for different samples; (2) criterion Q-sort—overall summarizing comparison of Q-sorts to criterion definitions of various CRPR concepts (the correlations are used as the scores themselves); (3) factor analysis—the discernment of types or clusters of people and the correlation between group membership and independent sources of information; (4) scale construction—summing of scores on a number of CRPR items so as to generate a scale score.

Evaluation of administration procedures: *Strengths:* The CRPR is a clear and easily administered measure that can be administered to large groups of people at one time. A variety of scoring procedures is available. *Limitations:* It is not always clear which scoring method is the most appropriate.

EVALUATION OF CONSTRUCTS MEASURED

Reliability: Reliability was assessed in two test–retest studies, one conducted at a 1-year interval and the other at a 3-year interval. The cross-time correlations in both studies were very high: 1-year interval—$r = .71$ (third-person form), $N = 90$; 3-year interval—$r = .64$ (mothers), $r = .65$ (fathers) (third-person form), $N = 66$ (Block, 1965).

Validity: Criterion validity was measured in a study in which mothers were observed interacting with their children and then were given the CRPR 4 years later. The congruence between the interaction scores and the CRPR scores was evaluated, and an "appreciable coherence" was found between the observational and self-descriptive data sets. Predictive validity was measured in a study that found adults' agreement on the CRPR to predict subsequent continuation or termination of their marriage (Block, Block, & Morrison, 1981) and adolescents' under-control and antisocial behavior (Block & Gjerde, 1986).

Clinical utility: The CRPR can be used effectively by clinicians to assess and compare individual family members' perceptions of child rearing. Clinicians can tap into an existing parental child-rearing orientation system and determine salient parental child-rearing attitudes as a means for encouraging appropriate child-rearing orientations or for modifying inappropriate child-rearing attitudes.

Research utility: As a research tool, the CRPR has been used to assess the relationship between self-reported parental attitudes and observed parental behavior and the continuity and change in parents' child-rearing orientations.

SUMMARY EVALUATION

The CRPR is a strong, comprehensive measure of parental child-rearing orientations. It is a widely used assessment tool and is appropriate for cross-cultural studies. Though somewhat lengthy, the Q-sort format of the measure is one of its primary strengths. It is important to note, however, that the CRPR is measuring child-rearing *attitudes* rather than actual child-rearing *behaviors*.

REFERENCES

Block, J. H. (1965). *The Child-Rearing Practices Report (CRPR): A set of Q items for the description of general socialization attitudes and values.* Unpublished manuscript, University of California at Berkeley, Institute of Human Development.

Block, J. H., Block, J., & Morrison, A. (1981). Parental agreement–disagreement on childrearing orientations and gender-related personality correlates in children. *Child Development, 52,* 965–974.

Block, J. H., & Gjerde, P. F. (1986). Distinguishing between antisocial behavior and undercontrol. In D. Olweus, J. Block, & M. Radke-Yarrow (Eds.), *Development of antisocial and prosocial behavior: Research theories and issues* (pp. 177–206). New York: Academic Press.

Roberts, G. C., Block, J. H., & Block, J. (1984). Continuity and change in parents' child-rearing practices. *Child Development, 55,* 586–597.

AUTHOR'S RESPONSE

The preceding description of the CRPR is quite correct, although abbreviated. It should be noted that a far more extensive bibliography on the CRPR than is cited is available on request from Jack Block. Regarding the time-consuming nature of the CRPR, noted as a limitation, I suggest that the method requires subjects to be more thoughtful than is usually the case in formulating their responses. The CRPR items, because of the Q-sort methodology employed, compete with each other for the subject's endorsement. In that competition among items, and the subject's subsequent ordering of the items, discriminations are made that are not captured by other methods permitting unrestrained endorsement of items treated separately. For perspective on how to score or analyze CRPR data, the researcher should consult published CRPR articles and/ or the monograph by Jack Block: *The Q-sort Method in Personality Assessment and Psychiatric Research.*

PC-5
Child's Attitude Toward Mother (CAM)/
Child's Attitude Toward Father (CAF)

GENERAL INFORMATION

Date of publication: 1982.

Author: Walter W. Hudson.

Source/publisher: Hudson, W. W. (1982). *The Clinical Measurement Package,* Homewood, IL: Dorsey Press.

Availability: Available from Dorsey Press, 1818 Ridge Road, Homewood, Illinois 60430.

Brief description: The CAM and CAF are 25-item scales designed for use in assessing the severity or magnitude of a child's problem with his or her mother or father. The scales are two of nine scales included in the Clinical Measurement Package, which provides an assessment of the severity of a variety of personal and social problems.

Purpose: The purpose of the CAM and CAF scales is to provide clinicians and researchers with reliable and valid single-subject, repeated measures of the severity of parent–child relationship problems.

Theoretical base: Atheoretical clinical measurement focus; not compatible with behavioral viewpoint.

PHYSICAL DESCRIPTION OF QUESTIONNAIRE

Physical features: The CAM and CAF scales include 25 items, each of which is responded to on a 5-point Likert (scale ranging from 1 = ''rarely or none of the time'' to 5 = ''most or all of the time.'' Items are both positively and negatively worded to reduce response bias. Items on the CAM and CAF scales are identical except for the substitution of the word *mother* or *father* on the appropriate scale. The reading level of the scales permits their use with children and adults aged 12 and above. The CAM and CAF are available in Chinese, French, German, and Spanish.

Unit of study: Mother–child or father–child dyad.

Respondent: Child.

Scales and dimensions: The CAM and CAF are unidimensional, with one problem severity score derived.

Manual: A comprehensive manual has been published (see ''source/publisher,''above), including information on purpose, use, administration, and scoring and reliability and validity data.

Standardization and norms: Normative data are available, based on a representative sample of 2,419 junior and senior high school students ranging in age from 11 to 19 (Saunders & Schuchts, 1987).

Evaluation of physical description of questionnaire: *Strengths:* The CAM and CAF are clearly written, easily and quickly administered, supported by a comprehensive manual, and available in several languages. *Limitations:* Lack of normative or descriptive data in the manual.

ADMINISTRATIVE PROCEDURES

Directions: Directions for completion are clearly stated on the scale.

Ease of use: The CAM and CAF are very straightforward and simple to use.

Training for administration and scoring: Straightforward directions for administration and scoring are provided in the manual. No special training for administration is required. Given the clinical nature of the scales, some clinical experience is appropriate for interpretation.

Scoring procedures: Scales are first reverse-scored for the positively worded items, then summed across items minus 25, which produces a score range from 0 to 100. A score of 30 has been determined to be the clinical cutoff indicative of severe problems.

Evaluation of administrative procedures: *Strengths:* The CAM and CAF are easily administered, completed, scored, and interpreted. *Limitations:* None noted.

EVALUATION OF CONSTRUCTS MEASURED

Reliability: Internal consistency of the CAM and CAF has been determined in three studies. Cronbach's alpha coefficients are as follows:

	$N = 664$	$N = 408$	$N = 2,419$
CAM	.94	.93	.95
CAF	.95	.95	.97

Test–retest reliability has not been determined. It is deemed by the author to be inappropriate for a measure intended to be sensitive to change in a relationship.

Validity: The CAM and CAF scales were found to significantly discriminate clinician-identified problem and nonproblem groups (Hudson, 1982) and to converge with a second self-report of parent–child problems (Hudson, 1982; Saunders and Schuchts, 1987).

Clinical utility: The CAM and CAF scales have demonstrated utility as a reliable measure of problem severity in the parent–adolescent relationship. The ease of use and brevity of the scales also permit their use as a repeated measure in single-subject research designs that are optimal for clinical settings.

Research utility: The research utility of the CAM and CAF is unknown, although the excellent reliability of the scales suggests potential usefulness.

SUMMARY EVALUATION

The CAM and CAF scales are short, easily used measures of the severity of problems in the parent–child relationship as viewed by the child. The scales are two of nine scales included in a broader assessment package, the Clinical Measurement Package. Internal consistency of the unidimensional CAM and CAF scales is excellent. Validity data are limited, but promising, at this time. Normative data are available. The major shortcoming of the CAM and CAF is their susceptibility to social desirability, which has neither been explored in research nor controlled in test construction.

REFERENCES

Hudson, W. W. (1982). *The Clinical Measurement Package*. Homewood, IL: Dorsey Press.
Saunders, B. E., & Schuchts, R. A. (1987). Assessing parent–child relationships: A report of normative scores and revalidation of two clinical scales. *Family Process, 26,* 373–381.

AUTHOR'S RESPONSE

No additional comments.

PC-6
Child's Report of Parental Behavior
Inventory (CRPBI)

GENERAL INFORMATION

Date of publication: 1971.

Authors: E. S. Schaefer (1965, original author); revision by G. K. Burger and J. A. Armentrout.

Source/publisher: G. K. Burger, Department of Psychology, University of Missouri, 8001 Natural Bridge, St. Louis, MO 63121.

Availability: Available from the author (see above).

Brief description: This version of the CRPBI is a 56-item, six-scale questionnaire assessing children's and adolescents' self-reports of parents' child-rearing behaviors and attitudes.

Purpose: The CRPBI is designed to investigate the influence that children's and adolescents' perceptions of their parents' child-rearing behaviors have on their social/personality development.

Theoretical base: Phenomenology, cognitive-developmental psychology. It is assumed that children's perceptions of their parents' behavior toward them are important influences on their personality development.

PHYSICAL DESCRIPTION OF QUESTIONNAIRE

Physical features: The CRPBI has been revised a number of times since its original 260-item version was reviewed (Schaefer, 1965). This revision consists of 56 items to which children respond whether their parent is "like," "somewhat like," or "not like" each of the statements listed. There are separate forms for the mother and father (Margolies & Weintraub, 1977).

Unit of study: Child, adolescent.

Respondent: Individual child, adolescent.

Scales and dimensions: There are six scales, one with 16 items and five with 8 items: Acceptance, Control through Guilt, Childcenteredness, Instilling Persistent Anxiety, Nonenforcement, and Lax Discipline. Through factor analyses, these six scales formed three factors; Acceptance versus Rejection, Psychological Autonomy versus Psychological Control, and Firm Control versus Lax control (Burger & Armentrout, 1971; Margolies & Weintraub, 1977).

Manual: None available.

Standardization and norms: None available.

Evaluation of physical description of questionnaire: *Strengths:* The shortness of the CRBPI is a considerable advantage over the original instrument. Items are written in behaviorally specific terms. *Limitations:* The reading level may be too high for some children, especially at lower grade levels.

ADMINISTRATIVE PROCEDURES

Directions: Children are asked to rate the extent to which each of their parents is like each of the statements on the questionnaire (Margolies & Weintraub, 1977). The instrument may be administered individually or to small groups of children.

Ease of use: The CRPBI instructions appear to be straightfoward.

Training for administration and scoring: No training is required.

Scoring procedures: Scoring appears to be done manually. Scores are derived by summing responses to individual items that comprise each of the three dimensions: "not like" = 1, "somewhat like" = 2, and "like" = 3 (Litovsky & Dusek, 1985).

Evaluation of administrative procedures: *Strengths:* The Instructions for completing the CRPBI seem to be simple, the 56 items are well within testing limits for even younger children. The 3-point response scale may be easier for younger children to comprehend. *Limitations:* The wording of some statements may be too difficult for some children at lower grade levels. Items that comprise each dimension are not provided. Manual scoring is time-intensive.

EVALUATION OF CONSTRUCTS MEASURED

Reliability: Internal consistency data are not reported for this version of the CRPBI. Test–retest reliability coefficients of the factors for the mother and father forms range from .66 to .93 over 1-week and 5-week test–retest intervals. One-week test–retest reliability coefficients for grades 4, 5, and 6 range from .62 to .96. (Margolies & Weintraub, 1977).

Validity: *Construct:* Factorial studies of different versions of the CRPBI have yielded the same three factors over samples varying in age and cultural background (e.g., Armentrout & Burger, 1972; Burger & Armentrout, 1971; Margolies & Weintraub, 1977; Schludermann & Schludermann, 1983). *Criterion:* Litovsky and Dusek (1985) report that parents of high-self-esteem adolescents are reported as more accepting, using less psychological control, and not as firm in making and enforcing rules than the parents of low-self-esteem adolescents.

Clinical utility: The CRPBI is specifically designed as a research instrument.

Research utility: The research utility of the CRPBI appears promising, given the consistent factorial validation of three child-rearing factors across different ages and cultural samples and limited, although acceptable, test–retest reliability data.

SUMMARY EVALUATION

The CRPBI is a 56-item self-report questionnaire that assesses children's and adolescents' perceptions of their parents' child-rearing behavior. Instructions are simple and test length is appropriate. The reading level of some items may be too high for children in lower grades. The three factors have factorial validity across different ages and cultural groups and limited, but acceptable, reliability data.

REFERENCES

Armentrout, J. A., & Burger, G. K. (1972). Factor analyses of college students' recall of parental childrearing behaviors. *Journal of Genetic Pscyhology, 121,* 155–161.

Burger, G. K., & Armentrout, J. A. (1971). A factor analysis of fifth and sixth graders' reports of parental child-rearing behavior. *Developmental Psychology, 4,* 483.

Litovsky, V. G., & Dusek, J. B. (1985). Perceptions of child rearing and self-concept development during the early adolescent years. *Journal of Youth and Adolescence, 14,* 373–387.

Margolies, P. J., & Weintraub, S. (1977). The revised 56-item CRPBI as a research instrument: Reliability and factor structure. *Journal of Clinical Psychology, 33,* 472–476.

Schaefer, E. S. (1965). Children's reports of parental behavior: An inventory. *Child Development, 36,* 413–424.

Schludermann, S., & Schludermann, E. (1983). Sociocultural change and adolescents' perceptions of parent behavior. *Developmental Psychology, 19,* 674–685.

AUTHOR'S RESPONSE

No additional comments.

PC-7
Child's Report of Parental Behavior
Inventory (CRPBI)—Revised

GENERAL INFORMATION

Date of publication: 1970, 1983.

Authors: E. S. Schaefer (1965, original author); revision by S. Schludermann and E. Schludermann.

Source/publisher: S. and E. Schludermann, Department of Psychology, University of Manitoba, Winnipeg, Manitoba, Canada R3T 2N2.

Availability: Available from authors (see above).

Brief description: This version of the CRPBI is a 108-item, 18-scale questionnaire assessing children's and adolescents' self-reports of parents' child-rearing behaviors and attitudes across different cultures.

Purpose: The CRPBI is designed to investigate the influence that children's and adolescents' perceptions of their parents' child-rearing behaviors have on their social/personality development.

Theoretical base: Phenomenology, cognitive-developmental psychology. It is assumed that children's perceptions of their parents' behavior toward them are important influences on their personality development.

PHYSICAL DESCRIPTION OF QUESTIONNAIRE

Physical features: This revision of Schaefer's 1965 measure consists of 108 items to which children respond whether their parent is "like," "somewhat like," or "not like" each of the statements listed. Separate mother and father forms are available.

Unit of study: Child, adolescent.

Respondent: Individual child, adolescent.

Scales and dimensions: There are 18 scales, with five to eight items per scale: Acceptance, Control through Guilt, Childcenteredness, Instilling Persistent Anxiety, Nonenforcement, Lax Discipline, Possessiveness, Rejection, Control, Enforcement, Positive Involvement, Intrusiveness, Hostile Control, Inconsistent Discipline, Acceptance of Individuation, Hostile Detachment, Withdrawal of Relations, Extreme Autonomy. Through factor analyses, these 18 scales formed three factors; Acceptance versus Rejection, Psychological Autonomy versus Psychological Control, and Firm Control versus Lax Control (Schludermann & Schludermann, 1970, 1983).

Manual: None available.

Standardization and norms: Means, standard deviations, and percentile tables are based on Canadian high school ($n = 364$) and university ($n = 1,192$) samples and are provided by sex for each factor.

Evaluation of physical description of questionnaire: *Strengths:* The shortened version has a considerable advantage over the original CRPBI. Percentile norms are available from the authors. Items are written in behaviorally specific terms. *Limitations:* The reading level may be too high for some children, especially at lower grade levels.

ADMINISTRATIVE PROCEDURES

Directions: Children are asked to rate the extent to which each of their parents is like each of the statements on the questionnaire (Schludermann & Schludermann, 1970, 1983). The instrument may be administered individually or in small groups.

Ease of use: The CRPBI instructions appear to be straightforward.

Training for administration and scoring: No training is required.

Scoring procedures: Scoring is done manually. The authors recommend machine-scoring. Scores are derived by summing responses to individual items that comprise each of the scales. Scores for the scales comprising each factor are summed and divided by the respective number of scales.

Evaluation of administrative procedures: *Strengths:* Instructions for completing the CRPBI seem to be simple. The 3-point response scale may be easier for younger children to comprehend. *Limitations:* The wording of some statements may be too difficult. The 108 items may approach testing limits for younger children. Manual scoring is time-intensive.

EVALUATION OF CONSTRUCTS MEASURED

Reliability: No reliability data are reported. Item reliabilities for items in the original measure (Schaefer, 1965) were used in scale construction.

Validity: *Construct:* Factorial studies of different versions of the CRPBI have yielded the same three factors over samples varying in age and cultural backgrounds (e.g., Armentrout & Burger, 1972; Burger & Armentrout, 1971; Margolies & Weintraub, 1977; Schludermann & Schludermann, 1983). *Criterion:* Traditional adolescents reported more firm and psychological control by parents than modern adolescents did. Younger adolescents reported more firm and psychological control than older adolescents did (Schludermann & Schludermann, 1983).

Clinical utility: The CRPBI is designed as a research instrument.

Research utility: The research utility of the CRPBI appears promising, given the consistent factorial validation of three child-rearing factors across different ages and cultural samples. The lack of reliability data is a serious shortcoming.

SUMMARY EVALUATION

This CRPBI version is a 108-item cross-cultural self-report questionnaire designed to assess children's and adolescents' perceptions of their parents' child-rearing behaviors. Instructions are simple, but the reading level of some items may be too high for younger children. It is one of the few research-oriented instruments with normative data (based on Canadian samples). The three factors have been replicated across different ages and cultural groups, but the lack of reliability data is a major problem.

REFERENCES

Armentrout, J. A., & Burger, G. K. (1972). Factor analyses of college students' recall of parental childrearing behaviors. *Journal of General Psychology, 121,* 155–161.

Burger, G. K., & Armentrout, J. A. (1971). A factor analysis of fifth and sixth graders' reports of parental child-rearing behavior. *Developmental Psychology, 4,* 483.

Margolies, P. J., & Weintraub, S. (1977). The revised 56-item CRPBI as a research instrument: Reliability and factor structure. *Journal of Clinical Psychology, 33,* 472–476.

Schaefer, E. S. (1965). Children's reports of parental behavior: An inventory. *Child Development, 36,* 413–424.

Schludermann, S., & Schludermann, E. (1970). Replicability of factors in Children's Report of Parent Behavior (CRBPI). *Journal of Psychology, 39,* 39–52.

Schludermann, S., & Schludermann, E. (1983). Sociocultural change and adolescents' perceptions of parent behavior. *Development of Psychology, 19,* 674–685.

PC-8
Cornell Parent Behavior Inventory
(CPBI)

GENERAL INFORMATION

Date of publication: 1969 (revised); Bronfenbrenner Parent Behavior Questionnaire.

Authors: E. C. Devereux, Jr., U. Bronfenbrenner, and R. R. Rodgers.

Source/publisher: U. Bronfenbrenner, Department of Human Development and Family Relations, Cornell University, Ithaca, NY 14850.

Availability: Available from the author (see above).

Brief description: The revised CPBI is a 30-item children's self-report questionnaire that assesses children's perceptions of their parents on 14 aspects of child-rearing attitudes and behavior.

Purpose: The CPBI is designed to measure children's perceptions of parental behavior toward them.

Theoretical base: Phenomenology, cognitive-developmental psychology. It is assumed that children's perceptions of their parents' attitudes and behavior influence their personality development.

PHYSICAL DESCRIPTION OF QUESTIONNAIRE

Physical features: The CPBI is a self-report questionnaire that consists of 30 items distributed over 14 scales. It has been used with children 8 years of age, with adolescents, and with adults. Respondents indicate how frequently their parents do each of the behaviors described on the questionnaire with three different five-item response scales: (1) "never," "only once in a while," '"sometimes," "usually," "almost always"; (2) "never," "only once in a while,," "sometimes," "often," "very often"; and (3) "never," "only once or twice a year," "about once a month," "about once a week," "almost every day.'' A short form that has been used in other research consists of a single item for each dimension (see Devereaux et al., 1974).

Unit of study: Child.

Respondent: Individual child.

Scales and dimensions: There are 14 scales: Nurturance, Principled Discipline, Instrumental Companionship, Consistency of Expectation, Encouragement of Autonomy, Indulgence, Prescription of Responsibilities, Achievement Demands, Control, Protectiveness, Affective Punishment, Deprivation of Privileges, Scolding, and Physical Punishment. Through factor analyses (Aguilino, 1986), the scales were associated with three major factors: support, discipline, and covert control.

Manual: None available.

Standardization and norms: None available.

Evaluation of physical description of questionnaire: *Strengths:* The CPBI items are written clearly in behaviorally specific terms. *Limitations:* The reading level may be too high for children at younger ages. The response format could be confusing to respondents.

ADMINISTRATIVE PROCEDURES

Directions: Children are asked to rate the extent to which each of the behaviors described on the questionnaire is true of how their parents act toward them (Buriel, 1981). The instrument may be administered to small groups of children.

Ease of use: The CPBI instructions are simple, but caution is needed because the response scale changes and may be confusing to some children.

Training for administration and scoring: No guidelines are provided other than the instructions on the test form.

Scoring procedures: Scoring appears to be done manually. Scores are derived by summing responses to individual items for each subscale. The scoring ranges from 1 ("almost always," "very often," "almost every day") to 5 ("never"), so that a high final score indicates affirmation of a given parental behavior and a low score indicates denial of a behavior (Devereux, Bronfenbrenner, & Rodgers, 1969). Items associated with each of the 14 scales are identified.

Evaluation of administrative procedures: *Strengths:* The CPBI instructions are simple, and 30 items are well within testing limits for children of this age. *Limitations:* Guidelines for interpretation and scoring are not provided. Manual scoring could become time-intensive, depending on the number of children examined.

EVALUATION OF CONSTRUCTS MEASURED

Reliability: Internal consistency for the three factors—support, discipline, and covert control—for mother and father forms of the CPBI ranged from .70 to .82 (Aguilino, 1986). Internal consistency data for the original scale are reported in Siegelman (1965). Test–retest reliability data were not reported.

Validity: *Construct:* The three factors identified by Aguilino (1986)—support, discipline, and covert control—consist of scales that are consistent with factors identified for the original version (Siegelman, 1965). Responses of English and American children to the CPBI were consistent with observational measures of parent–child interactions in both cultures (Barker & Barker, 1963, reported in Devereux et al., 1969). *Criterion:* Aguilino (1986) reports that children's perceptions of the parent–child relationship are strongly influenced by the quality of marital adjustment. Maternal demandingness and support related positively to internal locus of control for Anglo- and Mexican-American children. Internal control varied by ethnic group for paternal control and demandingness (Buriel, 1981).

Clinical utility: None demonstrated.

Research utility: With the exception of subscale reliability data, the research utility of the CPBI would appear to be promising. The rearing factors identified through factor analysis agree with those found in the original version and are consistent with other measures of the same constructs.

SUMMARY EVALUATION

The CPBI is a 30-item self-report questionnaire that has been used to assess children's, adolescents, and young adults' perceptions of their parents' child-rearing behavior toward them. Instructions are simple, and testing time is appropriate even for the younger age groups. The reading level of some items may be too high for younger children, and the changes in response formats are potentially confusing. The support, discipline, and covert control factors are consistent with children's perceptions of both parents and agree with the factors identified on the original version of the instrument. Reliability data are not reported for the individual scales, however, which limits the usefulness of this version of Bronfenbrenner's questionnaire.

REFERENCES

Aguilino, W. S., (1986). Children's perceptions of marital interaction. *Child Study Journal, 16,* 159–172.

Buriel, R. (1981. The relation of Anglo- and Mexican-American children's locus of control beliefs to parents' and teachers' socialization practices. *Child Development, 52,* 104–113.

Devereux, E. C., Bronfenbrenner, W., & Rodgers, R. R. (1969). Child-rearing in England and the United States: A cross-cultural comparison. *Journal of Marriage and the Family, 31,* 257–270.

Devereux, E. C., Shouval, R., Bronfenbrenner, U., Rodgers, R., Kav-Venaki, S., Kiely, E., & Karson, E. (1974). Socialization practices of parents, teachers and peers in Israel: The kibbutz versus the city. *Child Development, 45,* 269–281.

Siegelman, M. (1965). Evaluation of Bronfenbrenner's questionnaire for children concerning parental behavior. *Child Development, 36,* 163–174.

AUTHOR'S RESPONSE

No additional comments.

PC-9
Family–Peer Relationship Questionnaire
(FPRQ)

GENERAL INFORMATION

Date of publication: 1983.

Author: Edythe S. Ellison.

Source/publisher: Edythe S. Ellison, RN, EdD, College of Nursing, 845 South Damon Ave., University of Illinois at Chicago, Chicago, IL, 60612.

Availability: Available from the author (see above).

Brief description: The FPRQ is a two-part self-report measure developed for children aged 7 to 12 and their parents. The measure is designed to assess the quality of parental support and the quality of a child's peer relations. Parental support is conceptualized as parental availability, companionship and nurturance, and parents' activities in mediating between the child and the wider community. The child's peer relations are also assessed by both the child and the parent but are not considered part of the parental support construct.

Purpose: The purpose of the FPRQ is to assess the quality of parental support as perceived by both the parent and the child. A secondary purpose of the measure is to assess children's peer relations.

Theoretical base: Social support, ecological model.

PHYSICAL DESCRIPTION OF QUESTIONNAIRE

Physical features: The FPRQ is self-report attitudinal inventory. Part I measures quality of parental support; Part II gathers information on the peer relations of the child. Both parents and children complete a form of the measure. The majority of the FPRQ responses appear in a 5-point Likert format (from 1 = low frequency of a particular behavior to 5 = high frequency of a particular behavior). Some questions ask for estimates of time spent with the parent or child under various conditions (weekday, weekends, alone, with others) and information about peer relationships (names, length of friendship).

Unit of study: The parent–child relationship and the child's peer relations.

Respondent: The parent and the child.

Scales and dimensions: Three components exist in the Parent domain: Togetherness (32 items), Nurturance–Disclosure (14 items), and Peer Relationships (20 items). Similar components are included in the Child domain: Togetherness (32 items), Nurturance–Disclosure (15 items), and Peer Relations (13 items).

Manual: No manual is available, but the scoring procedures are available from the author.

Standardization and norms: None are available at this time.

Evaluation of physical description of questionnaire: *Strengths:* A primary strength of the FPRQ is its dual perspective. The measure assesses *both* parents' and children's perceptions of parental support. The measure is clear and easy to complete. *Limitations:* Children at the lower end of the respondent age range may have difficulty distinguishing between response points (i.e., 1–15 minutes or 16–30 minutes).

ADMINISTRATIVE PROCEDURES

Directions: Directions are clearly indicated on the test booklet.

Ease of use: The FPRQ appears easy to use.

Training for administration and scoring: No special training is required for administration or scoring of this measure.

Scoring procedures: All of the items are scored on a 1–5 scale, with 1 generally indicating very low frequency of a behavior and 5 indicating high frequency. The parental availability questionnaires that ask for time estimates are converted into a score that also ranges from 1 to 5. The item scores are then combined to form the component scores.

Evaluation of administration procedures: *Strengths:* The measure is easily administered and easily scored. *Limitations:* The younger children may have some difficulty with the reading level of the FPRQ Child form.

EVALUATION OF CONSTRUCTS MEASURED

Reliability: Cronbach's alpha coefficients were high, ranging from .65 to .86 for the mother–child, child–mother components and from .72 to .92 for the father–child, child–father components (Ellison, 1985a). Test–retest reliability for the children's report of Togetherness and Nurturance is .64 and .85, respectively (Ellison et al., undated).

Validity: *Construct:* The children's report of Nurturance was significantly related to feeling informed and reassured about their mother's illness. The children's Togetherness scores were negatively related to lack of information and fears, questions, and concerns about their mothers' illness (Ellison, Kieckhefer, Houck, & Wallace, undated). *Criterion:* Predictive validity studies are in progress (Ellison, 1985b).

Clinical utility: The FPRQ was developed primarily for use in health care settings. As an assessment tool, it can be used to measure the impact of an acute or chronic illness in a family member on the quality of the parent–child relationship. Studies using the FPRQ are in progress to explore the parent–child relationship within the health care environment. Data obtained from these studies can be used to plan and deliver health services to the family more effectively.

Research utility: As a research tool, the FPRQ can be used to examine how the quality of parental support changes over time in response to a family illness. Outside the health care environment, the FPRQ can be used to assess the relationship between parental support and children's achievement and competence, as mediated by parents' and children's gender and age. Further research needs to be conducted to demonstrate the research utility of the FPRQ.

SUMMARY EVALUATION

The FPRQ is designed primarily to measure the quality of parental support as perceived by both the parent and the child. The primary strength of the FPRQ lies in its dual perspective. The measure recognizes and addresses the importance of the inclusion of the child's perspective in the emotional health of the family environment. The measure is concise and easy to administer, making it a valuable tool to use in a health care setting. Continued work regarding the measure's validity would strengthen the FPRQ as both a clinical and a research assessment tool.

REFERENCES

Ellison, E. S. (1983). Parental support and school-aged children. *Western Journal of Nursing Research, 5*(2), 145–153.

Ellison, E. S. (1985a). A multidimensional, dual-perspective index of parental support. *Western Journal of Nursing Research, 7*(4), 401–424.

Ellison, E. S. (1985b). *Nursing research emphasis grant final report*. University of Washington, School of Nursing.
Ellison, E. S., Kieckhefer, G., Houck, G., & Wallace, K. (undated). *Child's perception of mother's illness*. Unpublished manuscript, University of Washington, School of Nursing.

AUTHOR'S RESPONSE

No additional comments.

PC-10
Home Environment Questionnaire
(HEQ-1R and HEQ-2R)

GENERAL INFORMATION

Date of publication: 1983.

Author: J. O. Sines.

Source/publisher: Psychological Assessment and Services, P.O. Box 1031, Iowa City, IA 52244.

Availability: Available from publisher (see above).

Brief description: The HEQ-1R and HEQ-2R are parent self-report questionnaires for one-parent and two-parent families, respectively, that assess the psychosocial environments of children. Each measure consists of 10 subscales measuring achievement, aggression (external, home, and total), supervision, change, affiliation, separation, sociability, and socioeconomic status.

Purpose: The measure is designed to determine the portion of children's clinically relevant behavior that can be accounted for by the environmental conditions to which they are exposed (Sines, Clarke, & Laner, 1984).

Theoretical base: Physical and psychosocial aspects of children's environments account for their behavior beyond the influence of personality characteristics. The theoretical base includes environmental press (Murray, 1938) and interactionism (Bowers, 1973; Ekehammar, 1974).

PHYSICAL DESCRIPTION OF QUESTIONNAIRE

Physical features: The HEQ-1R and HEQ-2R contain 91 and 123 items, respectively. There are 10 scales for each version of the instrument. The instrument is suitable for use with children in fourth to sixth grade in one- and two-parent families. Respondents (mothers) indicate whether the behavior described by the statement is true or false for their children.

Unit of study: Individual parent.

Respondent: Parent (mothers responded in validation sample).

Scales and dimensions: The scales of the HEQ-2R and HEQ-1R and the number of items, respectively, per scale are Achievement (8, 8), Aggression—External (10, 10), Aggression—Home (14, 14), Aggression—Total (24, 24), Supervision (9, 9), Change (19, 14), Affiliation (25, 10), Separation (9, 5) Sociability (4, 3), and Socioeconomic Status (25, 18).

Manual: The manual contains administration, scoring, and psychometric information for both test versions.

Standardization and norms: Data for the HEQ-2R were gathered in a small midwestern city from a sample of 544 Anglo mothers (292 boys and 252 girls) with a mean income of $18,000. Seventy-six mothers (42 boys, 36 girls) comprised the norming sample for the HEQ-1R. Means and standard deviations are reported for each sex. Data on clinical and nonclinical populations are currently being collected.

Evaluation of physical description of questionnaire: *Strengths:* Items are behaviorally specific. Although mothers were used in the norming sample, fathers could respond to items with equal facility. *Limitations:* The HEQ-1R norming sample is small. The language of some items seems extreme for true–false responding and may invite socially desirable responses.

ADMINISTRATIVE PROCEDURES

Directions: Respondents are asked to reach each statement and indicate whether the item is true or false for themselves or their children. Scale items concern the mother's, child's, or husband's behavior in the home environment (depending on the scale used).

Ease of use: Instructions are straight forward, and the true–false format is easy to follow.

Training for administration and scoring: Some experience with scoring templates is necessary.

Scoring procedures: Hand-scoring templates are applied to the HEQ answers to derive scale scores.

Evaluation of administrative procedures: *Strengths:* A manual for administration and scoring is available. Templates for scoring are provided. *Limita-*

tions: To facilitate scoring, items of each scale occur together on the test, which may lead to a response bias. Hand-scoring is time-intensive.

EVALUATION OF CONSTRUCTS MEASURED

Reliability: Six of the 10 scales of the HEQ-2R demonstrate adequate internal consistency for both sexes (Achievement, Aggression—External, Aggression—Home, Aggression—Total, Change, Affiliation, and Socioeconomic Status; KR-20 r's range from .69 to .85). The remaining four scales (Separation, Affiliation, Sociability, and Supervision) are low (KR-20 r's range from .27 to .49). Interscale correlations for both sexes are moderate to low, though statistically significant, given the sample size. When sexes are combined into a total sample ($n = 544$), the pattern and sign of interscale correlations remains similar to those found for each sex, suggesting that the scales are assessing similar constructs for both sexes. Sex differences were found, however, for a clinical sample. (Laing & Sines, 1982).

The internal consistency of the HEQ-1R scales is more variable. KR-20 r's ranging from .60 to .79 are found for Aggression—External, Aggression—Home, Aggression—Total, Affiliation, and Socioeconomic Status. The internal consistency coefficients for the remaining scales range from .04 to .59 (mean KR-20 $r = .36$). Interscale correlations are low and nonsignificant for both sexes (3 of 45 and 5 of 45 intercorrelations for boys and girls, respectively) and mostly involve the aggression subscales. Thus, subscales of HEQ-2R and HEQ-1R that show low reliability should be used with caution.

Validity: *Criterion:* Mothers' HEQ scale scores and ratings of children's behavior problems are significantly related (Laing & Sines, 1982). The age of the child is unrelated to assessed behaviors; however, the authors report that a social desirability response bias exists across samples (Laing & Sines, 1982; Sines et al., 1984).

Clinical utility: None reported.

Research utility: Few measures provide information on single-parent households. Thus, this measure could provide useful information once its psychometric properties have been improved.

SUMMARY EVALUATION

The HEQ-2R (123-items) and HEQ-1R (91 items) are true-false self-report parent questionnaires designed to measure the psychosocial environment of children to determine what portion of their clinically relevant behavior can be attributed to the environmental conditions to which they are exposed. Although these measures hold promise for clinicians and researchers, their utility is limited at present by inadequate psychometric development and test validation. Low internal consistency and a social desirability response set are particular weaknesses. Thus, although the instruments provide information on a potentially useful aspect of family functioning for two-parent and single-parent households, further psychometric development is needed.

REFERENCES

Bowers, K. (1973). Situationism in psychology: An analysis and a critique. *Psychological Review, 80,* 307–336.
Ekehammar, B. (1974). Interactionism in personality from a historical perspective. *Psychological Bulletin, 81,* 1026–1048.
Laing, J. A., & Sines, J. O. (1982). The Home Environment Questionnaire: An instrument for assessing several behaviorally relevant dimensions of children's environments. *Journal of Pediatric Psychology, 77,* 425–449.
Murray, H. A. (1938). *Explorations of personality.* New York: Oxford University Press.
Sines, J. O., Clarke, W. M., & Lauer, R. M. (1984). Home Environment Questionnaire. *Journal of Abnormal Child Psychology, 12,* 521–529.

AUTHOR'S RESPONSE

No additional comments.

PC-11
Index of Parental Attitudes (IPA)

GENERAL INFORMATION

Date of publication: 1982.

Author: Walter W. Hudson.

Source/publisher: Hudson, W. W. (1982). *The Clinical Measurement Package,* Homewood, IL: Dorsey Press.

Availability: Scale is printed in cited source.

Brief description: The IPA is a 25-item self-report questionnaire designed to measure the degree, severity, or magnitude of a problem in a parent–child relationship. The measure is one of nine short-form scales that make up the Clinical Measurement Package.

Purpose: The IPA assesses parental attitudes regarding the degree of contentment present within the parent–child relationship.

Theoretical base: Atheoretical.

PHYSICAL DESCRIPTION OF QUESTIONNAIRE

Physical features: The IPA is a 25-item questionnaire to which parents respond on a 5-point Likert scale ranging from "rarely or none of the time" to "mostly or all of the time."

Unit of study: Parent–child relationship.

Respondent: Parent.

Scales and dimensions: The IPA consists of a single scale of problem severity within the parent–child relationship.

Manual: The manual includes information on all the Clinical Measurement Package scales, of which the IPA is a part. The manual is comprehensive, well organized, and easy to use and includes information on test development, scoring procedures, and validation.

Standardization and norms: None available.

Evaluation of physical description of questionnaire: *Strengths:* The inventory is short and easy to use. The response format is clear, and the reading level is simple. *Limitations.* None noted.

ADMINISTRATIVE PROCEDURES

Directions: Respondents are asked to place a rating number beside each of the 25 items. The respondent chooses *one* child to be the target child throughout the completion of the questionnaire.

Ease of use: The IPA is very easy to use.

Training for administration and scoring: Minimal training is required to use the IPA. The manual provides clear instructions for administering the IPA scale, and self-training exercises are provided for those who have no prior experience administering a clinical measurement tool. Scoring consists of simply summing the rating scores on the 25 items.

Scoring procedures: A total score of problem severity is derived by the summation of the rating scores on the 25 items. The clinical cutoff score for the IPA is 30. A score above 30 indicates more severe problems; a score below 30 indicates the relative absence of problems.

Evaluation of administrative procedures: *Strengths:* The IPA is easy to administer and score. *Weaknesses:* The IPA scores falling just above and just below the established cutoff score can result in an ambiguous determination of the degree of problem severity in the parent–child relationship. As with all self-report questionnaires, social desirability responses can be a problem.

EVALUATION OF CONSTRUCTS MEASURED

Reliability: The IPA scale reliability (Cronbach's alpha) was .97 (Hudson, Wung, & Borge, 1980). Use of test–retest reliability for the IPA, which purports to be sensitive to change over time, was considered irrelevant by the author, so no test–retest reliability estimates are available.

Validity: A discriminant validity score of .88 was obtained between criterion groups (therapy clients with/without parent–child relationship problems) and

IPA scores (Nurius & Hudson, 1982). The IPA was positively related to scores on the Psycho-Social Screening Package (PSS), as predicted (r = .42 and .76) (Hudson, 1982).

Clinical utility: According to the author, the IPA is most beneficial and when used as an evaluation tool, and it can act as a monitoring device during the implementation and modification of a treatment regimen. The author cautions against using the IPA as a diagnostic screening device.

Research utility: The IPA is designed primarily as a clinical instrument; however, recent studies are indicating that the IPA may be useful in assessing experimental effects or surveying group differences. Continued work is necessary to determine the research utility of the IPA.

SUMMARY EVALUATION

The IPA is a 25-item self-report questionnaire developed to measure the problem severity present in a parent–child relationship. The IPA scale is a unidimensional measure of a personal or social problem and should not be taken as an assessment of cause, type, or origin of a problem. Although further psychometric validation is necessary for the IPA, the existing data indicate that the Index of Parental Attitudes scale is both a reliable and a valid measure for use in monitoring and assessing certain client problems in clinical settings. The IPA, like any self-report instrument, is susceptible to social desirability in responding.

REFERENCES

Hudson, W. W. (1982). *The Clinical Measurement Package: A field manual,* Homewood, IL: Dorsey Press.

Hudson, W. W., Wung, B., & Borge, M. (1980). Parent–child relationship disorders: The parent's point of view. *Journal of Social Service Research, 3*(3), 283–294.

Nurius, P. S., & Hudson, W. W. (1982). *The assessment of peer discord in clinical practice.* Unpublished manuscript, Florida State University School of Social Work, Tallahassee.

AUTHOR'S RESPONSE

No additional comments.

PC-12
Inventory of Parent and Peer Attachment
(IPPA)

GENERAL INFORMATION

Date of publication: 1986.

Authors: G. C. Armsden and M. T. Greenberg.

Source/publisher: G. C. Armsden, Department of Psychology, NI-25, University of Washington, Seattle, WA 98195.

Availability: Available from the authors (see above).

Brief description: The IPPA is a 75-item self-report questionnaire that measures adolescents' perceptions of the quality of their attachment with their parents and friends.

Purpose: The IPPA is designed to assess the nature of adolescents' feelings toward attachment figures.

Theoretical base: Ethological-organizational attachment theory (Bowlby, 1973; Sroufe & Waters, 1977).

PHYSICAL DESCRIPTION OF QUESTIONNAIRE

Physical features: Adolescents 16 to 20 years of age are asked to rate their feelings about their relationship with their mother, father, and close friends on a 5-point Likert-type scale (''almost never or never true'' to ''almost always or always true''). There are 75 items on the questionnaire (25 items repeated for the mother, father, and close friends).

Unit of study: Individual adolescent.

Respondent: Individual family member in mid to late adolescence.

Scales and dimensions: The three scales for the parent and peer sections of the IPPA are Trust, Communication, and Alienation. These scales were developed through factor-analytic techniques.

Manual: None available.

Standardization and norms: None available. The IPPA was developed with a sample of 179 16- to 20-year-old undergraduates (mean age, 18.9 years). Females comprised 63% of the sample.

Evaluation of physical description of questionnaire: *Strengths:* Items are written appropriately for respondents. *Limitations:* Although factor analyses were used to develop the Trust, Communication, and Alienation scales, their stability is questionable because of the low subject–item ratio. A manual and normative data are unavailable.

ADMINISTRATIVE PROCEDURES

Directions: Respondents are instructed to circle "how true" each statement describes their relationship with their parent or close friends. Brief instructions precede each section for the mother, father, and close friends. Individuals complete the scales separately.

Ease of use: Directions and items are self-explanatory, although in multiparent families (e.g., stepparents), the examiner should remember to instruct respondents to pick the parent who has had the most influence on them. The IPPA can be administered individually or in groups.

Training for administration and scoring: No training is required.

Scoring procedures: None available. Scoring appears to involve simply summing respondents' ratings (from 1 to 5) for each item for each of the three scales. Items associated with each scale are available from the authors.

Evaluation of administrative procedures: *Strengths:* Instructions are easy to follow. No training is required for administration. Testing time is brief. *Limitations:* Because the parent and peer items are on the same questionnaire, respondents may be inclined to compare their ratings for parents and peers.

EVALUATION OF CONSTRUCTS MEASURED

Reliability: Internal consistency (Cronbach's alpha) for the Trust, Communication, and Alienation scales on the parent (mother and father versions combined) and peer versions of the IPPA range from $r = .72$ to $r = .91$. Intercorrelations both between and within the parent and peer IPPA scales are high, indicating that the scales are not distinct and are measuring the same construct. Test–retest reliability ($n = 27$) was $r = .93$ and $r = .86$ for the parent and peer measure, respectively.

Validity: A multitrait-multimethod approach was used. *Convergent:* Parent and peer attachment scores are significantly related to several family measures: (1) the Family Self and Social Self concept subscales of the Tennessee Self-concept Sale; (2) the Cohesion, Expressiveness, and Conflict subscales of the Family Environment Scale (only the Expressiveness subscale was related to the peer measure); and (3) an author-developed measure of communication among family members. *Concurrent:* Parent and peer measures of attachment accounted for statistically significant portions of the variance in self-esteem and life satisfaction scores, as well as individuals' self-reported depression/anxiety and resentment/alienation on Bachman's (1970) Affective States Index. *Construct:* Individuals classified as secure in attachment scored higher in self-esteem and life satisfaction scores, and reported fewer negative life changes than insecure individuals. Further, quality of parent attachment was significantly related to individuals' coping strategies in challenging, threatening, and loss situations (Armsden, 1986).

Clinical utility: The IPPA has potential use in assessing adolescents' perceptions of the quality and security of their relationships with their parents and peers. Correlations between individuals' low scores on the IPPA and clinically relevant affective states (e.g., depression/anxiety, guilt, irritability/anger, resentment/alienation) and physical symptomatology further attest to the usefulness of this construct in the treatment of adolescents and their families. However, the authors would have to provide guidelines for classifying individuals into high versus low attachment groups as well as standardization and normative data.

Research utility: Strong validity data suggest that the instrument has definite promise in studying the role of attachment quality in adolescent relationships with others and its relation to other personality and social development issues involving adolescents. Several cautions are warranted, however. First, the IPPA needs standardization and normative data. Second, the high interscale correlations between and within parent and peer scales (Trust, Communication, Alienation) suggest that they are measuring the same attachment construct (not different aspects). Finally, the overclassification of females into the secure attachment group suggests the possibility of sex bias in test items.

SUMMARY EVALUATION

The original 77-item IPPA was developed from the Inventory of Adolescent Attachment (Greenberg, Siegel, & Leitch, 1983). The current IPPA consists of

25 items in which adolescents rate their attachment to their mother, father, and close friends (75 items total). Instructions are straightforward and easy to follow. Reliability and validity data are good, although high interscale correlations suggest that the three scales are assessing aspects of the same attachment construct, and combining scale scores may be more appropriate than using the subscales separately (which the authors have done in some studies). Standardization and normative data are needed to facilitate classification of individuals in terms of attachment quality. This information would greatly imrprove the utility of the instrument for both clinical and research purposes.

REFERENCES

Armsden, G. G., (1986, March). *Coping strategies and quality of parent and peer attachment in late adolescence*. Paper presented at the First Biennial Meeting of the Society for Research on Adolescence, Madison, WI.

Armsden, G. G., & Greenberg, M. T. (1984). *The Inventory of Parent and Peer Attachment: Individual differences and their relationship to psychological well-being in adolescence*. Unpublished manuscript, University of Washington, Seattle, Department of Psychology.

Bachman, J. G. (1970). *Youth in transition: The impact of family background and intelligence on tenth-grade boys* (Vol. 2). Ann Arbor, MI: Blumfield.

Bowlby, J. (1973). *Attachment and loss: Vol. 2. Separation*. New York: Basic Books.

Greenberg, M. T., Siegel, J. M., & Leitch, C. J. (1983). The nature and importance of attachment relationships to parents and peers during adolescence. *Journal of Youth and Adolescence, 12*(5), 373–386.

Sroufe, L. A., & Waters, E. (1977). Attachment as an organizational construct. *Child Development, 48,* 1184–1199.

PC-13
Maryland Parent Attitude Survey (MPAS)

GENERAL INFORMATION

Date of publication: 1966.

Author: Donald K. Pumroy.

Source/publisher: D. K. Pumroy, College of Education, University of Maryland, College Park, MD 20742.

Availability: The MPAS and its scoring key and I-score table are available from the author (see above).

Brief description: The MPAS is a research instrument designed to measure parent attitudes toward child rearing while controlling for the effects of social desirability. The instrument consists of 95 forced-choice items that correspond to one of four types of parenting styles: Disciplinarian, Indulgent, Protective, and Rejecting. The items are appropriate for use with either sex.

Purpose: The MPAS is designed to provide a measure of parenting styles that is free from the influence of social desirability.

Theoretical base: The four types of parenting styles assessed on the MPAS correspond to styles generally considered important in the research literature (e.g., Maccoby, 1980). The assumption is that these rearing styles/attitudes influence children's social and personality development.

PHYSICAL DESCRIPTION OF QUESTIONNAIRE

Physical features: Unlike other instruments assessing parenting styles (e.g., the Parent Attitude Research Instrument), the forced-choice item format of the MPAS minimizes parents' tendencies to chose socially desirable responses on the test. For each of the 95 paired items, respondents indicate which of the choices is most representative of their child-rearing attitude. Answers are written on the questionnaire or on IBM answer sheets. There are 45 statements depicting each type of parenting style (the first five pairs are not scored).

Unit of study: Parents' parenting styles.

Respondent: Parent—mother or father.

Scales and dimensions: The MPAS measures four parenting styles: Disciplinarian, Indulgent, Protective, and Rejecting (Pumroy, 1966).

Manual: No manual is available.

Standardization and norms: The instrument was standardized on a group of 197 male and 186 female college students (mean age and age range: 20.8 years and 16–37 years for males; 18.5 years and 16–44 years for females). Means and standard deviations were calculated for each of the four parenting styles and were used in the development of T-scores.

Evaluation of physical description of questionnaire: *Strengths:* Items are easy to read and understand. *Weaknesses:* The questionnaire is long. Norms are based on a college population, whose child-rearing attitudes may not be representative of the population of parents.

ADMINISTRATIVE PROCEDURES

Directions: Instructions for completing the MPAS are given at the top of the first page of each questionnaire.

Ease of use: The MPAS is very easy to use. Respondents select the child-rearing attitude from each pair of statements that is most consistent with their views.

Training for administration and scoring: No training is needed for anyone with minor experience in test scoring, although it is not explicitly stated how the raw scores are summed and then used on the T-score conversion table for each parenting style.

Scoring procedures: A scoring key is provided by the author, along with a T-score conversion table. A subject apparently receives a raw score of 1 each time he or she chooses one of the four types of parenting attitudes. These raw scores are converted to T-scores on the conversion table for each parenting style. Separate tables are provided for mothers and fathers.

Evaluation of administrative procedures: *Strengths:* Instructions are easy to follow. The MPAS is simple to administer and score. No special training is required. It could be administered to groups of parents. *Limitations:* None quoted.

EVALUATION OF CONSTRUCTS MEASURED

Reliability: A 3-month test–retest reliability on 54 college students yielded coefficients ranging from .62 to .73 for the four parenting styles. Split-half (Spearman-Brown) reliability coefficients ranged from .67 to .84 in a separate sample of 90 male and female college students. Reliability data are not available for a population consisting solely of parents. The correlations between the Indulgent and Disciplinarian and Rejecting scales are $-.39$ and $-.56$ between the Protective and Rejecting scales. Although the interscale correlations are consistent with theory, the high correlations indicate that the scales are not independent of one another; that is, they may represent different aspects of the same construct (Tolor, 1967).

Validity: *Concurrent:* Brody (1964, cited in Pumroy, 1966) found that mothers who were high on Disciplinarian ratings were more directing and restricting in their interactions with their children. Further, mothers' prohibitions were positively related to their scores on the Rejecting scale. However, it should be cautioned that males' and females' scores on the MPAS correspond somewhat to typical sex role socialization patterns; that is, females score higher on the Indulgent scale and males score higher on the Disciplinarian scale (Pumroy, 1966). Correlations between the MPAS scales and the Edwards Social Desirability Scale range from $-.17$ to .19; significance levels are not reported (Tolor, 1967).

Clinical utility: The MPAS was designed for research purposes; it is not intended to be used clinically.

Research utility: The MPAS was designed for research purposes; however, its utility is limited by the high interscale correlations, which indicate that the scales are measuring different facets of the same construct. The chief advantage is that it appears to reduce respondents' tendencies to chose socially desirable responses, which is an important test feature in this kind of research.

SUMMARY EVALUATION

The MPAS provides information on parents' indulgent, disciplinarian, protective, and rejecting child-rearing attitudes. It is easy to administer and score, although test length may affect the validity of respondents' choices. Its chief advantage is its forced-choice format, which reduces the likelihood of respondents choosing the most socially appropriate responses. The lack of a representative norming sample limits the adequacy of reported reliability and validity data.

REFERENCES

Maccoby, E. E. (1980). *Social development: Psychological growth and the parent–child relationship.* New York: Harcourt-Brace.

Pumroy, D. K. (1966). Maryland Parent Attitude Survey: A research instrument with social desirability controlled. *Journal of Psychology, 64,* 73–78.

Tolor, A. (1967). An evaluation of the Maryland Parent Attitude Survey. *Journal of Psychology, 67,* 69–74.

PC-14
Parent Attitude Research Instrument
(PARI Q⁴)

GENERAL INFORMATION

Date of publication: 1971.

Authors: E. S. Schaefer and R. Q. Bell (1958); revised by S. Schludermann and E. Schludermann.

Source/publisher: S. Schludermann and E. Schludermann, Department of Psychology, The University of Manitoba, Winnipeg, Manitoba, Canada R3T 2N2.

Availability: Available from authors (see above).

Brief description: The PARI Q^4 is a self-report questionnaire that assesses parental attitudes toward child-rearing and family life.

Purpose: The PARI Q^4 is designed to assess parental attitudes that are hypothesized to be relevant to their child-rearing practices.

Theoretical base: Social and developmental psychology. It is assumed that parental socialization practices influence the child's personality development.

PHYSICAL DESCRIPTION OF QUESTIONNAIRE

Physical features: The PARI has been revised a number of times previous to this version (see Becker & Krug, 1965; Sims & Paolucci, 1975). The PARI Q^4 has forms for the father (115 items) and the mother (130 items). Each form consists of 23 scales and incorporates items from the original PARI developed by Schaefer and Bell (1958) and Zuckerman's (1958) modifications to reduce response bias. The response format consists of a 4-point Likert scale on which respondents indicate whether they strongly agree, mildly agree, mildly disagree, or strongly disagree with each attitude statement.

Unit of study: Individual parent.

Respondent: Individual mother or father.

Scales and dimensions: The 23 scales of the mother and father forms differ somewhat in content. In factor analyses, the scales of the mother and father forms loaded (either positively or negatively) on two major factors: Authoritarian Control and Family Disharmony, and Democratic Attitudes and Paternal Detachment, respectively.

Manual: None available.

Standardization and norms: Means and development deviations for the scales and factor scores for separate male ($n = 387$) and female ($n = 425$) samples are available from the authors.

Evaluation of physical description of questionnaire: *Strengths:* Test scales are comprehensive and cover a variety of child-rearing attitudes for both mother and father. *Limitations:* Normative data are limited and are based on college samples, which may not be representative of the parent population. Statements are often written in absolute terms (e.g., "You must always . . ."), which may be related to the extreme response bias found with the test (Becker & Krug, 1965; Schludermann & Schludermann, 1974, 1977).

ADMINISTRATIVE PROCEDURES

Directions: Instructions are listed on the top of each questionnaire. Respondents are asked to read each attitude statement and circle the letter indicating their level of agreement or disagreement with it.

Ease of use: No special administration procedures are required. The PARI Q[4] can be administered to individuals or groups. Directions are clear and simple to follow. Items are written clearly.

Training for administration and scoring: No training is required for administration or scoring, although the scorer must know which scales are associated with the factors described previously and whether to add or subtract a scale when summing the scales for a total score for each factor.

Scoring procedures: Procedures are available from the authors. Responses are summed to obtain scores for each scale. These scale scores are then summed (or subtracted if they load negatively) for each factor to obtain total factor scores for the factors of the mother and father forms. Authors recommend machine scoring and using computer programs to expedite scoring.

Evaluation of administrative procedures: *Strengths:* The PARI Q[4] is simple to administer and easy to read. Items are worded clearly. *Limitations:* The instrument is somewhat long, which may affect the parents' responses. Scoring differs for the mother and father forms and will take time to learn, whether done manually or by computer.

EVALUATION OF CONSTRUCTS MEASURED

Reliability: Test–retest reliability coefficients (Pearson r) for the scales of the father form range from .57 to .75; for the mother form, from .52 to .81. Factor score reliabilities range from .75 to .87. (Specific scale reliabilities are available from the authors.)

Validity: Little is available on the PARI Q[4]. In a study of response bias, social desirability effects, and the factor structure of the PARI Q[4], 425 female and 387 male college students completed the instrument (mean age, 18.5 years). The influence of acquiescence or opposition response sets on the PARI Q[4] is reduced, but it remains affected by an extreme response set for mother and father forms (Schludermann & Schludermann, 1974, 1977). Females' social desirability is moderately negatively related to the Family Disharmony factor and unrelated to the Authoritarian Control factor, whereas the males' responses appear unaffected by social desirability. (Becker and Krug, 1965 provide an extensive review of validity studies with the original PARI—Schaefer & Bell, 1958).

Clinical utility: Few differences were found in the self-reports of normal versus schizophrenic mothers or among mothers of children with various disabling conditions (Becker & Krug, 1965) with the original PARI. No clinical studies have been conducted with PARI Q[4].

Research utility: Research utility is unknown because of the lack of validity data and the presence of an extreme response set.

SUMMARY EVALUATION

The PARI Q[4] is a self-report questionnaire that assesses parents' attitudes about child-rearing, parent–child relationships, and roles of family members. The 23 scales of the questionnaire are associated with two primary factors for each form: Authoritarian Control and Family Disharmony (mother form); Democratic Attitudes and Paternal Detachment (father form). Items are clearly written and appear to cover relevant aspects of child-rearing attitudes, and the instructions are easy to understand. Although this instrument is not affected by acquiescence or opposition response sets, as are earlier versions, an extreme response set bias remains. Scoring is time-consuming if done manually. Adequate norms have not been developed. Test–retest reliability of the scales and factors is satisfactory. The current lack of psychometric data limits the utility of the instrument for clinical or research purposes.

REFERENCES

Becker, W. C., & Krug, R. S. (1965). The Parent Attitude Research Instrument: A research review. *Child Development, 36,* 329–365.

Schaefer, E. S., & Bell, R. Q. (1958). Development of a parental attitude research instrument. *Child Development, 29,* 339–361.

Schludermann, S., & Schludermann, E. (1970a) Conceptual frames of parental attitudes of fathers. *Journal of Psychology, 75,* 193–204.

Schludermann, S., & Schludermann, E. (1970b) Conceptualization of maternal behavior. *Journal of Psychology, 75,* 205–215.

Schludermann, S., & Schludermann, E. (1971) Response set analysis of a parental Attitude Research instrument (PARI). *Journal of Psychology, 79,* 205–215.

Schludermann, S., & Schludermann, E. (1974) Response set analysis of mother's form of Parental Attitude Research Instrument (PARI). *Journal of Psychology, 86,* 327–334.

Schludermann, S., & Standardization, E. (1977) A methodological study of a revised maternal attitude research instrument: PARI Q⁴. *Journal of Psychology, 95,* 77–86.

Sims, L. S., & Paolucci, B. (1975). An empirical examination of the Parent Attitude Research Instrument (PARI). *Journal of Marriage and the Family, 37,* 724–732.

Zuckerman, M. (1958). Reversed scales to control acquiescence response set in the Parental Attitude Research Instrument. *Child Development, 30,* 523–532.

AUTHOR'S RESPONSE

No additional comments.

PC-15
Parent Perception Inventory
(PPI)

GENERAL INFORMATION

Date of publication: 1983.

Authors: Ann Hazzard and Andrew Christensen.

Source/publisher: Andrew Christensen, Department of Psychology, University of California, Los Angeles, CA, 90024.

Availability: Available from the author (see above).

Brief description: The PPI is an 18-item self-report questionnaire designed to measure children's perceptions of positive and negative parental behaviors.

Purpose: The purpose of the PPI is to provide a measure of children's perceptions of their family environment through the use of a short measure (36 items) containing behaviorally relevant concepts.

Theoretical base: Social learning theory.

PHYSICAL DESCRIPTION OF QUESTIONNAIRE

Physical features: The PPI includes 18 items, each of which is responded to on a 5-point Likert scale from "never" to "a lot." For younger children, pictures of thermometers are used to represent the five response points. The 18 parental behaviors concepts are first assessed for mother and then for father.

Unit of study: Parent.

Respondent: Child.

Scales and dimensions: The PPI consists of two nine-item dimensions: positive parental behaviors and negative parental behaviors. The positive parental behaviors include: positive reinforcement, comfort, talk time, involvement in decision making, time together, positive evaluation, allowing independence, assistance, and noverbal affection, and the negative parental behaviors include: privilege removal, criticism, command, physical punishment, yelling, threatening, time-out, nagging, and ignoring. Based on the 18 parental behavior classes, four Parent Perception Inventory subscales are derived for each child: Mother Positive, Mother Negative, Father Positive, and Father Negative.

Manual: No manual is available. The directions for scoring the PPI are available from the author.

Standardization and norms: Hazzard, Christensen, and Margolin (1983) report means and standard deviations for small samples of boys and girls in distressed and nondistressed families.

Evaluation of physical description of questionnaire: *Strengths:* The items in the measure seem to cover a wide range of behaviorally relevant concepts. A number of descriptions and examples are given for each concept. The 5-point Likert scale provides ease of response. *Limitations:* The descriptions and examples within each item do not always appear to be representing the same concept (e.g., the concept of independence is described by "lets you do what other kids do" and "lets you do things on your own"). Because it is a verbal report measure, it could be subject to social desirability response bias. Distinguishing between the response points could be challenging for young children (e.g., "a little" vs. "sometimes"); however, the scoring sheet does include pictures of thermometers, filled to varying degrees, above each of the five response points to further clarify the response points for the young children.

ADMINISTRATIVE PROCEDURES

Directions: Directions are clearly indicated on the questionnaire sheet.

Ease of use: The PPI is easy to use, and no special equipment is required.

Training for administration and scoring: Administration and scoring require no special training.

Scoring procedures: All items are scored 0 to 4 ("never" to "a lot"). Each child receives six scores per measure: a positive and negative score for both mother and father and a total score—the positive score minus the negative subscore (negative score minus scores for items 2, 14, 18—for both mother and father. Either the subscale scores or the total scores can be used for clinical purposes, depending on the particular clinical purpose. For example, in working with parents who were deficient in positive interaction with their child, one might look at positive subscales only. However, for a broader overview of parent–child interaction from the child's perspective, one might use a total score.

Evaluation of administrative procedures: *Strengths:* The PPI is easy to administer, complete, and score. *Limitations:* It is unclear whether all six scores are valuable as outcome variables or just the total scores.

EVALUATION OF CONSTRUCTS MEASURED

Reliability: Internal reliability of the PPI was calculated by computing item–total correlations for each item and the subscale to which the item contributed; r's ranged from .34 to .83. Cronbach's alpha was also computed for each of the four subscales: Mother Positive = .84; Mother Negative = .78; Father Positive = .88; Father Negative = .80. Alphas were calculated separately on two groups of children on all four subscales. For older children (ages 10–13), alphas ranged from .74 to .89. For younger children (ages 5–9), alphas ranged from .81 to .87 (Hazzard, Christensen, & Margolin, 1983).

Validity: *Convergent:* Correlations were computed between the four subscales and (1) a child's self-concept measure (Piers-Harris or McDaniel-Piers scales) and (2) a parental measure of child conduct disorder (CBC Externalizing Score). Correlations between self-concept and the four subscales were Mother Positive = .36; Mother Negative = −.51; Father Positive = .27; Father Negative = −.41. Correlations between conduct and the subscales were Mother Positive = −.18; Mother Negative = .50; Father Positive = .08; Father Negative = .40 (Hazzard, Christensen, & Margolin, 1983). *Discriminant:* Correlations were computed between the four subscales and two measures that were not expected to be highly related: (1) the child-completed WRAT and (2) the Becker Intellectual Inadequacy Scale. Correlations between the four subscales and the WRAT were Mother Positive = −.22; Mother Negative = −.01; Father Positive = −.04; Father Negative = −.17. Correlations between the subscales and intellectual deficiency were Mother Positive = −.12; Mother Negative = .23; Father Positive = .02; Father Negative = .18 (Hazzard, Christensen, & Margolin, 1983).

Clinical utility: The PPI could be used as an assessment and outcome instrument in family therapy studies. It could be used to target problematic parent behaviors and to assess increases or decreases in the frequency of these behaviors. No studies have as yet demonstrated its clinical usefulness.

Research utility: One study has suggested that the PPI may be used to demonstrate that perceived parental similarity may be related to distressed versus nondistressed families (Hazzard, Christensen, Margolin, 1983). More studies need to be conducted to demonstrate the measure's research utility.

SUMMARY EVALUATION

The Parent Perception Inventory is an efficient measure of children's perceptions of parental behaviors. It is a short measure for young children that taps specific accounts of parental behavior rather than global, attitudinal dimensions. The major strengths of this instrument are its ease of administration and scoring. Limitations include its response format, requiring greater precision than a young child is capable of, and its potentially misinterpreted item descriptions.

REFERENCE

Hazzard, A., Christensen, A., & Margolin, G. (1983). Children's perceptions of parental behaviors. *Journal of Abnormal Child Psychology, 2*(1), 49–60.

AUTHOR'S RESPONSE

Recently, a parent version of the Parent Perception Inventory was developed. With this form, parents answer the same questions about their behavior toward their child as their child does. If parents and children are both given the Parent Perception Inventory to complete independently, valuable information on convergence and divergence between parent and child perspectives can be obtained.

Currently, we are using the Parent Perception Inventory to gather data on three samples of families: families with a preadolescent boy diagnosed as having Attention Deficit Disorder, families undergoing divorce, and "normal" families. We will use the Parent Perception Inventory in the research to assess not only the level of parental positive and negative behavior but to assess family alliances (e.g., data from the Parent Perception Inventory could suggest more positive and less negative interaction between Dad and child than between Mom and child).

PC-16
Parent as a Teacher Inventory (PAAT)

GENERAL INFORMATION

Date of publication: 1984.

Author: Robert D. Strom.

Source/publisher: Scholastic Testing Service, Inc., 480 Meyer Rd., Bensenville, IL 60106.

Availability: Available from the publisher.

Brief description: The PAAT is a 50-item inventory designed to assess parents' attitudes about their role in their children's creativity, play, and learning and their levels of frustration and need for control over their children's behavior.

Purpose: The purpose of the scale is for parents to describe their feelings about several aspects of their interaction with their children, their standards for assessing the importance of certain aspects of child behavior, and their value preferences and frustrations concerning child behavior. It is intended for parents of children aged 3 to 9 and was initially developed for determining parents' needs in a parent education curriculum.

Theoretical base: Parental influence upon child development, with an emphasis on Torrance's work on creativity and Strom's work on the role of play in development.

PHYSICAL DESCRIPTION OF QUESTIONNAIRE

Physical features: The PAAT includes 50 items, each of which is responded to on a 4-point Likert scale ranging from "strong yes" to "strong no." The reading level is quite basic, but the questions can be presented orally if necessary. The PAAT has been translated into 15 languages, including Spanish, French, German, Greek, and Italian.

456

Unit of study: Parent–child dyad.

Respondent: Parent.

Scales and dimensions: Five subscales are assessed: Creativity, Frustration, Control, Play, and Teaching-Learning.

Manual: A detailed manual—including purpose, administration and scoring information, reliability and validity data, and references—is available from the publisher.

Standardization and norms: No norms are included in the manual, although the author has established a computer data bank for completed studies using the PAAT and will make comparative scores from various subpopulations available.

Evaluation of physical description of questionnaire: *Strengths:* The PAAT is clearly written and is easy to administer and respond to in a short period of time. The comprehensive manual provides useful documentation for the measure. *Limitations:* Norms are not included in the manual.

ADMINISTRATIVE PROCEDURES

Directions: Directions are clearly indicated on the test booklet.

Ease of use: The PAAT appears to be quite straightforward. No special equipment is needed. Foreign-language versions and versions for nonverbal responses are provided.

Training for administration and scoring: Administration requires no special training. Straightforward scoring instructions are provided in the manual.

Scoring procedures: Subscale scores are computed by reversing the scoring on designated items and summing response codes, as outlined in the manual. The Parent as a Teacher Profile is intended to accompany the PAAT as a guide for feedback to individual respondents and for program planning. The profile restates all 50 PAAT items in an abbreviated and positive form for uniformity of interpretation. In addition to its value in helping individual parents identify their child-rearing strengths and needs, the profile can also be used to recognize discrepant expectations between a child's mother and father or parent surrogates.

Evaluation of administrative procedures: Strengths: The PAAT is easy to administer, complete, and score. *Limitations:* None noted.

EVALUATION OF CONSTRUCTS MEASURED

Reliability: Reliability alpha coefficients ranged from .71 to .88 across 17 studies listed in the manual. No test–retest data were presented.

Validity: Validity was established by comparing parents' written responses on the PAAT to their behavior as observed in their homes. Johnson (1975) found that there was consistency between parental expression and behavior 66% of the time. In a subsequent study by Panetta (1980), consistency levels were found to be 75% and 85%. In a study of criterion-related validity, the PAAT was used as a pre–post assessment in a parent and child education project. Posttesting of the 88 parents in the program showed significant gains on all five subscales of the PAAT and on the total score (Strom & Johnson, 1978).

Clinical utility: The PAAT can be used to assist parent educators in designing programs and interventions.

Research utility: The PAAT can be used in pre–post test evaluation studies. It is also useful as an index of parental attitudes about the family as a learning context for the child.

SUMMARY EVALUATION

The PAAT is a useful, concise instrument that can be used in prevention and intervention programs as well as in research. Its reliability and validity have been established in a series of studies, and cross-study data are being systematically collected by the author.

REFERENCES

Johnson, A. (1975). *An assessment of Mexican-American parent child-rearing feelings and behaviors.* Unpublished doctoral dissertation Arizona State University.

Panetta, S. J. (1980). *An exploration and analysis of parental behaviors which may be related to a child's problem solving abilities.* Unpublished doctoral dissertation, University of Northern Colorado.

Strom, R. D. (1984). *Parent as a Teacher Inventory manual.* Bensenville, IL: Scholastic Testing Service.

Strom, R. D. (1987). Childrearing dilemmas of immigrants to the United States. *Journal of Experimental Research in Education, 24,* 91–102.

Strom, R., Escobar, I., & Daniels, S. (1986). Supporting Venezuelan families through parent attitude assessment. *Journal of Instructional Psychology, 13,* 147–152.

Strom, R. D., Fleming, S., & Daniels, S. (1984). Parenting strengths of single fathers. *Elementary School Guidance and Counseling, 19*, 77–87.

Strom, R., Goldman, R., Rees, R., & Daniels, S. (1984). A comparison of childrearing attitudes of parents of handicapped and nonhandicapped children. *Journal of Instructional Psychology, 11*, 89–103.

Strom, R., & Johnson, A. (1978). Assessment for parent education. *Journal of Experimental Education, 47*, 9–16.

Strom, R., & Slaughter, H. (1978). Measurement of childrearing expectations using the Parent as a Teacher Inventory. *Journal of Experimental Education, 46*, 44–53.

Strom, R., Slaughter, H., & Rees, R. (1981). Childrearing expectations of families with atypical children. *American Journal of Orthopsychiatry, 5*, 285–296.

AUTHOR'S RESPONSE

Research concerned with parental competencies has primarily emphasized differences between socioeconomic groups or educational levels, with the implicit assumption that advantage in child-rearing and parental behavior is solely a function of these dimensions. In several cross-cultural studies using the PAAT, we have examined the influence of *child access to parents' time,* a nontraditional variable that can be directly manipulated in ways that more traditional socioeconomic traits cannot be. We found that differences in access to parent's time seem to be more relevant than parent income or formal schooling. Parents who spent more time interacting with their youngsters were more accepting of typical child behavior than were parents who spent less time with sons and daughters. In order to augment the use of PAAT, two new instruments are currently undergoing psychometric assessment. These measures, the Parental Strengths and Needs Inventory and the Grandparent Strengths and Needs Inventory, are intended for families with children aged 7 to 18.

PC-17
Parental Acceptance–Rejection
Questionnaire—Adult Form

GENERAL INFORMATION

Date of publication: 1980.

Author: Ronald H. Rohner.

Source/publisher: Rohner, R. (1984). *Handbook for the study of parental acceptance and rejection* (rev. ed.). Storrs: University of Connecticut, Center for the Study of Parental Acceptance and Rejection.

Availability: Scale is printed in cited source.

Brief description: The Parental Acceptance–Rejection Questionnaire (PARQ)—Adult Form is a 60-item self-report questionnaire for the cross-cultural assessment of parents' perceptions of the accepting–rejecting rearing practices they experienced from their own mothers when they were children. *Note:* The PARQ-Adult is identical to the PARQ-Mother version except in tense and pronoun (e.g., Adult—''My mother said nice things about me''; Mother—''I say nice things about my child'').

Purpose: The PARQ-Adult is designed to measure cross-culturally adults' perceptions of their mothers' child-rearing practices toward them as children.

Theoretical base: Theory of socialization based in anthroponomy (worldwide principles of behavior), ethnography, social and developmental psychology. The theory is concerned with consequences of perceived parental acceptance–rejection on the behavioral, cognitive, and emotional functioning of adults.

PHYSICAL DESCRIPTION OF QUESTIONNAIRE

Physical features: The PARQ—Adult consists of 60 statements in which adults rate their perceptions of their mother's accepting–rejecting rearing behaviors in terms of ''almost always true,'' ''sometimes true,'' ''rarely true,'' and ''almost never true.'' Test items were screened for idiomatic American English and were translated into Bengalese, Czechoslovakian, Hindi, Korean, Swedish, Urdu, and Telugu (continents of the last two sites are not reported in the manual).

Unit of study: Parents' experience of accepting–rejecting rearing practices of their mothers.

Respondent: Individual mother (or father).

Scales and dimensions: The PARQ-Adult consists of four scales: Warmth/ Affection (20 items), Aggression/Hostility (15 items), Neglect/Indifference (15 items), and Undifferentiated Rejection (10 items).

Manual: The manual contains the PARQ-Adult, scale descriptions, directions for administration and scoring, and reliability and validity information.

Standardization and norms: The standardization sample consisted of 66 undergraduate students (even sex distribution). Ethnicity and socioeconomic status of sample subjects are not reported. Normative data are not available. Also, the size and demographic characteristics of relevant cross-cultural groups are not reported, although the author refers to survey research of 101 societies to identify common forms of accepting–rejecting behaviors (Rohner, 1975).

Evaluation of physical characteristics of questionnaire: *Strengths:* Items are written clearly in behaviorally specific terms. The scale can be modified easily for research with fathers. *Limitations:* The standardization sample is small and not sufficiently described. Undergraduates may not be representative of the population for which the instrument is designed to be used. Cross-cultural data are not reported.

ADMINISTRATIVE PROCEDURES

Directions: Each questionnaire has a title page with instructions for completing the items. Adults are instructed to reflect back to when they were 7 to 12 years of age and ask themselves if an item was basically true ("almost always" or "sometimes") or untrue ("rarely," "almost never") about the way their own parents treated them as children in terms of acceptance–rejection. Respondents are instructed to react from their perspective as 7- to 12-year-olds, not as they currently view their parents' practices. Responses are marked on the questionnaire. Completion of the questionnaire takes 10 to 15 minutes. Additional instructions for the examiner are given in the manual.

Ease of use: The PARQ-Adult instructions are straightforward, although the examiner should ensure that mothers are responding in terms of how they experienced their mothers' practices when they were 7 to 12 years of age.

Training for administration and scoring: Guidelines for administration and scoring are outlined in the manual (Rohner, 1984). No special training is needed.

Scoring procedures: Items reflecting each scale are arranged on a scoring sheet and scored as follows: "almost always true" = 4; "sometimes" = 3; "rarely" = 2; "almost never" = 1. Instructions for scoring of items on the scales are provided and must be done manually by the examiner. Scores for each scale are obtained by summing the item scores. A total PARQ score is obtained by summing across the four scales (with reverse scoring of the Warmth/Affection scale total score; a table is provided). Author recommends but does not provide a table to convert the four scale scores into z-scores before summing the scores to form a total composite score.

Evaluation of administrative procedures: *Strengths:* Directions are straight-forward, but the examiner should ensure that respondents react to their parents' practices with them when they were from 7 to 12 years of age. *Limitations:* The lack of answer sheets means reproducing the questionnaires for successive administrations, although instructions could be modified easily for answer sheets. Standard score conversion is recommended, but tables are not provided.

EVALUATION OF CONSTRUCTS MEASURED

Reliability: The author indicates that items on the current questionnaire have been revised on an ongoing basis since the original norming in 1973. How-ever, the nature of these changes and relevant sample information are not re-ported. Reliability data were gathered from a sample of 147 male and female undergraduates. Internal consistency coefficients (Cronbach's alpha) for the four scales ranged from .86 to .95. In a second sample of 58 undergraduate stu-dents, the alpha coefficients ranged from .83 to .96, with a median coefficient of .90. Reliabilities on the Spanish version of the scale ranged from .71 to .96, with a median of .84, for a sample of 91 Puerto Rican adolescents. Interscale correlations are high and statistically significant, suggesting that the scales are assessing the same construct (the range is from −.43 to .89), as posited by the author (i.e., parental acceptance–rejection). Consistent with theory, the Warmth/ Affection scale is negatively correlated with the Rejection, Neglect/Indiffer-ence, and Aggression/Hostility scales (−.43, −.71 and −.45, respectively).

Validity: Several of the most relevant studies are reported here (see Rohner, 1984, for further validity data).
   Concurrent and convergent: High and statistically significant correlations are reported between the PARQ-Adult Warmth/Affection scale, Neglect/Indiffer-ence scale, and Rejection scale and the Child Report of Parent Behavior Inven-tory (CRPBI) (Schaefer, 1964) scales of Acceptance, Hostile Detachment, and Rejection (r = .90, .86, and .81, respectively). The PARQ Aggression/Hostil-ity scale was positively correlated with the Physical Punishment Scale of the

Bronfenbrenner Parent Behavior Questionnaire (BP) ($r = .81$) (Siegelman, 1965).

Discriminant: The PARQ Neglect/Indifference and Warmth/Affection scales correlate more highly with their respective validation scales (cited above) than other PARQ scales. Interscale correlations between PARQ Aggression/Hostility and Rejection scales and noncriterion scales are equivalent to their correlations with their validation scales.

Factor analyses of PARQ items yielded two factors relevant to the author's parental acceptance–rejection theory. Factor I consisted of items from the Aggression/Hostility, Neglect/Indifference, and Rejection scales, denoting rejection. Factor II consisted of items from the Warmth/Affection scale, denoting acceptance. The intercorrelation of the factors is .55, indicating that they are not independent and may represent bipolar ends of a single dimension. The subject–item ratio is very small, however, and the results of the factor analysis may not be stable.

Construct: In a Spanish version of the PARQ-Adult, Saavedra (1980) found that adolescents' perceptions of self-esteem and self-adequacy correlated positively with maternal and parental warmth.

Clinical utility: The author suggests that, consistent with child abuse literature, parents who experienced rejection as children are more likely to reject their own children (Parke & Collmer, 1975; Rohner, 1984). Also, since parental rejection has been implicated in a variety of children's individual psychiatric and behavioral disorders (Rohner & Nielsen, 1978), the PARQ would be relevant to professionals working with families of abused and rejected children. Further validation of the scale with clinical populations would increase its utility.

Research utility: The author reports that from a survey of 101 societies, adults in societies where children tend to be rejected are more emotionally unresponsive and emotionally unstable and have a more negative world view than adults in societies where children are accepted (Rohner 1975; Rohner, Berg, & Rohner, 1982; Rohner & Rohner, 1981, 1982). Thus, the instrument appears to be relevant to cross-national studies of the impact of parents' perceptions of their own parents' accepting–rejecting rearing practices and their development of social and personality dispositions.

SUMMARY EVALUATION

The PARQ-Adult is a 60-item self-report questionnaire concerning adults' perceptions of their child-rearing histories. The measure is easy to administer, and the items are easy to comprehend. The instrument demonstrates promising discriminant and construct validity for the American sample and appears well founded in theory. The standardization sample and reliability/validity data are based on undergraduate students in the United States, which may be unrepresentative of parent populations, especially those in other cultures. High interscale correlations suggest that the scales are not independent but represent facets of a single acceptance–rejection construct. Although the author claims that the instrument is suitable for cross-cultural use and has published a number of related articles, cross-cultural data are not reported.

REFERENCES

Parke, R. D., & Collmer, C. W. (1975). Child abuse: An interdisciplinary analysis. In E. M. Hetherington (Ed.), *Review of child development research* (Vol. 5, pp. 509–590). Chicago: University of Chicago Press.

Rohner, R. P. (1975). *They love me, they love me not: A worldwide study of the effects of parental acceptance and rejection.* New Haven, CT: HRAF Press.

Rohner, R. P. (1984). *Handbook for the study of parental acceptance and rejection* (rev. ed.). Storrs: University of Connecticut, Center for the Study of Parental Acceptance and Rejection.

Rohner, R. P., Berg, S., & Rohner, E. C. (1982). Data quality control in the standard cross-cultural sample: Cross-cultural codes. *Ethnology, 21,* 359–369.

Rohner, R. P., & Frampton, S. (1982). Perceived parental acceptance–rejection and artistic preference: An unexplained contradiction. *Journal of Cross-Cultural Psychology, 13,* 250–259.

Rohner, R. P., & Nielsen, C. C. (1978). *Parental acceptance–rejection: A review and annotated bibliography of research and theory.* New Haven, CT: HRAF Press.

Rohner, R. P., & Rohner, E. C. (1981). Parental acceptance–rejection and parental control: Cross-cultural codes. *Ethnology, 20,* 245–260.

Rohner, R. P., & Rohner, E. C. (1982). Enculturative continuity and the importance of caretakers: Cross-cultural codes. *Behavior Science Research, 17,* 91–114.

Saavedra, J. M. (1980). Effects of perceived parental warmth and control on the self-evaluation of Puerto Rican adolescent males. *Behavior Science Research, 15,* 41–53.

Schaefer, E. S. (1964). *Child's Report of Parent Behavior Inventory.* Washington, DC: National Institutes of Health.

Siegelman, M. (1965). Evaluation of Bronfenbrenner's questionnaire for children concerning parental problems. *Child Development, 36,* 163–174.

AUTHOR'S RESPONSE

No additional comments.

PC-18
Parental Acceptance–Rejection
Questionnaire—Child Form

GENERAL INFORMATION

Date of publication: 1980.

Author: Ronald H. Rohner.

Source/publisher: Rohner, R. (1984). *Handbook for the study of parental acceptance and rejection* (rev. ed.) Storrs: University of Connecticut, Center for the Study of Parental Acceptance and Rejection.

Availability: Scale is printed in cited source.

Brief description: The Parental Acceptance–Rejection Questionnaire (PARQ)—Child Form is a 60-item self-report questionnaire for the cross-cultural assessment of 9 to 11-year-old children's perceptions of parental accepting–rejecting behaviors. *Note:* The PARQ-Child items are identical to those in the Mother and Adult versions, except that items were rephrased or simplified to be relevant from a child's perspective.

Purpose: The PARQ-Child is designed to measure children's perceptions of parental acceptance–rejection rearing behaviors cross-culturally and to determine the impact of these perceptions on their social and personality development.

Theoretical base: Theory of socialization based in anthroponomy (worldwide principles of behavior), ethnography, social and development psychology.

PHYSICAL DESCRIPTION OF QUESTIONNAIRE

Physical features: The PARQ-Child consists of 60 statements about parental accepting–rejecting behaviors that the child rates in terms of "almost always true," "sometimes true," "rarely true," and "almost never true." The PARQ-Child has been translated into Bengalese, Czechoslovakian, Hindi, Korean, Spanish (Mexican and Puerto Rican versions), Telugu, and Tiv (Nigeria).

Unit of study: Individual child's perceptions of parents' rearing behaviors.

Respondent: Individual child.

Scales and dimensions: The PARQ-Child consists of four scales: Warmth/ Affection (20 items), Aggression/Hostility (15 items), Neglect/Indifference (15 items), Undifferentiated Rejection (10 items).

Manual: The manual contains the PARQ-Child, scale descriptions, directions for administration and scoring, and reliability and validity information.

Standardization and norms: The sample consisted of 220 fourth- and fifth-grade students (9–11 years old) in three metropolitan Washington, D.C., elementary schools. There were no significant age or sex differences in responses to test items. Sample demographics are not reported. The size and demographic characteristics of other cultural groups for which the instrument has been translated are not reported. Normative data are not reported.

Evaluation of physical characteristics of questionnaire: *Strengths:* Items are written clearly, in behaviorally specific terms and in language easily understood by children. *Limitations:* The standardization and cross-cultural sample are not described well enough to know the population for which the instrument is designed to be used. The reading level may be too high for children in lower age ranges.

ADMINISTRATIVE PROCEDURES

Directions: Each questionnaire has a title page with instructions for completing the items, along with a sample item. Children are instructed to ask themselves if the statement is basically true ("almost always" or "sometimes") or untrue ("rarely," "almost never") about the way their mother treats them. Responses are marked on the questionnaire. Completion time of the questionnaire depends on the reading skill of the children. In the norming group, directions were read aloud to the fourth-grade children. Additional instructions for the examiner are in the manual.

Ease of use: The PARQ-Child instructions are straightforward, although the examiner should ensure that the children understand that they are to indicate how their mothers are treating them currently. Otherwise, the instrument appears easy to use and to follow.

Training for administration and scoring: Guidelines for administration and scoring are outlined in the manual (Rohner, 1984). No special training is required.

Scoring procedures: Items reflecting each scale are arranged on a scoring sheet and scored as follows: "almost always true = 4; "sometimes" = 3; "rarely" = 2; "almost never" = 1. Instructions for scoring of items on the scales are provided and must be done manually by the examiner. Scale scores are obtained by summing item scores for each scale. A total PARQ score is obtained by summing across the four scales (with reverse scoring of the Warmth/Affection scale total score; a table is provided). Author recommends but does not provide a table to convert the four scale scores into z-scores before summing the scores to form a total composite score.

Evaluation of administrative procedures: *Strengths:* Directions are straightforward, but the examiner should ensure that children are responding how they feel their mothers are currently treating them. *Limitations:* The lack of answer sheets means reproducing the questionnaires for successive administrations, although modifications could be made easily to use answer sheets. Standard score conversion is recommended, but tables are not provided.

EVALUATION OF CONSTRUCTS MEASURED

Reliability: Reliability data were gathered from a sample of 220 male and female fourth- and fifth-grade children. Internal consistency coefficients (Cronbach's alpha) for the four scales ranged from .72 to .90.

Validity: *Concurrent/convergent:* High and statistically significant correlations are reported between the PARQ-Child Warmth/Affection scale, Neglect/Indifference scale, and Rejection scale with the Acceptance, Hostile Detachment, and Rejection Scales of the Child Report of Parent Behavior Inventory (Schaefer, 1964) ($r = .83, .64$ and $.74$, respectively). The PARQ Aggression/Hostility scale was positively correlated with the Physical Punishment scale of Bronfenbrenner's Parent Behavior Questionnaire (BPB) (Siegelman, 1965) ($r = .55$).

Construct: The author (Rohner, 1975), in a survey of over 100 societies, reports that rejected children are more hostile, aggressive, or passive-aggressive and evaluate themselves more negatively than accepted children. Rohner and Pettengill (1985) found that Korean children's reports of maternal warmth, hostility, and undifferentiated rejection were positively related to maternal but not parental control. This pattern was interpreted as consistent with culturally prescribed roles of authority in Korean families and as different from findings associated with cultural beliefs concerning control and parental aggression/hostility in American children.

Discriminant: PARQ scales have not clearly been demonstrated to measure separate constructs. Interscale correlations are high and statistically significant (the range is from $-.40$ to $.80$), suggesting that the scales are assessing aspects of the same construct, as posited by the author (i.e., parental acceptance–rejection). Consistent with theory, the Warmth/Affection scale is negatively correlated with the Rejection, Neglect/Indifference, and Aggression/Hostility scales ($r = -.40$, $-.72$, and $-.50$, respectively) (Rohner, 1984).

Factor analyses of PARQ items yielded two factors consistent with the author's parental acceptance–rejection construct. Factor I, rejection, consisted of items from the Aggression/Hostility, Neglect/Indifference, and Rejection scales of the PARQ and related CRPBI and BPBQ scales. Factor II consisted of items from the PARQ Warmth/Affection scale and the CRPBI Acceptance scale, denoting acceptance. The intercorrelation of the factors is .50, indicating that they are not independent but may represent bipolar ends of a single dimension. The results of the factor analysis may not be stable, however, as the subject–item ratio is low.

Clinical utility: Parental rejection has been implicated in a variety of children's individual psychiatric and behavioral disorders (Rohner & Nielsen, 1978). Thus, the assessment of parental behaviors described on the PARQ would be relevant to professionals working with families. Further validation of the scale with clinical populations would increase its utility.

Research utility: The instrument would appear to be useful for examining cultural differences in parental acceptance–rejection practices and the impact of such practices on children's social and personality development.

SUMMARY EVALUATION

The PARQ-Child is a 60-item self-report questionnaire concerning children's perceptions of their parents' warmth/affection, aggression/hostility, neglect/indifference, and rejection (undifferentiated). Instructions are straightforward, and the test is easy to administer. Although data on test development are reported, the samples are not sufficiently described, and normative data are unavailable. Also, the author does not provide information on instrument development conducted in other cultures. Nevertheless, the instrument demonstrates convergent and concurrent validity for the American sample and construct validity for cross-cultural samples. High interscale correlations suggest that the scales are not independent and represent facets of the same acceptance–rejection construct, as posited by the author.

REFERENCES

Rohner, R. P. (1975). *They love me, they love me not: A worldwide study of the effects of parental acceptance and rejection.* New Haven, CT: HRAF Press.

Rohner, R. P. (1980). Worldwide tests of parental acceptance–rejection theory. *Behavior Science Research, 15,* 1–21.

Rohner, R. P. (1984). *Handbook for the study of parental acceptance and rejection* (rev. ed.). Storrs: University of Connecticut, Center for the Study of Parental Acceptance and Rejection.

Rohner, R. P., & Nielsen, C. C. (1978). *Parental acceptance–rejection: A review and annotated bibliography of research and theory.* New Haven, CT: HRAF Press.

Rohner, R. P., & Pettengill, S. M. (1985). Perceived parental acceptance–rejection and parental control among Korean adolescents. *Child Development, 56,* 524–528.

AUTHOR'S RESPONSE

No additional comments.

PC-19
Parental Acceptance–Rejection
Questionnaire—Mother Form

GENERAL INFORMATION

Date of publication: 1980.

Author: Ronald H. Rohner.

Source/publisher: Rohner, R. (1984). *Handbook for the study of parental acceptance and rejection* (rev. ed.). Storrs: University of Connecticut, Center for the Study of Parental Acceptance and Rejection.

Availability: Scale is printed in cited source.

Brief description: The Parental Acceptance–Rejection Questionnaire (PARQ)—Mother is a 60-item self-report questionnaire designed to assess mothers' accepting–rejecting behaviors toward their children. *Note:* The PARQ-Mother is identical to the PARQ-Adult except in tense and pronoun (e.g., Adult—"My mother said nice things about me"; Mother—"I say nice things about my child").

Purpose: The PARQ-Mother is designed to measure parental acceptance–rejection behaviors toward children in different cultures.

Theoretical base: Theory of socialization based in anthroponomy (worldwide principles of behavior), ethnography, social and developmental psychology. It is concerned with the consequences of parental acceptance–rejection on the behavioral, cognitive, and emotional development of children cross-nationally.

PHYSICAL DESCRIPTION OF QUESTIONNAIRE

Physical features: The PARQ-Mother consists of 60 statements depicting parental accepting–rejecting behaviors. Responses to each statement are made on a 4-point scale: "almost always true," "sometimes true," "rarely true," and "almost never true." The PARQ-Mother has been translated into Bengalese, Czechoslovakian, Hindi, Korean, and Telugu (African).

Unit of study: Mothers' rearing attitudes.

Respondent: Individual parent (typically the mother).

Scales and dimensions: The PARQ-Mother consists of four scales: Warmth/Affection (20 items), Aggression/Hostility (15 items), Neglect/Indifference (15 items), and Undifferentiated Rejection (10 items).

Manual: The manual contains the PARQ-Mother, scale descriptions, directions for administration and scoring, and reliability and validity information.

Standardization and norms: None reported.

Evaluation of physical characteristics of questionnaire: *Strengths:* Items are written clearly, in behaviorally specific terms. *Limitations:* No normative data are available.

ADMINISTRATIVE PROCEDURES

Directions: Each questionnaire has a title page with instructions for completing the items. Mothers are instructed to ask themselves if a statement about a particular accepting–rejecting behavior is basically true ("almost always" or "sometimes") or untrue ("rarely," "almost never") regarding the way they are currently treating their children. Responses are marked on the questionnaire. Completion of the questionnaire will take 10 to 15 minutes. Additional instructions for the examiner are given in the manual.

Ease of use: The PARQ-Mother instructions are straightforward, although the examiner should ensure that respondents rate their overall reactions toward their child *currently* (versus a retrospective account). Otherwise, the instrument appears easy to use. A separate scale would have to be completed for each child in the family if a total family assessment were desired.

Training for administration and scoring: Guidelines for administration and scoring are outlined in the manual (Rohner, 1984). No special training is required.

Scoring procedures: Items reflecting each scale are arranged on a scoring sheet and scored as follows: "almost always true" = 4; "sometimes" = 3; "rarely" = 2; "almost never" = 1. Instructions for scoring of items on the scales are provided and must be done manually by the examiner. Scores for each scale are obtained by summing the item scores. A total PARQ score is obtained by summing across the four scales (with reverse scoring of the Warmth/Affection scale total score; a table is provided). Author recommends but does not provide a table to convert the four scale scores into z-scores before summing the scale scores to form a total composite score.

Evaluation of administrative procedures: *Strengths:* Directions are straightforward, but the examiner should ensure that respondents are reacting to items in terms of their overall *current* relationship with their children. *Limitations:* The lack of answer sheets means reproducing the questionnaires for successive administrations, although test instructions could be altered easily for using answer sheets. Standard score conversion is recommended, but tables are not provided.

EVALUATION OF CONSTRUCTS MEASURED

Reliability: No published data.

Validity: No published data.

Clinical utility: Parental rejection has been implicated in a variety of children's psychiatric and behavioral disorders (Rohner & Nielsen, 1978), so the PARQ would appear to be useful in identifying parents' accepting–rejecting profiles. However, validation studies are lacking.

Research utility: The author reports that from a survey of 101 societies, adults in societies where children tend to be rejected are more emotionally unresponsive and emotionally unstable and have a more negative world view than adults in societies where children are accepted (Rohner, 1975). Thus, the instrument would appear to be useful in identifying parental accepting–rejecting behaviors that influence children's social and personality development. But again, validation studies are needed.

SUMMARY EVALUATION

The PARQ-Mother is a 60-item self-report questionnaire concerning mothers' overall interactions with their children in terms of warmth/affection, aggression/hostility, neglect/indifference, and rejection (undifferentiated). The instructions are straightforward. Although the measure is easy to use and well written, reliability and validity data are not reported, which is a serious drawback. However, the reliability and validity data on the Adult version of the PARQ is adequate and promises similar results for this version. The author claims that the instrument is suitable for cross-cultural use and has published a number of related articles. However, the apparent lack of relevant normative data reduces the utility of the instrument for such purposes.

REFERENCES

Rohner, R. P. (1975). *They love me, they love me not: A worldwide study of the effects of parental acceptance and rejection.* New Haven, CT: HRAF Press.

Rohner, R. P. (1980). Worldwide tests of parental acceptance–rejection theory. *Behavior Science Research, 15,* 1–21.

Rohner, R. P. (1984). *Handbook for the study of parental acceptance and rejection* (rev. ed.). Storrs: University of Connecticut, Center for the Study of Parental Acceptance and Rejection.

Rohner, R. P., & Nielsen, C. C. (1978). *Parental acceptance–rejection: A review and annotated bibliography of research and theory.* New Haven, CT: HRAF Press.

AUTHOR'S RESPONSE

No additional comments.

PC-20
Parenting Stress Index (PSI)

GENERAL INFORMATION

Date of publication: 1983.

Author: Richard R. Abidin.

Source/publisher: Pediatric Psychology Press, 320 Terrell Road West, Charlottesville, VA 22901

Availability: Available from the publisher (above): specimen set, containing manual, test booklets, 10 answer sheets; manual; test booklets; answer sheets; profile sheets. A computer-scoring and report-generating program is also available.

Brief description: The Parenting Stress Index is a 101-item self-report questionnaire designed for screening and diagnosis of parental stress in parents of children under age 10. It assesses stressful child, parental, and situational characteristics.

Purpose: The PSI is designed to identify parent–child systems under stress and families at risk for dysfunctional parenting and emotional pathology. According to the author, the PSI is useful for early identification screening, individual diagnostic assessment, pre–post measures of intervention effectiveness, and research on effects of stress.

Theoretical base: Attachment theory, temperament theory, stress theory.

PHYSICAL DESCRIPTION OF QUESTIONNAIRE

Physical features: The PSI includes 101 items, each of which is responded to on a 5-point Likert scale from "strongly agree" to "strongly disagree." The PSI also includes 19 optional items that assess the presence of specific stressful family events.

Unit of study: Individual parent and child; parent–child dyad.

Respondent: Parent.

Scales and dimensions: In the child domain, the subscales include Adaptability, Acceptability of the Child to the Parent, Child Demandingness, Child Mood, Child Distractibility/Hyperactivity, and Child Reinforces Parent. In the Parent domain, subscales include Parent Depression or Unhappiness, Parent Attachment, Restrictions Imposed by the Parental Role, Parent's Sense of Competence, Social Isolation, Relationship with Spouse, and Physical Health.

Manual: A comprehensive manual is available from Pediatric Psychology Press (see above.)

Standardization and norms: Percentile rankings are given for scale scores based on a sample of 600 parents of both normal and problem children visiting small-group pediatric clinics in central Virginia. The norm group was predominantly white and included a range of family income and parental age.

Evaluation of physical description of questionnaire: *Strengths:* The PSI is clearly written; it is easy to administer and respond to in a short period of time. The comprehensive manual provides useful documentation for the measure. *Limitations:* The norm group is not entirely representative of the U.S. population; thus, claims about generalizability must be made with caution.

ADMINISTRATIVE PROCEDURES

Directions: Directions are clearly indicated on the test booklet.

Ease of use: The PSI appears to be quite straightforward. No special equipment is needed.

Training for administration and scoring: Administration requires no special training. Scoring instructions are included in the manual.

Scoring procedures: Subscale scores are computed by adding the weights of the numbers found above the answers selected on the answer sheet. Information about norms and clinical interpretations are provided in the manual.

Evaluation of administrative procedures: *Strengths:* The PSI is easy to administer, complete, and score. *Limitations:* None noted.

EVALUATION OF CONSTRUCTS MEASURED

Reliability: Test–retest correlations in the Parent domain were .71, .91, and .69 and in the Child domain, .82, .63, and .77, for intervals of 3 weeks, 1–3 months, and 3 months, respectively. Alpha reliabilities ranged from .62 to .70 for the subscales of the Child domain and .55 to .80 for the subscales of the Parent domain; alpha for the total Child domain score was .89, and alpha for the Parent domain was .93. Total stress score alpha was .95.

Validity: The manual details numerous studies that have successfully demonstrated the PSI's content, construct, and criterion-related validity. For example, the PSI successfully discriminated between samples of physically abusive and nonabusive mothers (Mash, Johnston, & Kovitz, 1983). Significant decreases were found in parental stress in two groups of parents who were receiving parent training courses (Lafferty et al., 1980). Factor-analytic studies demonstrated that the factors are not completely independent but that most items load primarily on the appropriate subscales.

Clinical utility: The PSI can be used as a screening device to help identify patients at risk. It may also be used in a pre–post test format for establishing the effectiveness of intervention programs and to help formulate treatment plans. According to literature on the measure, the PSI is currently being used in more than 300 medical centers, mental health clinics, and programs that serve families.

Research utility: The PSI can be used in pre–post test evaluation studies. The measure also shows promise for research studies investigating links between parenting stress and outcomes for children and parents.

SUMMARY EVALUATION

The PSI is a straightforward measure that is easy to administer and score. It has multiple potential uses and has been used successfully in screening, diagnosis, and pre–post testing following interventions. Substantial evidence regarding the instrument's reliability and validity has accrued. Weaknesses of the measure include its nonrepresentative norm group.

REFERENCES

Abidin, R. R. (1982). Parenting stress and utilization of pediatric services. *Children's Health Care, 11,* 70–73.
Abidin, R. R. (1983). *Parenting Stress Index manual.* Charlottesville, VA: Pediatric Psychology Press.
Burke, W. T., and Abidin, R. R. (1980). Parenting Stress Index (PSI): A family system assessment approach. In R. R. Abidin (Ed.), *Parent education and intervention handbook.* Springfield, IL: Charles C Thomas.
Cowan, P. A., & Cowan C. P. (1986). Men's involvement in parenthood:

Identifying the antecedents and understanding the barriers. In P. Berman & F. A. Pederson (Eds.), *Fathers' transitions to parenthood.* Hillsdale, NJ: Erlbaum.

Kazak, A. E., & Marvin, R. S. (1984). Differences, difficulties, and adaptation: Stress and social networks in families with a handicapped child. *Family Relations, 33,* 1–11.

Lafferty, W., Cote, J., Chafe, P. Kellar, L., & Robertson, H. (1980). *The use of the Parenting Stress Index (PSI) for the evaluation of Systematic Training for Effective Parenting (STEP) programme.* Unpublished manuscript, Beechgrove Regional Children's Center, Toronto, Ontario, Canada.

Lloyd, B. H., & Abidin, R. R. (1984). Revision of the Parenting Stress Index. *Journal of Pediatric Psychology, 10*(2), 169–177.

Mash, E. J., & Johnston, C. (1983a). Parental perceptions of child behavior problems, parenting self-esteem and mothers' reported stress in younger and older hyperactive and normal children. *Journal of Consulting and Clinical Psychology, 51,* 86–99.

Mash, E. J., & Johnston, C. (1983b). The prediction of mothers' behavior with their hyperactive children during play and task situations. *Child and Family Behavior Therapy, 5,* 1–14.

Mash, E. J., Johnston, C., & Kovitz, K. (1983). A comparison of the mother–child interactions of physically abused and non-abused children during play and task situations. *Journal of Clinical Child Psychology, 12,* 337–346.

McKinney, B., & Peterson, R. A. (1987). Predictors of stress in parents of developmentally delayed children. *Journal of Pediatric Psychology, 12,* 133–150.

AUTHOR'S RESPONSE

No additional comments.

PC-21
Perceived Parenting Questionnaire
(PPQ)

GENERAL INFORMATION

Date of publication: 1971 (adaptation of Bronfenbrenner's Parent Behavior Questionnaire, Siegelman, 1965).

Authors: U. Bronfenbrenner (see Siegelman, 1965); revision by A. P. MacDonald, Jr.

Source/publisher: MacDonald, A. P., Jr. (1971). Internal–external locus of control: Parental antecedents. *Journal of Consulting and Clinical Psychology, 37,* 141–147.

Availability: Available in published source (see above).

Brief description: The PPQ is a 21-item questionnaire that assesses adolescents' perceptions of their parents' child-rearing behaviors in nine domains.

Purpose: The PPQ is designed to investigate young adults' perceptions of their parents' parenting styles and the relationship of these perceptions to their social, cognitive, and personality development.

Theoretical base: Phenomenology, cognitive-developmental psychology. It is assumed that adolescents' perceptions of their parents' child-rearing practices influence their personality development.

PHYSICAL DESCRIPTION OF QUESTIONNAIRE

Physical features: The PPQ consists of 21 items on which adolescents or young adults rate the frequency of their parents' behavior toward them in terms of three different 5-point response scales: (1) "never," "only once or twice a year," "about once a month," "about once a week," "almost every day"; (2) "never," "only once in a while," "sometimes," "often," "very often"; and (3) "never," "only once in a while," "sometimes," "usually," "almost always." There are separate forms for the mother and father (MacDonald, 1971).

Unit of study: Young adult, adolescent (i.e., his or her perception of parental child-rearing attitudes and behavior).

Respondent: Individual adolescent or young adult.

Scales and dimensions: Various numbers of PPQ items and scales have been used (e.g., see Gfellner, 1986; Halpin, Halpin, & Widdon, 1980; Marquis & Detweiler, 1985). The original adaptation consists of 21 items forming one five-item and eight two-item scales: Instrumental Companionship, Nurturance, Principled Discipline, Predictability of Standards, Protectiveness, Physical Punishment, Achievement Pressure, Deprivation of Privileges, Affective Punishment. Through factor analysis with the 21-item version, three factors consistent with the literature were identified: Loving, Demanding, and Punishment (after Siegelman, 1965). The fourth factor, Maternal Control, differentiated maternal control and induction from the above practices (Gfellner, 1986).

Manual: None available.

Standardization and norms: None available.

Evaluation of physical description of questionnaire: *Strengths:* The PPQ can be completed quickly but covers key aspects of the parent–child relationship. Items are written in behaviorally specific terms. *Limitations:* The multiple response formats may be confusing to adolescents and may confound scale interpretation with type of response format.

ADMINISTRATIVE PROCEDURES

Directions: Children are asked to rate the extent to which each of their parents engages in certain rearing behaviors (MacDonald, 1971). The instrument may be administered individually or in small groups.

Ease of use: PPQ instructions are not available.

Training for administration and scoring: No training is required. No guidelines are provided.

Scoring procedures: Scoring appears to be done manually. Scores are derived by summing responses to individual items that comprise each of the nine scales (e.g., "almost always" = 5; "usually" = 4; "sometimes" = 3; "once in a while" = 2; "never" = 1).

Evaluation of administrative procedures: *Strengths:* Administration time for the PPQ is short. *Limitations:* Special instructions for the different response scales would seem advisable, especially for younger respondents.

EVALUATION OF CONSTRUCTS MEASURED

Reliability: Internal consistency for the mothers' form ranges from .50 to .82; for the fathers' form, the range is .48 to .81 across the nine scales (MacDonald, 1971). Halpin et al. (1980) report coefficients from .38 to .84 across the nine scales. Test–retest reliability data are not reported.

Validity: *Construct:* Factorial studies of this adaptation, the original Bronfenbrenner instrument (Siegelman, 1965), and a slightly longer form (Devereux, Bronfenbrenner, & Rodgers, 1969) yield similar factors over samples varying in age and cultural background (e.g., see Aguilino, 1986; Gfellner, 1986). *Criterion:* Gfellner (1986) reports that the Loving factor is positively related and the Demanding factor is negatively related to adolescents' ego development. Among Indian and white adolescents, self-ratings of self-esteem were positively related to perceptions of parental instrumental companionship, nurturance, and principled discipline. Parental punishment was negatively related to adolescents' locus of control and self-esteem (Halpin et al., 1980).

Clinical utility: None demonstrated.

Research utility: The PPQ is potentially useful as a research tool. Its factorial consistency with other similar instruments (see the CRBPI) and the larger scale (Devereaux et al., 1969) is a strong point. Additional reliability data are need to demonstrate consistency of measurement of the nine constructs assessed by the questionnaire, especially since there are so few items per scale.

SUMMARY EVALUATION

The PPQ is a 21-item self-report questionnaire that assesses adolescents' perceptions of their parents' parenting styles, either in the past or currently. Instructions are simple and test length is very short, but three different response scales add to the complexity of scale administration. Three factors have factorial validity across different ages and cultural groups, but test–retest reliability data are not reported and are needed.

REFERENCES

Aguilino, W. S. (1986). Children's perceptions of marital interaction. *Child Study Journal, 16,* 159–172.

Devereux, E. C., Bronfenbrenner, U., & Rodgers, R. R. (1969). Child-rearing in England and the United States: A cross-national comparison. *Journal of Marriage and the Family, 31,* 257–270.

Gfellner, B. M. (1986). Changes in ego and moral development in adolescents: A longitudinal study. *Journal of Adolescence, 9,* 281–302.

Halpin, G., Halpin, G., & Whiddon, T. (1980). The relationship of perceived parental behaviors to locus of control and self-esteem among American Indian and white children. *Journal of Social Psychology, 11,* 189–195.

MacDonald, A. P., Jr. (1971). Internal–external locus of control: Parental antecedents. *Journal of Consulting and Clinical Psychology, 37,* 141–147.

Marquis, K. S., & Detweiler, R. A. (1985). Does adopted mean different? An attributional analysis. *Journal of Personality and Social Psychology, 48,* 1054–1066.

Siegelman, M. (1965). Evaluation of Bronfenbrenner's questionnaire for children concerning parental behavior. *Child Development, 36,* 163–174.

PC-22
Perceptions of Parental Role Scales
(PPRS)

GENERAL INFORMATION

Date of publication: 1982.

Authors: Lucia A. Gilbert and Gary R. Hanson.

Source/publisher: Marathon Consulting and Press, P.O. Box 09189, Columbus, OH 43209-0189.

Availability: Available from the publisher.

Brief description: The PPRS is designed to measure perceived parental role responsibilities. The measure contains 78 items assessing 13 parental areas in three major domains: teaching the child (e.g., cognitive development, social skills), meeting the child's basic needs (e.g., health care, child's emotional needs), and serving the interface role between the child and the family and other social institutions (e.g., social institutions, family unit).

Purpose: The purpose of the PPRS is to provide a comprehensive measure of perceived parental role responsibilities that reflects the views of both male and female working parents.

Theoretical base: Role theory.

PHYSICAL DESCRIPTION OF QUESTIONNAIRE

Physical features: The PPRS is a 78-item self-report attitudinal inventory. Individuals respond to the 78 items by circling a response that best reflects their perceptions of the parental role. The responses appear in a 5-point Likert format ranging from 1 ("not at all important as a parental responsibility") to 5 ("very important as a parental responsibility").

Unit of study: Parent.

Respondent: Parent.

Scales and dimensions: The 78-item inventory consists of 13 parental scales in three major domains. Although the 13 scales are moderately intercorrelated (median intercorrelation = .56), only 25% to 30% of the variance associated with any two scales is shared, indicating that each scale represents a relatively independent dimension of perceived parental role responsibilities. The dimensions assessed include the following (the numbers of items in each domain and scale are included in parentheses):

Teaching (42)
  Cognitive Development(6)
  Social Skills (7)
  Handling of Emotions (6)
  Physical Health (6)
  Norms and Social Values (6)
  Personal Hygiene (5)
  Survival Skills (6)
Basic Needs (25)
  Health Care (7)
  Food, Clothing, and Shelter (5)
  Child's Emotional Needs (7)
  Child Care (6)
Family as an Interface with Society (11)
  Social Institutions (6)
  Family Unit (5)

Manual: The manual includes a brief introduction to the PPRS, development of the scales, and administration and scoring procedures. It also includes reliability and validity statistical data. Uses and interpretation of the measure are provided at the end of the manual.

Standardization and norms: No norms are available at this time.

Evaluation of physical description of questionnaire: *Strengths:* The inventory covers a wide range of parental role responsibilities. *Limitations:* The parental role responsibilities span the various stages of child rearing, resulting in confusion as to which stage of child rearing each responsibility is addressing. A parent may feel that "introducing a child to family traditions" is less important for a young child but very important for an older child.

ADMINISTRATIVE PROCEDURES

Directions: Directions are clearly indicated on the test booklet.

Ease of use: The PPRS appears easy to use.

Training for administration and scoring: No special training is required for the administration or scoring of this instrument.

Scoring procedures: Mean item scores are calculated for each of the 13 scales (i.e., the sum of responses for all items comprising the scale divided by the number of items responded to on that scale). Since the PPRS was developed primarily as a research instrument, group mean scores, rather than individual scores, are usually reported. However, for purposes of use in educational and counseling settings, plotting individual mean scores on a profile form is appropriate.

Evaluation of administrative procedures: *Strengths:* The instrument is easy to administer and score. *Limitations:* The inventory requires at least an eighth-grade reading level for respondents. A lack of adequate English reading knowledge would decrease the validity of the scores.

EVALUATION OF CONSTRUCTS MEASURED

Reliability: The coefficient alpha estimates for the 13 scales ranged from .81 to .91, indicating a high internal consistency. The 1-month, test–retest reliability coefficients were also high, ranging from .69 to .91, with a median of .82 (Gilbert & Hanson, 1982).

Validity: *Criterion:* Women scored significantly higher than men on a majority of the parenting responsibilities (Gilbert & Hanson, 1982). *Construct:* Median correlation among the scales is .56, suggesting that the scales are measuring aspects of the same construct.

Clinical utility: Although the PPRS was primarily developed for use as a research instrument, the comprehensive characteristic of the instrument makes it useful in educational and counseling settings. The PPRS has provided useful information to working parents, expectant fathers, and primary care nursing programs. The PPRS would also be useful in identifying similarities and differences in couples' parental perceptions.

Research utility: As a research tool, the PPRS has been used to explore the changing perceptions of the parental role (Gilbert & Hanson, 1982) and society's role in parenting (Gilbert & Gram, 1984). The PPRS would be useful in examining the relationship between parental role responsibilities and stress and coping and those mediating variables (personal and situational) that modify the relationship between parenting and stress. The data collected from the PPRS could also be used to test and clarify current theoretical assumptions regarding the differential parenting role enactment for mothers and fathers.

SUMMARY EVALUATION

The Perceptions of Parental Role Scales is designed as a measure of working parents' perceived parental role responsibilities. The primary strengths of the PPRS lie in the comprehensiveness of the measure. A wide variety of parental role perceptions in *dual-working* families are addressed. It is important to remember that this measure assesses perceptions rather than actual behaviors and that the relationship between parental role perceptions and parental role behaviors is still unclear. The PPRS was developed from the responses of middle-class, white, working parents employed in a university setting, so caution must be taken when making generalizations from the measure.

REFERENCES

Gilbert, L. A., & Gram, A. (1984, August). *Parental satisfaction and responsibilities in dual-earner and traditional families: Are there differences?* Paper presented at the annual meeting of the American Psychological Association, Toronto.

Gilbert, L. A. & Hanson, G. R. (1982). *Manual for Perceptions of Parental Role Scales.* Columbus, OH: Marathon Consulting and Press.

Gilbert, L. A. & Hanson, G. R. (1983). Perceptions of parental role responsibilities among working people: Development of a comprehensive measure. *Journal of Marriage and Family, 45,* 203–212.

AUTHOR'S RESPONSE

An important criterion in the scale's construction was that the items reflect parental role responsibilities agreed to by both women and men for rearing a child, *regardless of the child's gender*. This is a unique and key aspect of the PPRS.

PC-23
Pleasure-Arousal and Dominance-Inducing Scales of Parental Attitudes (PADSPA)

GENERAL INFORMATION

Date of publication: 1979.

Authors: C. A. Falender & A. Mehrabian.

Source/publisher: Albert Mehrabian, Department of Psychology, University of California at Los Angeles, 405 Hilgard Ave., Los Angeles, CA 90024.

Availability: Available from author (see above).

Brief description: The PADSPA is a 46-item questionnaire that assesses parental attitudes hypothesized to induce in children feelings of pleasure, arousal, or being dominated.

Purpose: The PADSPA is designed to measure parental attitudes regarding child-rearing that create an emotional climate for their children.

Theoretical base: It is assumed that parental attitudes create an emotional climate characterized by three orthogonal dimensions: pleasure–displeasure, arousal–nonarousal, and dominance–submissiveness (Mehrabian, 1980; Russell & Mehrabian, 1977).

PHYSICAL DESCRIPTION OF QUESTIONNAIRE

Physical features: On a separate answer sheet, parents indicate their agreement or disagreement with 46 items concerning child rearing on a 9-point Likert-type scale (+ 4 "very strong agreement"; 0, "neither agree nor disagree"; − 4, "very strong disagreement"). Statements are worded in positive and negative terms to control for response bias, although many are stated in absolute terms.

Unit of study: Child.

Respondent: Individual parent (norms are available only for mothers).

Scales and dimensions: Emotional climate is measured on three scales: Pleasure–Displeasure (18 items), Arousal–Nonarousal (12 items), and Dominance–Submissiveness (16 items).

Manual: The manual, available from the author, provides scoring information and normative data.

Standardization and norms: Means and standard deviations are provided for each scale, based on a sample of 246 mothers who were participating in child observation classes. No other demographic information is reported.

Evaluation of physical description of questionnaire: *Strengths:* Items are stated clearly. The questionnaire is relatively short. *Limitations:* Items often are stated in absolute terms, which may induce response bias to agree or disagree. Although some normative data are available, age, ethnicity and socioeconomic information concerning the sample is needed.

ADMINISTRATIVE PROCEDURES

Directions: As written, the directions assume some test-taking knowledge on the part of the respondents. Mothers are instructed to respond in terms of one child. Completion time is about 5 to 10 minutes.

Ease of use: The instructions and questionnaire items are clearly written and easy to follow for educated respondents. Mothers with no test-taking experience may need to have the instructions reviewed for them.

Training for administration and scoring: No training is required.

Scoring procedures: Procedures are available from the author. For each scale, the sum of negatively worded items is subtracted from the sum of positively worded items. Separate scores are obtained for each scale.

Evaluation of administrative procedures: *Strengths:* Directions and items are easy to read and understand. No specialized training is needed to administer and score the questionnaire. *Limitations:* Mothers without test-taking experience may need assistance in using the existing test format.

EVALUATION OF CONSTRUCTS MEASURED

Reliability: Internal consistency (KR-20) coefficients for the Arousal–Nonarousal, Pleasure–Displeasure, and Dominance–Submissiveness scales are .62, .79, and .77, respectively.

Validity: *Construct:* Interscale correlations are low (range, .03 to − .14), suggesting that the scales are assessing independent dimensions of parental child-rearing attitudes.

Clinical utility: None reported.

Research utility: None reported, but the concept of an emotional climate created through child-rearing practices merits further validation work.

SUMMARY EVALUATION

The PADSPA is a 46-item, 9-point Likert-type questionnaire that assesses the emotional climate created for children by parental child-rearing attitudes. Instructions and items are easy to read. Items are positively and negatively worded to reduce response bias, although many items are stated in extreme terms, which may promote either general agreement or disagreement. Although the concept of an emotional climate created by child-rearing attitudes is theoretically interesting, the psychometric properties of the instrument need further development, and validity studies are needed, as the authors suggest, to confirm its research and/or clinical utility.

REFERENCES

Falender, C. A., & Mehrabian, A. (1980). The emotional climate for children as inferred from parental attitudes: A preliminary validation of three scales. *Educational and Psychological Measurement, 40,* 1033–1042.
Mehrabian, A. (1980). *Basic dimensions for a general psychological theory.* Cambridge, MA: Oelgeschlager, Gunn & Hain.
Russell, J. A., & Mehrabian, A. (1977). Evidence for a three-factor theory of emotions. *Journal of Research in Personality, 11,* 273–294.

Section IX
Indexes to Abstracts

Index of Measures by Type

For page numbers, see "Index of Measure Titles" beginning on page 492.

INTERACTION CODING SCHEMES

Affective Style Measure: I-1
Defensive and Supportive Communication Interaction System: I-2
Developmental Environments Coding System: I-3
Family Conflict and Dominance Codes: 3 Variations: I-4
Family Constraining and Enabling Coding System: I-5
Family Interaction Code: I-6

Family Interaction Coding System: I-7
Family Interaction Scales: I-8
Family Task: I-9
Individuation Code: I-10
Interaction Process Coding Scheme: I-11
Parent–Adolescent Interaction Coding System: I-12
Structural Analysis of Social Behavior: I-13

RATING SCALES

Beavers-Timberlawn Family Evaluation Scale: R-1
Centripetal/Centrifugal Family Style Scale: R-2
Clinical Rating Scale for the Circumplex Model of Marital and Family Systems: R-3

FAM Clinical Rating Scale: R-4
Family Interaction Q-Sort: R-5
Global Coding Scheme: R-6
Global Family Interaction Scales: R-7
McMaster Clinical Rating Scale: R-8

SELF-REPORT QUESTIONNAIRES: WHOLE-FAMILY FUNCTIONING

Children's Version of the Family Environment Scale: W-1
Colorado Self-Report Measure of Family Functioning: W-2
Conflict Tactics Scale: W-3
Family Adaptability and Cohesion Evaluation Scales III: W-4
Family APGAR: W-5

Family Assessment Measure: W-6
Family Environment Scale: W-7
Family Evaluation Form: W-8
Family Functioning in Adolescence Questionnaire: W-9
Family Process Scales, Form E: W-10
Family Relationship Questionnaire: W-11
Index of Family Relations: W-12

SELF-REPORT QUESTIONNAIRES: FAMILY STRESS AND COPING

SELF-REPORT QUESTIONNAIRES: PARENT–CHILD RELATIONSHIPS

Index of Measure Titles

Bold numbers indicate page numbers in this volume.

Index of Authors

For page numbers, see "Index of Measure Titles" beginning on page 492.

Index of Variables

For page numbers, see "Index of Measure Titles" beginning on page 492.

Acceptability of the Child to the Parent: PC-7

Acceptance: I-5, PC-6, PC-7

Acceptance of Individuation: PC-7

Acceptance vs. Rejection: PC-3, PC-7

Accord: FC-7

Achievement: PC-10

Achievement Demands: PC-8

Achievement Orientation: W-7

Achievement Pressure: PC-21

Acknowledgment: I-11

Acquiring Social Support: FC-1

Active-Recreational Orientation: W-2, W-7

Active Understanding/Empathy: I-5

Actively Resist or Threaten: I-3

Adaptability: R-3, PC-20

Adaptation, or Family Problem Solving: W-5

Affect: I-4, W-9, W-11

Affection: W-5, PC-3

Affective Conflict: I-3

Affective Constraining: I-5

Affective Enabling: I-5

Affective Expression: W-6

Affective Involvement: R-8, W-6, W-14

Affective Punishment: PC-8, PC-21

Affective Quality of Parent–Child Interaction: PC-4

Affective Responsiveness: R-8, W-14

Affiliation: I-13, PC-10

Affiliative Orientation vs. No Affiliative Orientation: R-5

Aggression Communication: I-4

Aggression—External: PC-10

Aggression—Home: PC-10

Aggression—Total: PC-10

Aggression/Hostility: PC-17, PC-18, PC-19

Aggressive/Assertive Behaviors: R-2

Agree/Assent: I-12

Agree/Disagree: I-8

Agreement: I-6, R-7

Alienation: PC-12

Alliances: I-9

Allowing Independence: PC-15

Antagonism: I-6

Appraisal: I-12

Appropriate Topic Change: R-7

Approval: I-7

Arousal–Nonarousal: PC-23

Asks for Opinion: I-6

Asks for Orientation: I-6

Asks for Suggestion: I-6

Assistance and Nonverbal Affection: PC-15

Attack: R-7

Attempted Interruptions: I-4

Attention: I-7

Authoritarian Control: PC-4, PC-14

Authoritarian Family Style: W-2

Avoidance: I-3

Basic Needs—Child Care: PC-22

Basic Needs—Child's Emotional Needs: PC-22

Basic Needs—Family as an Interface with Society: PC-22

Basic Needs—Family Unit: PC-22

Basic Needs—Food, Clothing, and Shelter: PC-22

Basic Needs—Health Care: PC-22

Basic Needs—Social Institutions: PC-22

Bedtime: FC-6

Behavior Control: R-8, W-9, W-14

Benign Criticism: I-1

Change: PC-10

Childcenteredness: PC-6, PC-7

Child Demandingness: PC-20

Child Distractibility/Hyperactivity: PC-20

Child Mood: PC-20